PUNCHING ABOVE
THEIR WEIGHT

Edward Bofen
31. 07. 13

PUNCHING ABOVE THEIR WEIGHT

The Winchester University Press
NEW PERSPECTIVES ON VETERINARY HISTORY

The early twenty-first century has seen a dramatic growth in both scholarly and public interest in all aspects of the health and illness of domesticated animals. The aim of this series is to provide an international forum of academic publications that explore veterinary history from a range of multidisciplinary perspectives. By doing so, the series sheds new light on various aspects of veterinary history and makes a contribution to the growing scholarship in this area.

PUNCHING ABOVE
THEIR WEIGHT

The British Veterinary Association

1882–2010

Edward Boden

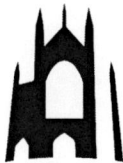

WINCHESTER
UNIVERSITY PRESS

Published by the Winchester University Press 2013

First Published in Great Britain in 2013 by
The Winchester University Press
University of Winchester
Winchester SO22 4NR

British Library Cataloguing-in-Publication Data
A CIP catalogue record for this book is available
from the British Library.

ISBN: 978-1-906113-10-0

Printed and Bound in Great Britain

CONTENTS

Preface   *viii*
Acknowledgements   *ix*
List of Illustrations   *x*
List of Abbreviations and Acronyms   *xi*

Chapter 1
   Making a start   1
   The National Veterinary Association   8
   Veterinary Record launched   14

Chapter 2
   Clinical considerations   22
   Vaccines   26
   Municipal appointments   34
   'Amalgamation' of local divisions   38
   Hunting dies   43

Chapter 3
   War breaks out   46
   'New epoch' predicted   50
   Money matters   53
   Armistice   56
   The *Veterinary Record* acquired   58

Chapter 4
   A troubled decade   74
   Aims and objects   77
   Administering the Association   80
   The NVMA and its divisions   82

Chapter 5
   Foot-and-mouth disease: the first major outbreak   90
   FMD returns   94
   Another outbreak   96
   FMD's most serious outbreak   98

CONTENTS

Chapter 6
State Veterinary Service proposed 102
Government proposals 'a travesty' 107
Negotiations resumed 110
A new president and another war 114
Wartime animal health schemes 117
Veterinary education plans 122

Chapter 7
After hostilities 127
Vets and the animal charities 137
Unregistered practice and the 1948 Act 144

Chapter 8
A home of their own 154
BVA initiates new Anaesthetics Act 158
Practice communications 160

Chapter 9
New ideas, new enthusiasms 163
Another look at veterinary education 171
Welfare implications of intensification 172
Growth of small animal practice 174
Some presidents of the 1960s and 1970s 180
Inflationary problems 188
The profession under scrutiny 191

Chapter 10
Another Swann report 196
Furore of threat to veterinary schools 204

Chapter 11
The Association's centenary 211
Behind the scenes 214
'No confidence' motion 225

CONTENTS

Chapter 12

    Tendering for veterinary contracts   229

    Conflicting views on managing meat hygiene   233

    Towards a centralised service   241

Chapter 13

    Disease control   248

    Tuberculosis, bovine and human   248

    Aujeszky's disease eradication; a case history   257

    Newcastle disease   261

    Brucellosis   263

    BSE: A devastating new disease   264

Chapter 14

    Veterinary pharmaceutical products   269

    Animal medicines and advertising   271

    Medicines supply investigation   275

    Advertising veterinary services   279

    The question of gender   285

Chapter 15

    Decline of farm practice   297

    Company practices   304

    The millennium   309

    What of the future?   311

Notes   316

Select Bibliography   338

Appendices

    British Veterinary Association (BVA) Presidents   340

    BVA Divisions   342

    Financial Status and Membership   346

Index   348

PREFACE

In 1882, a small group of veterinary surgeons decided to form an association that would, they hoped, protect the interests and support the scientific and clinical aspirations and social aims of their young profession. They had large ambitions but few resources. The new, over-arching body, built on the strengths of existing local veterinary associations, became the British Veterinary Association. For some thirty years the Association survived as an annual meeting of practitioners, academics and public health veterinarians. The advent of war in 1914 brought concentration on supplying the needs of army horses and government recognition of the Association as a negotiating body. The acquisition of its own journal increased both membership and negotiating influence; the decline in horse numbers, the establishment of practitioner-based engagement in a State Veterinary Service and the rise of small animal practice all shaped the growth of the Association and the way it, and veterinary practice itself, was administered. The acceptance of women in the profession, at first grudging, then overwhelming, brought a different dimension to the social aspects of veterinary work. The final outcome was a self-governing body collating numerous individual specialist associations into a cohesive democratic whole. The BVA has sought to serve the interests of the veterinary profession and influence government and industry in furtherance of its role as guardians of the health and welfare of the nation's animal population. In engaging with political forces much larger than their own, the Association and its members have always fought above their weight.

The way the British Veterinary Association flourished carries a message that has universal resonances.

ACKNOWLEDGEMENTS

Among the many people who have provided help, information and advice in the preparation of this book are John Tandy, who helped launch the project; several past presidents of the BVA who generously shared their experiences; members of the staff of the Association, particularly the secretary-general, Henrietta Alderman, and Helena Cotton and her colleagues of the secretariat; James Baird, formerly the Association's chief executive; Elizabeth Shaw of the Wellcome Trust; Clare Boulton and her colleagues from the RCVS Charitable Trust Library, and the staff of the Harold Cohen Library, Liverpool University.

The work owes a great deal to the knowledge and guidance of Dr Abigail Woods of Imperial College, London, who mentored the project and suggested lines of additional research.

A grant from the Wellcome Trust funded research for the project; the BVA contributed some word processing costs.

The index was compiled by Catherine Shingler; Mark Shingler advised on technical presentation of the manuscript.

I am extremely grateful to all those individuals and organisations, and to the many others whom I have been unable formally to acknowledge.

EB

ILLUSTRATIONS

1. George Fleming (RCVS Charitable Trust Library) 4

2. Students at the Royal Veterinary College, London 17

3. George Amos Banham (*Veterinary Record*) 20

4. One of the first covers of *Veterinary Record* 28

5. Dublin conference outing, 1904 (*Veterinary Record*) 33

6. William Hunting (*Veterinary Record*) 44

7. Horses returning from the front in the 1914–1918 war 49

8. Orlando Charnock Bradley 62

9. Sir Stewart Stockman (*Veterinary Record*) 92

10. Harry Steele-Bodger (*Veterinary Record*) 115

11. Dr W. R. 'Reg' Wooldridge (*Veterinary Record)* 121

12. George Gould (*Veterinary Record*) 131

13. Alasdair Steele-Bodger (*Veterinary Record*) 152

14. *Veterinary Record* cover from the 1950s 157

15. Mary Brancker (*Veterinary Record*) 182

16. Dr Storie-Pugh (RCVS Charitable Trust Library) 184

17. Her Majesty at BVA HQ in 1982 (*Veterinary Record*) 213

18. Aileen Cust (RCVS Charitable Trust Library) 286

19. Dame Olga Uvarov (RCVS Charitable Trust Library) 289

The cover depicts the Headquarters of the British Veterinary
Association, Mansfield Street, London

ABBREVIATIONS AND ACRONYMS

ARC	Agricultural Research Council
BSAVA	British Small Animal Veterinary Association
BSE	Bovine Spongiform Encephalopathy
BVA	British Veterinary Association
BVHA	British Veterinary Hospitals Association
DEFRA	Department of the Environment, Food and Rural Affairs
EFRACom	Environment, Food and Rural Affairs Committee
EHO	Environmental Health Officer
EHOA	Environmental Health Officers Association
FRCVS	Fellow of the Royal College of Veterinary Surgeons
FSA	Food Standards Agency
FVE	Federation of Veterinarians of the EEC
HEFC	Higher Education Funding Council
LVI	Licensed Veterinary Inspector
MAF	Ministry of Agriculture and Fisheries
MAFF	Ministry of Agriculture Fisheries and Food
MHS	Meat Hygiene Service
MRCVS	Member of the Royal College of Veterinary Surgeons
NCDL	National Canine Defence League (name changed to Dogs Trust)
NFU	National Farmers Union
NVA	National Veterinary Association
NVMA	National Veterinary Medical Association
OFT	Office of Fair Trading
OVS	Official Veterinary Surgeon
PDSA	Peoples Dispensary for Sick Animals
RANA	Registered Animal Nursing Auxiliary
RCVS	Royal College of Veterinary Surgeons
RN	Registered Nurse

ABBREVIATIONS AND ACRONYMS

RSPCA	Royal Society for the Prevention of Cruelty to Animals
RVC	Royal Veterinary College (London)
SPVS	Society of Practising Veterinary Surgeons
SVP	Society of Veterinary Practitioners
UFAW	Universities Federation for Animal Welfare
UGC	Universities Grants Committee
VMD	Veterinary Medicines Directorate
VN	Veterinary Nurse
VPC	Veterinary Products Committee
WSAVA	World Small Animal Veterinary Association
WVA	World Veterinary Association

CHAPTER ONE

MAKING A START

In the mid 19th century, British veterinarians were a disparate and disorganised group. The title 'veterinary surgeon' had been adopted in 1791 by founders of the Royal Veterinary College, Britain's first veterinary school. It was intended to demarcate the school's formally trained diploma holders from the mass of other animal healers.[1]

A corporate body, the Royal College of Veterinary Surgeons (RCVS), had received its Royal Charter in 1844, which meant a register of members (MRCVS) could be established.[2] However, the charter had no statutory effect; there were no exclusive rights to the title and anyone could call himself (there were no women vets) a veterinary surgeon. Moreover, William Dick, who had founded a second veterinary school in Edinburgh in 1828, refused to support the RCVS and to submit his students to its examinations. Instead, they received a certificate from the Highland and Agricultural Society (HAS). The Scottish diploma was not generally accepted in London and there were in effect two cadres of 'qualified' vets.[3]

The disastrous cattle plague (rinderpest) epidemic of the 1860s threw into prominence the shortcomings of many qualified practitioners in treating any animal except the horse: they frequently demonstrated their incompetence, failing to diagnose (or misdiagnosing) rinderpest, taking no action when needed, and causing disruption at other times.[4]

Qualified vets also faced growing competition from unqualified individuals. Although they had no college training, many of these 'vets' had completed apprenticeships or learned on the job. Consequently, they were often as good, if not better, at managing animal injuries and ailments than qualified vets, whose training was largely theoretical.

Sporadic attempts to improve the regulatory and educational system for entrants to the veterinary profession had had little effect, not least because vets themselves could not agree on a future vision for the profession. While all sought higher status for the profession, improved incomes and an improved standard of competence, 'in a rapidly changing society, veterinary surgery stood at a crossroads. Should it seek to join medicine as a learned, scientific profession, bound by gentlemanly modes of conduct, or did advancement depend upon a more practical, businesslike orientation? Was self-improvement sufficient to convince society that qualified vets were superior to unqualified, or was a legal monopoly required?'[5]

In 1866 the RCVS promoted a Veterinary Surgeons Bill, with the aim of achieving statutory recognition of the MRCVS qualification and the prevention of unqualified practice. The Bill was withdrawn as it had no chance of being accepted: a main reason was the lack of unity among the profession, particularly between the Scottish and English practitioners, and the lack of general support, in particular that of the chief medical officer J. R. Simon and H. R. Bruce, vice-president of the Privy Council, who did not think that the state of veterinary science at the time 'was sufficiently advanced to entitle the members of the College to a monopoly of the practice'.[6]

The situation of the veterinary profession at the time was not unlike that in medicine fifty years earlier, when the fledgling British Medical Association (BMA) came into being as the Provincial Medical and Surgical Association. Then, and indeed until the passing of the Medical Act of 1858, which the BMA had long struggled to see into law, the organisation of medical practice in Britain was chaotic.

2

Anyone could set up in practice and call himself a doctor. The Act set up a medical register, established the General Medical Council and aimed to bring some uniformity of standards to the training provided by the various colleges and institutions offering medical and surgical qualifications.[7] By 1879, holders of the Highland certificate had become eligible for membership of the RCVS, the HAS having withdrawn its certificate in favour of the RCVS exams. Thus, the 'single portal' qualification was established: the diploma examination of the RCVS.

The growing unity of the profession paved the way for the passage of a Veterinary Surgeons Act in 1881, a development actively worked for by George Fleming (1833–1901) and by T. A. Dollar, an Edinburgh (HAS) qualified vet who had, after a struggle, become well established and influential in London veterinary circles. Fleming, RCVS president 1881–83,[8] had himself passed the examinations of both bodies. His career saw him progress from farrier's forge-boy to pioneering veterinary scientist, author, explorer, and director-general of the Army Veterinary Department. He was one of a metropolitan veterinary elite who modelled the profession's future on that of the medical profession: 'The days of the so-called "practical man" have gone by . . . the veterinarian must now be an educated scientific man.'[9] He felt that in demarcating qualified from unqualified vets, legislation would promote the status and prospects of the profession and encourage a higher standard of entrants.

The passing of the 1881 Act, achieved against considerable opposition, was due in large measure to the efforts of Fleming. He lobbied for the Bill, attending Parliament every day for five weeks when the Bill was before the House. Taking advantage of an unexpected hiatus in the proceedings to persuade a cabinet minister with whom Fleming was acquainted to present it, the Bill was passed – largely because none of its opponents happened to be present.[10] The Act, at last, restricted the title 'veterinary surgeon' to qualified vets whose names appeared on the register of the RCVS. However, anyone who could demonstrate that they had practised as a veterinarian for the

3

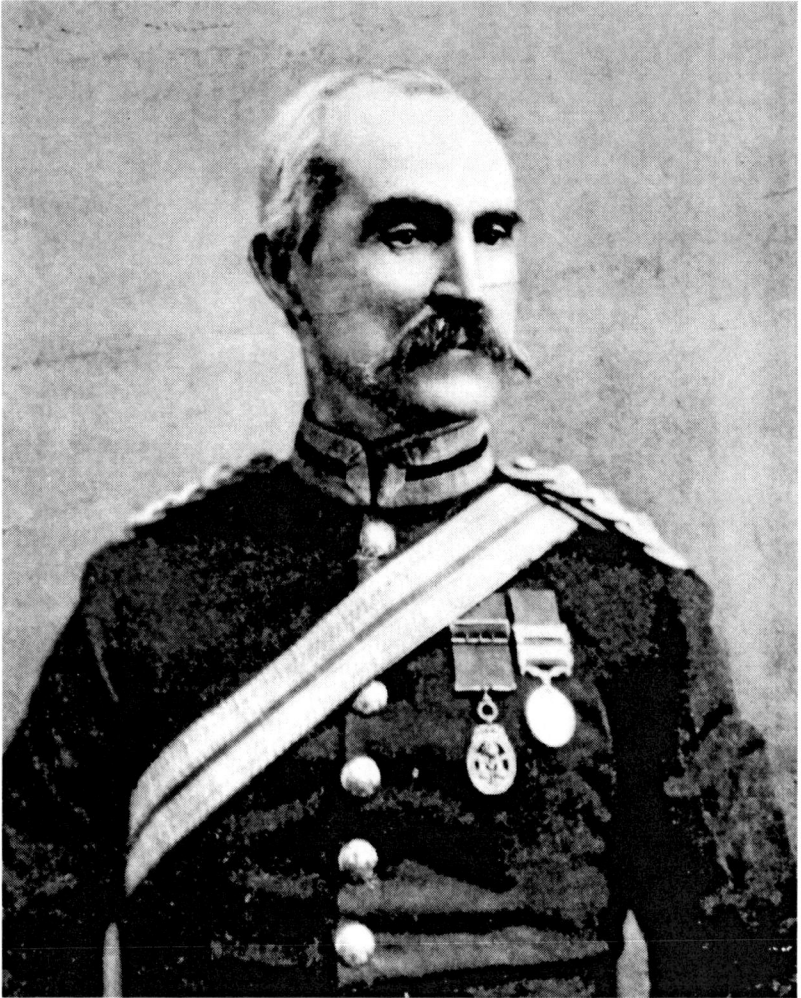

Figure 1. George Fleming, who rose from farrier's forge boy to become director of the Army Veterinary Service. As president of the RCVS, he was a major supporter of the initiative to establish the National Veterinary Association.

previous five years was permitted to retain the title, and admitted to an RCVS supplementary register on payment of three guineas (£3. 3s.).

While one of the effects of the Act was to encourage qualified vets to 'see themselves in newly corporate terms, as a breed apart from unqualified non-members',[11] some had already begun to cooperate with qualified colleagues in neighbouring practices through the formation of local veterinary associations. Established particularly in the provinces (see table below), they met two or three times a year, mainly to discuss clinical matters. Most of them also held annual dinners. This social element was (and remains) an important part of veterinary meetings, giving a rare opportunity for the members of a scattered profession to meet together and foster a sense of unity, with shared interests and concerns.

Veterinary associations founded before 1900

1858	West of Scotland
1861	Lancashire
1863	Yorkshire
1863	North of England
1866	Midland Counties
1868	Eastern Counties
1873	Central
1873	Southern Counties
1882	Lincoln
1883	Scottish Metropolitan
1883	Royal Counties
1884	Western Counties
1888	Ayrshire
1894	North of Scotland

The value of professional solidarity had been demonstrated in the 1860s in a commercial way during a Manchester strike of shoeing smiths; farriery was then an important part of the service provided by many veterinary practices. Members of the Lancashire Veterinary Medical Association banded together to share stocks of shoes, scoured the country for replacement smiths and eventually broke the strike.[12] Such a countrywide action was, of course, made possible by the development of a countrywide railway service which by the 1850s had grown to link all cities and most provincial towns with one another. The railways made it practicable for individuals in almost all parts of the country to travel conveniently to a given location to attend meetings, something essential if any nationwide association was to be a reality.

The idea of a national veterinary association, to represent and speak for all registered practitioners, took shape in 1880, after a few veterinary surgeons attended the BMA annual meeting in Cambridge. There was a shared interest (and some rivalry) between vets and medical men because both were involved in public health inspections, particularly meat hygiene, and some vets would attend the relevant sessions of the BMA conference.[13]

One of those attending the Cambridge conference was a young man called George Amos Banham. Banham was not a typical veterinary practitioner. Born in Cambridge in 1853, the son of a presumably prosperous tailor, he undertook an 'articled pupilage' with a veterinary surgeon, following which he qualified from the Royal Veterinary College, where he was a brilliant student. He won the First Fitzwygram Prize (awarded to the most academically outstanding student from UK veterinary schools) in a year in which fellow student Sir John McFadyean (who became Britain's leading veterinary scientist and principal of the Royal Veterinary College)[14] came second. Banham continued his studies in Berlin, then the world leader in scientific research. On returning to London he was appointed veterinary surgeon to the Brown Animal Sanatory (sic) Institution, a veterinary hospital and research institute – with ambitions to emulate the Pasteur Institute – under the University of London. In this post, Banham worked with the eminent medical scientist, C. S. Roy.[15]

In 1881, shortly before the BMA meeting took place, Banham moved to Cambridge where he took over a busy practice which he further expanded by acquiring a second vet's practice (Sparrow's), which was situated in the stable block of the Bird Bolt hotel.[16]

As well as running the practice, which grew into a large and prosperous one, he wrote a textbook, *Tables of veterinary posology and therapeutics* (Baillière, Tindall &

Cox: London, 1887), which became a standard work. In addition, he authored numerous papers, one of which is probably the most comprehensive account of contemporary horse-shoeing techniques, materials and economics written.[17] Although he sold his practice in 1907 (to J. G. Runciman), for over forty years Banham remained closely involved in national veterinary politics, sometimes controversially. He was a member of the RCVS council from 1902 until 1922, being vice-president in 1902, 1908 and 1920; but he was never elected president. His obituarist described him as 'a short man, of cultured appearance and sensitive mien' but also 'showing signs of certain temperamental defects which made him over sensitive to criticism'.[18]

Impressed by the conference and no doubt by the strength of the BMA's united approach to matters of professional interest, Banham took the lead in founding a National Veterinary Congress, held in London the following year, 1882. At that congress he presented a paper, 'A scheme for forming a British National Veterinary Association'. He said: 'The existing local veterinary societies should look upon the national association as a connecting link between them, although the association claimed no connection with their individual rights and constitutions.' The proposal found immediate support from senior members of the profession including George Fleming (still president of the RCVS), who chaired the meeting, and William Hunting, a leading London practitioner who later founded the journal *Veterinary Record.*

Fleming arranged to set up a steering committee to plan the proposed association and draw up rules. Selection of the committee's membership was left to Banham, assisted by J. H. Steel. Steel was attached to the Army Veterinary Department; he was appointed principal of the Bombay Veterinary College in May 1886 and took no further part in the affairs of the Association. The steering committee elected Fleming as president; Banham and John Penberthy, a professor at RVC, were appointed joint honorary secretaries. The first general meeting was planned for 8 May 1883 at the Royal Society of Arts, John Street, London. All registered veterinary surgeons were sent written invitations to join the new national association and the secretaries of the local veterinary societies were asked to act as 'whips' and collect subscriptions – 10s. 6d. per member – 'which they had done with great zeal'.[19]

Fleming's involvement in this initiative is highly significant. It complemented his work in developing the 'top-down' veterinary surgeons act by promoting the 'bottom-up' development of veterinary identity and expertise. It also reveals his continuing conviction that the veterinary profession should model itself on the medical profession. In his presidential address at that first meeting, he argued that 'The medical profession many years ago recognised the necessity for such an institution as that which the veterinary profession are now starting and the advantages which that profession has derived from the British Medical Association can scarcely be too highly estimated.' In building on and extending the activities of local societies in 'the gathering and dissemination of knowledge and the interchange of ideas.' it was 'bound to effect a large amount of good, not only to the profession but to the public'.[20]

THE NATIONAL VETERINARY ASSOCIATION

It was agreed that the new body should be called the National Veterinary Association, and its aims should be limited 'for the present' to providing the means for general meetings of members of the Association in various parts of the kingdom 'to promote and advance veterinary science and maintain the honour and integrity of the profession'.

The Association's council, it was decided, should comprise the president of the RCVS, the principal of each of the veterinary schools, the principal veterinary surgeon of the Army Veterinary Department, the Professional Adviser to the Privy Council (government chief veterinary officer), the presidents and secretaries of each of the existing local associations 'in league with the [national] Association' and 'six others, residing in various parts of the Kingdom, (particularly those parts where Local Veterinary Medical Societies do not exist)'. In addition, the retiring president each year was elected an ex officio life member of council.

Unlike many other professional bodies, such as the RCVS, council was not a body elected by the membership as a whole. It was, rather, a branch representatives' gathering. That cumbersome structure then adopted remained little changed in essence (except for dropping the six local non-association members) until the 1970s. It would become increasingly unwieldy as the number of divisional societies, specialist divisions and past presidents grew.

The rules included provision that council should meet once a year at the time and place of the general meeting, and that those meetings should be held in various parts of the country, under the direction of a provincial (i.e. local) committee. And for many years the general meeting, held annually, was the only event in which all NVA members could participate and, indeed, virtually the sole perceived activity of the Association. Seventy-two members (out of a total of 102) attended the first meeting in 1883. At its conclusion, Thomas Greaves, a leading Manchester practitioner, was elected president for the ensuing year and George Banham general secretary, an honorary post he retained until 1890.

The first day's proceedings, which had begun with a paper on the soundness of the horse, concluded with a dinner at which 'there were no less than twelve toasts and fourteen speakers responded. In addition, there were songs and musical selections which went on until a late hour.'[21] That admixture of science and sociability was to be the recipe for veterinary conferences up to the present day.

The papers presented at the annual meetings tended, naturally, to reflect the clinical concerns of the day. Descriptions of quotidian problems faced by the practising vet, described as they developed over the years, were often mundane. But the knowledge gained from discussion by practitioners over the years did help to widen veterinary knowledge. Clinical matters, however, were not the new

Association's sole concern. Right from the start, socio-political and professional business matters also figured in the programmes. A description of the topics discussed at early meetings offer a flavour of the key veterinary concerns and opinions of the day.

At the 1883 meeting, as well as the business recorded above, the first paper presented was on 'Human and bovine tuberculosis; its communicability', by J. H. Cox, of the Army Veterinary Department: the second discussed 'The Contagious Diseases (Animals) Act and how far it may be extended and improved, coupled with human sanitation' by Professor W. Whalley, of Edinburgh.[22] Such topics reflected the desire of leading vets to carve out a greater veterinary role in preserving the public's health, and the development of what Hardy has described as 'municipal veterinary hygiene' in some provincial cities.[23] This theme was maintained the following year, when the NVA held its meeting at Manchester University. Ninety-one members (plus sixty-four guests) attended out of a membership which had increased to 221. The treasurer reported 'the Association is prospering!' and that there was a balance of £37 11s. 11d. after paying expenses. Papers discussed included 'Public health as affected by food supply obtained from animals' by James McCall, principal of Glasgow Veterinary College; a discussion on 'Trichina disease in man; cysticercus, rinderpest, foot-and-mouth disease, pleuropneumonia, anthrax, bovine tuberculosis, and swine plague' resulted in the recommendations 'that [meat] inspectors should be properly trained' and 'submitted to searching examinations'.

The topic 'The prevention of cruelty to animals' by a Mr T. Biggs (speaking for the RSPCA) produced a somewhat acrimonious debate. Vets accused the RSPCA of bringing unnecessary prosecutions for procedures such as tail docking of horses, at that time a common operation. A motion 'That this meeting condemns the indiscriminate and unnecessary docking of horses [tails]' was withdrawn. The following, rather more anodyne, amendment was passed: 'In the opinion of this meeting, the operation of docking horses as a means of averting danger to man is not cruel when shown to be necessary.' The proposer, William Hunting, later played a very significant role in the development of the NVA.[24] His motion gives an important insight into the prevailing veterinary belief that the ethics of animal treatment was a matter on which the profession, not laymen, should decide.[25]

In 1885 the general meeting was held in Birmingham. It was opened by a brilliant surgeon, Sampson Gamgee (1828–1886), principal of the Birmingham Medical Institute. He was a son of Joseph Gamgee (1801–1894), and a brother of John Gamgee (1834–1894), pioneering veterinary surgeon. Sampson Gamgee had qualified as a vet from the RVC but was immediately invited to study surgery at University College, London. He gained his MRCS in 1854 and devoted the rest of his life mainly to the practice of (human) surgery. However, he always retained a keen interest in veterinary matters.[26]

His opening address to the meeting was a wide ranging survey of comparative surgery in man and animals in which he emphasised the value of 'natural healing' – 'Antiseptics have their value but the greatest antiseptic is life.' He also noted the interest that the pioneering surgeon, John Hunter (1728–1793), had taken in veterinary education: Hunter had bought shares in the London veterinary college on its formation and fostered its influence. Gamgee said: 'What progress might have been made if Hunter's influence had been acted upon.'

Other papers discussed pleuropneumonia and swine plague, scheduled diseases which were proving difficult to control by means of the state's 'stamping out policy'. As members of the central government's Veterinary Department and as inspectors to the Local Authorities, vets were intimately involved in the making and execution of this policy.[27]

A presentation by Sir F. W. J. Fitzwygram on 'The origin of diseases' addressed a topic popular amongst scientific audiences following the discoveries of Pasteur and Koch.[28] It divided disease into 'specific' diseases, which arose 'from neglect of good sanitary precautions', and 'spontaneous' diseases, 'generally due to bad stable management'. The gathering agreed 'that this meeting is of the opinion that contagious diseases of animals do not arise spontaneously; that they are spread solely by contagion and may be stamped out by the adoption of proper measures.'[29]

The 1886 gathering was held in Scotland for the first time, at Edinburgh. The total attendance was eighty-nine; the membership had risen to 310 – still below 10 per cent of practising vets. Banham, the general secretary, was able to announce that the Association had rented accommodation at 10 Red Lion Square. The premises had recently been acquired by the RCVS as its own headquarters; a move made possible by the fact that wealthy London veterinary surgeon T. A. Dollar had advanced £500 for the purpose (the College was perennially short of funds – its only regular income coming from examination fees). The move no doubt suited both parties for reasons of convenience and economy (there was considerable overlap in the membership of the councils of both bodies.). Banham also scotched a rumour that the NVA was to start a new journal. It had, however, been proposed that 'at some time' the Association should, with local associations, publish their own proceedings.[30]

The programme included a paper by J. S. Hurndall, a London vet: 'Can experimental pathology be rendered useful in elucidating a definite system of veterinary therapeutics?' Hurndall called for renewed investigation into the action of drugs in the interest of 'true therapeutics'. He said that prescriptions were 'written daily for various forms of disease when the prescriber was quite in the dark as to the why or wherefore of his recommendations'. Hurndall proceeded to give examples of the use of aconite in bronchitis in horses, the improvement being measured by auscultation and observation of changes in clinical signs. He was critical of 'traditional remedies such as tartar emetic and phosphorus' and advocated the use of aconite in dilute solution for most lung conditions. It turned out that he was actually speaking of homoeopathic preparations in minute doses, for example five drops of tincture as the dose for a horse. One speaker in the discussion commented that he had had equally effective results with plain water, when he had found himself without aconite.[31]

Professor W. O. Williams, of the New Veterinary College, and R. Roberts presented the results of a survey on 'Anaesthetics and anaesthesia in relation to veterinary practice'. Although anaesthesia had rapidly entered human medicine following the initial use of ether in 1846, its use within veterinary practice had been more limited. By 1881 chloroform use was still not routinely taught at the RVC.[32] The authors had asked leading veterinarians in the European colleges about the anaesthetic techniques they used. The conclusion was that chloroform was the best general agent; for horses 'place a leather bag containing a sponge soaked in chloroform, secure it firmly round the face with a strap'. For dogs and cats, 'place [the animal] in a box or drawer containing a sponge soaked with a small quantity of chloroform.'[33] For many years the procedure was (at least anecdotally) performed by placing the animal patient inside a Wellington boot containing a chloroform-soaked wad of cotton wool.

It was at the Peterborough meeting in 1887 that George Banham gave the paper on shoeing mentioned above. The title was 'The horse-shoeing forge and its relations to the employer or master, the labourer or workman, and the public'. This comprehensive discourse described the various types of shoe, the cost of premises and materials, the number of shoes of different types that could be made from a hundredweight (cwt.) of new iron, and the number that could be made from old (reforged) shoes. The types and cost of ready-made shoes were given and the prices of nails, rasps, coal and coke were set out. The charge for making and fitting a set of four horseshoes was quoted as 5s. 6d. in London, 3s. 0d. in the country.[34]

During discussion of the paper, Professor Whalley said that 'all young veterinary surgeons should have experience in a shoeing forge' – but he thought that a 'trade paper' was 'not really appropriate for a professional meeting'. Vets' relationship with the forge had been a key point of dispute in 1870s discussions on professional advancement. For most practicing vets it was a valuable source of income: 'If Mr So and So brings his horse to be shod, he will bring it to be doctored; and therefore it is not what the forge pays, but the practice it brings which makes it answer.'[35] However, for aspirational vets like Fleming and Whalley, who were not reliant on veterinary practice for an income, it smacked of trade.[36]

VETERINARY RECORD LAUNCHED

The 1887 meeting resolved unanimously that 'the time has arrived for the profession to be represented by a Weekly Scientific Journal', published under the auspices of the National Veterinary Association – representing the Veterinary Medical Associations of Great Britain – and supported by a registered staff of contributors.'[37]

The following July, William Hunting launched just such a publication, the *Veterinary Record*. The *Veterinary Record* was not the first veterinary journal. *The Veterinarian* (founded 1828) and *The Veterinary Journal* (founded in 1875 by George Fleming) were well established and covered some of the same ground. However, these were monthly publications. Hunting's new journal was published every week and carried verbatim reports of council and local association meetings. This gave it an immediacy that the other publications could not match. He acted on his own initiative in introducing this competitor to Fleming's established *Veterinary Journal*. It is speculation to surmise that he wanted to pre-empt action by the Association but it would not have been surprising; and there may have been an element of personal rivalry with his eminent colleague.

William Hunting was an influential figure who had followed his father, Charles, into the profession. Charles Hunting had, from lowly beginnings, developed large veterinary and farming interests. William was one of a handful of graduates from the short-lived New Veterinary College, Edinburgh, which John Gamgee had set up to provide a more scientific education than the other two schools. He worked in practice, and as professor of veterinary science at the Royal Agricultural College, leaving to take up a professorial post offered by Gamgee, who was moving his college to London. That job was short-lived as Gamgee's institution, the Albert Veterinary College, Pimlico, closed down in 1865. Hunting resumed practice in London and was soon showing a keen interest in clinical investigations. One of his early and long standing interests was glanders, a zoonotic disease endemic among the equine population and consequently of serious economic and public health importance. He had contracts with the London County Council to provide health care to its vast stable of horses (he claimed to have performed 600 post mortems a year)[38] and also, at one time, the London Road Car Company. He was a prolific author of veterinary texts (including a book on glanders), a frequent speaker at veterinary meetings, and a member of the Board of Agriculture committee on glanders.

At 42, Hunting was already an experienced journalist when he established the *Veterinary Record*. The publication was launched with the aid of a loan of £50 (which he never repaid) from his colleague T. A. Dollar (who had also subsidised the RCVS move to Red Lion Square). However, he has been described as 'erratic but brilliant' as a student and as 'never having had any money'.[39]

He wrote in his first issue: 'We do not make our appearance under the auspices of the National Association, we cannot, *as yet* [my italics], claim to represent the Veterinary Associations of Great Britain and we are only supported by a voluntary staff of contributors'. In fact, it was to be thirty years before the Association bought the title and it became the official journal of the Association. The NVA might have acquired it after Hunting's death in 1913, but the intervention of the 1914–1918 war delayed the purchase until 1920. Today it is still the main journal of the veterinary profession in the UK.

Setting out his plan for the new journal, Hunting hoped it would earn the title of 'representative' by appealing to the whole profession and opening its pages to 'all who have the will to assist the progress of our corporate body'. 'Careful observation makes a skilful practitioner, but his skill dies with him. By recording his observations he adds to the knowledge of his profession,' said Hunting, urging his colleagues to submit clinical papers of the cases they saw. In addition, he promised to publish 'carefully written papers by experts, notes and news of interest to the whole profession and accounts of the existence and spread of contagious disease'.

Hunting said the *Record* would also cover the affairs of council (RCVS as well as NVA), educational matters, and the proceedings of the various veterinary medical societies: 'Not only is a scientific journal but a professional journal our idea of what is wanted.'[40] This was perhaps an allusion to Fleming and his *Veterinary Journal.* In earlier debates about the profession's future, William Hunting's father, Charles, had rejected Fleming's vision of a scientific profession in favour of a more utilitarian vision.[41]

By 1888 the pattern of meetings and the topics covered had become well established. 'The importance of the study of comparative pathology', by Dr H. E. Armstrong, medical officer of health for Newcastle-on-Tyne, was the first paper. It discussed the transmission of diseases from animals to man and the lack, at the time, of 'adequate procedures' in slaughterhouses. The meeting agreed that 'In the interests of Public Health it is desirable that all large towns should be provided with Public Abattoirs and that slaughtering of cattle, sheep and pigs on private premises should be abolished.' A worthy aim, perhaps, but not one that would be realised.

'Veterinary education and requirements', a recurring subject discussed on this occasion by E. Faulkner, stressed the need for veterinary students to have a good general education followed by a combination of academic ('collegiate') and professional education. He believed that intending students should spend one year with an established veterinary practice before starting an academic course. The first year of study should include basic anatomy (equine and comparative), chemistry, and botany. The

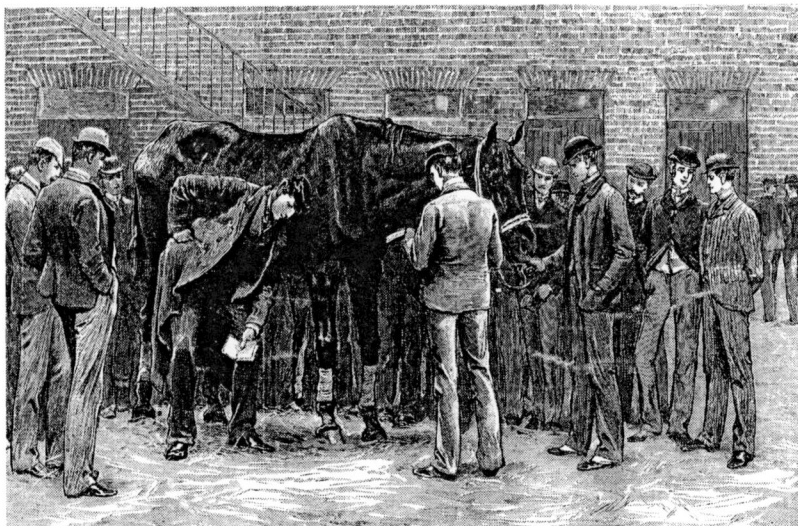

Figure 2. 'Students under the direction of a professor: free practice – sounding a horse'. Caption to an 1891 illustration produced on the centenary of the Royal Veterinary College. 'Sound' was one of the mechanical aids to diagnosis described by William Hunting.

five-month summer recess should be spent seeing practice with a qualified vet.

In the second year, the anatomy of the horse and other animals should be studied in more detail, together with physiology and histology. Again the summer should be devoted to seeing practice. The third, and final, year would add hygiene and general stock management and breeding, together with morbid anatomy and pathology, and micro-biology. Further education should be encouraged while the vet was working in practice. Examiners, said Faulkner, should be of a higher standard generally than was currently the case and the practice of appointing medical men as examiners (which had been the general rule when the RVC was founded, and was still followed for certain non-clinical subjects) discontinued. He also argued that 'after obtaining the MRCVS diploma it was essential that further experience should be gained ... On no account is it desirable to commence in [independent] practice before attaining this.'[42] The meeting was rounded off by a perennial conference topic, 'Some diseases of the foot of the horse', by Frederick Smith.

In 1889 the topic of vaccination included a paper on 'Natural and inoculated cowpox' by E. M. Crookshank, professor of bacteriology and comparative pathology at Kings College, London. It reflected the ongoing debate within medical scientific circles on the relationship between smallpox and cowpox and whether they were actually the same diseases. The answer had implications for the use of calves in the production of human smallpox vaccine.

Other subjects were 'the diseases of the urinary and generative organs' (E. A. MacGillivray) and 'Some contagious diseases of the horse' (Professor F. W. Alston Edgar). William Hunting gave an account of 'Mechanical aids to diagnosis'. Some of these were already well established within human medicine but others were relatively new inventions.[43] They included: probes; sounds (produced by percussion or pressure); specula, including mouth gags or balling irons; weights and measures, including specific gravity of body fluids and alteration in the size or form of body parts; thermometers; and stethoscopes. Although the straight stethoscope then common was 'inapplicable to animals' he predicted the binaural instrument (soon to become universal) would 'come to be useful with experience'. Hunting felt the ophthalmoscope of little value – 'Without considerable experience the superficial parts of the eye can be seen better without it.' The sphygmograph was 'useful as a recorder, but not many cases where it teaches the practitioner more than . . . a finger on the pulse'. However, 'every practitioner should be able to use a micro–scope' when identifying external parasites and examining milk, blood or urine. Finally, electricity was 'of value in providing light to examine body cavities'.[44]

It was decided to hold the following year's meeting – and to change the name of the occasion to 'annual general meeting' – in Dublin. Ireland was not, of course, divided at that time and the Irish Veterinary Medical Association was a division of the NVA. In accordance with custom, a member was proposed as president who lived in the locality in which the meeting would take place. It was not according to custom, however, that two Irish candidates were proposed: T. H. Simcocks and J. D. Lambert. After a debate, Simcocks was elected. It was to prove an unfortunate choice. Simcocks fell ill, and no arrangements were made for Dublin. A 'scratch' meeting was held in London on 2 October 1890. The only paper submitted was by Banham himself, who was still secretary of the Association. Membership, which had been struggling for some years, had fallen to 274 and a scant forty-three attended this special meeting. After the non-event, a critical editorial in the *Veterinary Record,* presumably written by its editor, William Hunting, wondered 'how the Association is to extricate itself from the mess into which it has been allowed to fall by the neglect of its officers'.[45] At the time Hunting, although a member of council, was not himself an officer.

Much of the blame was directed at Banham who, as general secretary, was the prime mover of the Association, although Simcocks, who was supposed to be the main organiser of the event, said Banham was in no way responsible for the debacle. Banham's conduct of the Association's affairs had been called into question the previous year. A special meeting of council in October 1889 had discussed the item 'The management of the Association and the general secretary's [Banham's] manner of conducting it'.

This had followed an exchange of correspondence with council member J. Sutcliffe Hurndall and others about Banham's failure to notify some council members of a meeting of the provisional committee for the next year's general meeting.[46] The correspondence ran for some weeks in the *Veterinary Record* until the editor drew it to a close, saying 'surely both sides had opportunity enough to exhaust the matter'.

Banham, however, was not proposing to let the matter drop; he said he intended to 'air the matter in another channel'.[47] Which he did in *The Veterinarian* and *The Veterinary Journal.*[48]

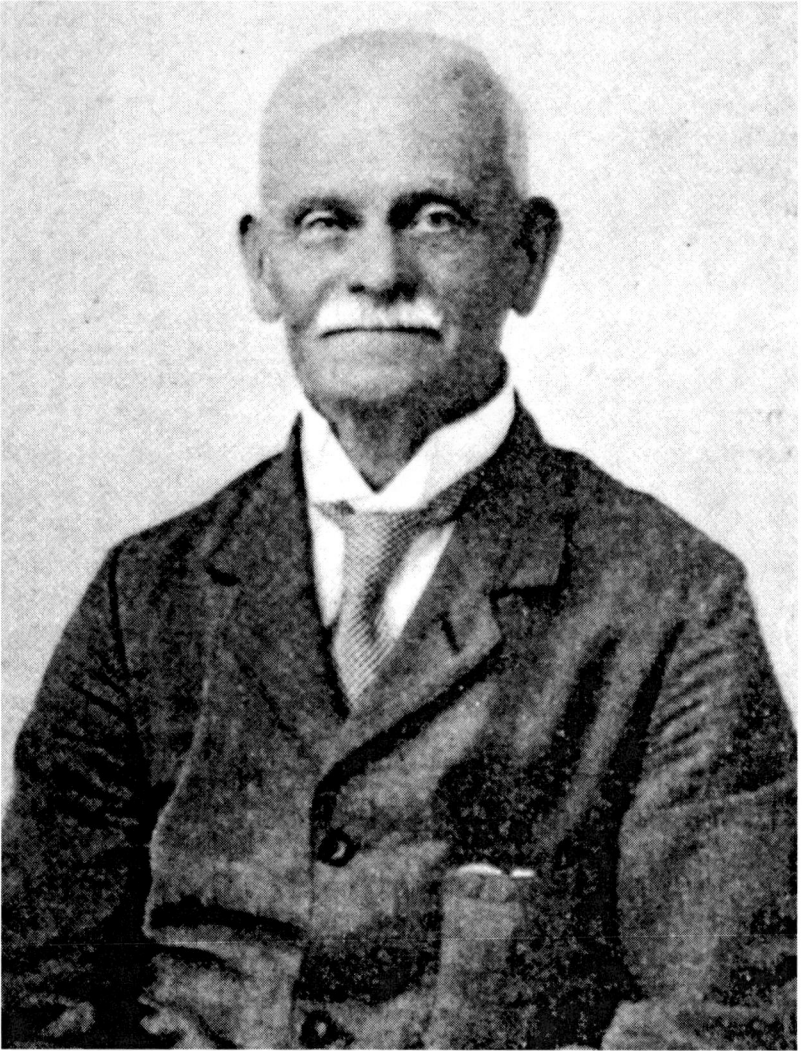

Figure 3. George Amos Banham, the 'touchy, sometimes difficult' man who was the catalyst for the formation of the National Veterinary Association and its mainstay for a decade.

The NVA council, at that special meeting, had considered that Banham had conducted the Association properly and had 'no instructions to offer for the secretary's future guidance'. At the 'scratch' general meeting in London, held in the wake of the failure of the Dublin meeting, the topic of the management of the Association was again raised, by

Banham himself, and the 'unfortunate correspondence' and the complaints made against Banham were discussed.49 The president, Simcocks, wrote that he was unable to be present; Professor Pritchard, who should have taken the chair in his stead, cancelled his attendance at a very late stage. The discussion was chaired by Professor W. O. Williams, who declared he was 'extremely sorry to find myself in the position of chairman today'. He said 'it was very much to be regretted' that the general meeting in Dublin had not taken place. But they would not reflect on the past nor find fault with anybody: Our duty is to do what we can to resuscitate this moribund Society.'

Banham resigned. In a vote of thanks for his services as secretary, although several members referred to 'differences' with him, all, including Hurndall, paid tribute to his work for the Association. Banham would have none of it, however. In response, he gave a lengthy rebuttal of the charges laid against him and vigorously attacked those who had criticised his conduct of affairs. He accused the speakers of hypocrisy. 'I have done more to build up the Association than any man in it,' he said. 'And now I trust that those who have brought it down will turn around and give as much energy in raising it to that standard we have ever wished to hold.' John Malcolm, municipal veterinary officer for Birmingham, was elected general secretary of the Association in his place[50] – unpaid, of course.

That was the end of Banham's ten-year stint as secretary, but he did not abandon his interest in veterinary political activities; he was a member of the RCVS council from 1902 to 1922.

CHAPTER TWO

CLINICAL CONSIDERATIONS

At the 1891 meeting in Doncaster, the perennial problem of members in arrears with their subscription payments was again to the fore. The NVA was, however, in fact far from the moribund body that the *Veterinary Record* had called it the previous year. A substantial effort by the new secretary, John Malcolm, had reduced the number of backsliders in paying their subscriptions from 113 to fifty. The income, £195 13s. 3d., allowed £119 5s. 11d. to be carried forward; there was in addition £200 invested.

Professor Wortley Axe presided over a programme that included a presentation on 'Tuberculosis of domestic animals' by John MacFadyean, professor of pathology and bacteriology at the Dick veterinary school, who had been asked by the Royal Commission on tuberculosis to conduct scientific enquiries into the effects of food infected with bovine tuberculosis.[1] Other papers reflected growing interest in the possibilities of vaccinating or inoculating livestock against infectious diseases. A paper on 'Blackquarter and its so-called preventives' by Professor John Penberthy of the Royal Veterinary College indicated that setons were commonly used. These were strips of fabric soaked in 'muscle juice' (serum) from an infected animal and threaded through a fold of skin of the animal being treated. Another measure again involved 'muscle juice', 'dried on powder sterilised on glass plates' and used as an inoculation. Both methods produced 'mixed' results. Professor W. Williams looked at the treatment of 'Influenza' and described experiments in preparing vaccines from 'muscle juice' taken from infected animals, again with 'varied results'.

The NVA returned north of the border, this time to Glasgow, for its AGM in 1892. This time, papers addressed some of the more economically important diseases encountered by vets in practice.

Professor J. M. McCall, the president, introduced a report by a committee appointed by the NVA to look into 'Parturient apoplexy, or milk fever'. This was a puzzling condition that caused cows to collapse around calving time. The report was in fact a series of case histories of the condition. Various treatments were employed, from opium to laxative drenches, none of which made an appreciable difference to the condition of the animal. He gave a similar report on 'Haemoglobinurea (azoturia)' in horses. This condition, which involved severe muscle cramps, stiffness and pain, was traditionally known as 'Monday morning disease' because it occurred in working horses following a day's rest on Sunday. McCall detailed a variety of therapies, including rubbing with turpentine liniment, purging, and dosing with chloral hydrate and alcohol – but no procedure seemed superior in its remedial properties to any other.

Another topic of great interest to practicing vets, owing to the frequency with which they performed it, was 'castration of the domestic animals'. Professor J. W. Dewar reviewed current methods, including cautery, ligature of the spermatic cord, compression by a wooden clamp 'with or without caustic', torsion, and the ecraseur (Burdizzo) as commonly used. William Hunting then addressed the meeting on 'The veterinarian, his position and his prospects'. He maintained that improved education was the key to a prosperous future for the profession and welcomed a proposed extension of the veterinary course to four years – a controversial move because of fears, which proved justified, that it would discourage recruitment. Hunting, however, believed the longer course would enable vets to become 'just as certain in the management of animals in health as in the treatment of animals in disease'. 'Have we

23

not neglected preventive medicine?' he asked. Although the horse was still the mainstay of the practitioner and its study the predominant interest of the veterinary colleges, other species were finding a place. First, cattle and sheep received Hunting's consideration. The dog, too, was now a regular patient. More recently, he said, 'the pig has been added to the list of animals brought under our hands'; not the individual animal, but it was becoming more common for professional advice to be sought for pedigree stock.

Hunting went on: 'There are two conditions, however, under which the pig becomes an important addition to our list of animals – in connection with contagious disease which affects the whole herd, and in connection with the transmission of disease to human beings.' Similar considerations, he noted, applied to birds. Those words were written well over a century before swine flu and bird flu had become a threat to man.[2]

An innovation at Glasgow was the conference excursion; a pleasure trip on Loch Lomond, rated an 'unqualified success'. The conference excursion was to become a popular feature of subsequent annual meetings.

Manchester was the location of the 1893 meeting, presided over by the president, E. Faulkner, a local practitioner. 'The inspection of animals intended for food, prior to and after death, with the most humane methods of slaughter' was a main topic. Sir John McFadyean described the practices current at the time. Cattle were most usually killed by stunning, often with a poleaxe, and bleeding out. Bleeding without stunning, as practiced under Mosaic law, was said to be 'cruel'; 'pithing' and shooting were other methods in use. Calves, sheep and pigs were 'almost invariably killed by bleeding without stunning'.[3] The paper was critical of British slaughterhouse procedures compared with those in Germany: inspection prior to slaughter, as was the practice in Germany, 'is nowhere carried out in this country', said the speaker. Manchester and Edinburgh, which had municipal abattoirs, and had appointed veterinary surgeons for meat inspection duties, were exceptions to the generally poor standards of privately owned operations. Inspectors should be present to witness the slaughtering, he said, although he acknowledged that would require an 'unreasonably large' number of inspectors. All slaughterhouses should be licensed, it was advocated.[4] Such calls for greater veterinary involvement in meat inspection would be repeated frequently in future years.[5]

The subject of anaesthesia was revisited, this time by E. Wallace Hoare, who reiterated the view expressed by Professor Williams in 1886 that chloroform was the most favoured anaesthetic for horses. Wallace Hoare later wrote the standard textbooks *Veterinary materia medica and therapeutics* and *A system of veterinary medicine.*

Hoare said he used the patented 'Carlisle's inhaler' for administration, and gave advice for introducing and monitoring anaesthesia. A dose of 1 oz chloroform for an adult horse was recommended to induce anaesthesia, with increments of ½ oz. to maintain it.[6] A comment in the *Veterinary Record* referred to recent press publicity in which it was argued that chloroform was cheap so there was no reason why it should be not used just as much in the veterinary practice as in human treatment. The article pointed out that, in fact, use of chloroform would add considerably to the cost because of the extra time and care that were needed both to administer the chloroform and to supervise the animal's recovery following its administration.[7] This was also the view of W. Pallin, who was awarded the RCVS's first fellowship by thesis in 1896. His report on horse castration claimed that 'the whole operation would be performed while the effect of the anaesthetic was in preparation.'[8]

William Hunting was president in 1894 for the AGM in London. His address celebrated the progress of the profession since the granting of the RCVS charter in 1844. 'Fifty years ago the practice of veterinary medicine might almost be said to consist of bleeding, physicking and blistering – with the aggravation of large and repeated doses of mercury and opium,' he said. Although they were still empirics, (working mainly from practical experience) vets now endeavoured to understand the morbid processes they treated. 'We base the selection of our remedies on better principles than simple faith.' Hunting summarised the benefits to animals and their owners brought by advances in surgery, such as the use of chloroform as an anaesthetic, the study of hereditary diseases, the growing knowledge of parasitic conditions and veterinary hygiene in improving health and longevity of their animal patients. He concluded: 'We no longer follow at a distance the work of medical research. We have struck out for ourselves and are independent pioneers in the field of comparative pathology and indispensable guides in the sciences of hygiene and preventive medicine.'[9] Hunting was a good orator and his optimistic words were more of a rhetorical aspiration than a statement of the actual situation. As already noted, anaesthetics were not widely used; vets were still generally looked down upon by doctors; there few were prospects or facilities for those who wished to conduct scientific research, and municipal appointments in veterinary hygiene were few and far between.[10]

As for the Association, the membership situation was once again serious. Of the 321 nominally listed, 107 members were in arrears with their subscriptions. 'It is very obvious that if the society [*sic*] is to maintain its position', said the treasurer, 'some steps must be taken to remedy this.'[11] He did not go on to identify what those steps might be.

VACCINES

A paper on 'Animal vaccines' by J. A. W. Dollar gave a history of inoculation and the development of attenuated vaccines. It was a very extensive survey of the state of knowledge at the time.[12] John Dollar was one of two sons of the leading – and wealthy – London veterinary surgeon T. A. Dollar (he who had funded the launch of Hunting's *Veterinary Record* and the establishment of RCVS and NVA headquarters at Red Lion Square). After qualifying from London in 1887, John had taken further courses in bacteriology at London University and in 1889 had visited the Alfort and Lyon veterinary schools and studied microbiology in Berlin, where he had also worked in Robert Koch's laboratory,[13] then the world's leading centre for microbiological research. This training enabled him to elucidate and discuss the mechanisms by which immunity developed.

'Pain: Its indications and significance in the domesticated animals' was a largely philosophical discourse on the nature of pain and how it is caused and exhibited in the animal. This was a topical issue owing to the ongoing controversy about the use of animals in scientific research. While the detrimental aspects of vivisection were advertised frequently by anti-vivisection societies,[14] the paper's author, Professor John Penberthy, felt that: 'The pain inflicted and the object in view must bear a proper relationship to each other ... If by feeding or inoculating two animals we can save the life and prevent the suffering of a herd, or a household or a city, we are surely justified' in inflicting pain.[15]

The following year's AGM at Birmingham, under the presidency of J. M. Parker, saw Professor J. McQueen, a man whose name was to feature in the leadership of the NVA for many years, elected general secretary in place of John Malcolm, who had resigned.

Extending their interest in public health from the promotion of meat hygiene to the production of safe milk, the meeting passed a resolution 'That we petition the proper authorities to take into their early and serious consideration the question of having veterinary inspection of all dairy cows'.[16] The stimulus to this resolution was the growing awareness – prompted by the work of the Royal Commission – that bovine tuberculosis could spread to humans via milk.

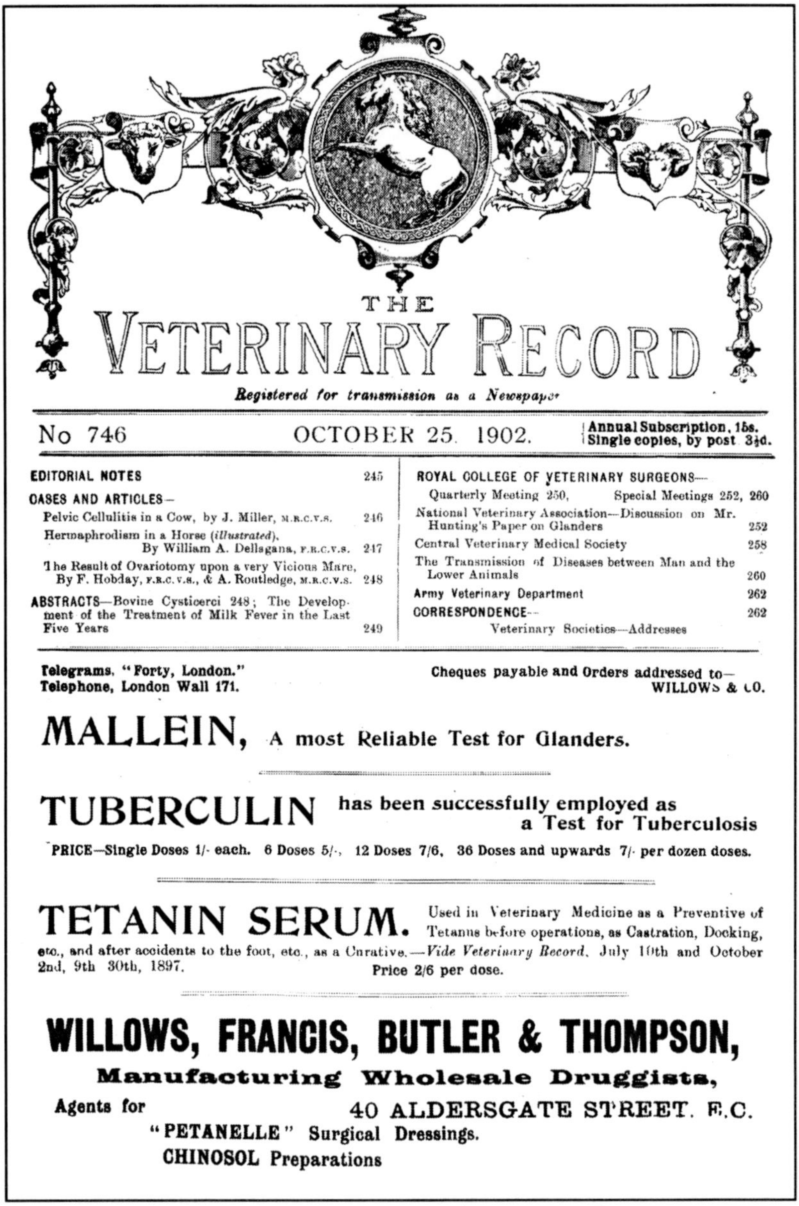

THE VETERINARY RECORD

Registered for transmission as a Newspaper

No 746   OCTOBER 25. 1902.   Annual Subscription, 15s.
                                                              Single copies, by post 3½d.

EDITORIAL NOTES 245	**ROYAL COLLEGE OF VETERINARY SURGEONS—**
OASES AND ARTICLES—	Quarterly Meeting 250, Special Meetings 252, 260
Pelvic Cellulitis in a Cow, by J. Miller, M.R.C.V.S. 246	National Veterinary Association—Discussion on Mr. Hunting's Paper on Glanders 252
Hermaphrodism in a Horse (*illustrated*), By William A. Dellagana, F.R.C.V.S. 247	Central Veterinary Medical Society 258
The Result of Ovariotomy upon a very Vicious Mare, By F. Hobday, F.R.C.V.S., & A. Routledge, M.R.C.V.S. 248	The Transmission of Diseases between Man and the Lower Animals 260
ABSTRACTS—Bovine Cysticerci 248 ; The Development of the Treatment of Milk Fever in the Last Five Years 249	Army Veterinary Department 262
	CORRESPONDENCE— 262
	Veterinary Societies—Addresses

Telegrams, "Forty, London."
Telephone, London Wall 171.

Cheques payable and Orders addressed to—
WILLOWS & CO.

MALLEIN, A most Reliable Test for Glanders.

TUBERCULIN has been successfully employed as a Test for Tuberculosis

PRICE—Single Doses 1/- each. 6 Doses 5/-, 12 Doses 7/6, 36 Doses and upwards 7/- per dozen doses.

TETANIN SERUM.

Used in Veterinary Medicine as a Preventive of Tetanus before operations, as Castration, Docking, etc., and after accidents to the foot, etc., as a Curative.—*Vide Veterinary Record*, July 10th and October 2nd, 9th 30th, 1897.

Price 2/6 per dose.

WILLOWS, FRANCIS, BUTLER & THOMPSON,

Manufacturing Wholesale Druggists,

Agents for   40 ALDERSGATE STREET. E.C.
"PETANELLE" Surgical Dressings.
CHINOSOL Preparations

Figure 4. One of the first covers of *Veterinary Record*, advertising early biological products.

Harry Olver delivered a paper on 'Abortion'; the main thrust being a survey of contagious or epizootic abortion and the means of controlling it. The isolation of aborting animals and disinfection of the premises they were kept in were advocated.[17]

Professor McQueen, discussing 'Abdominal surgery' mainly in the horse, gave a series of case histories. As the surgical procedures, often heroic, that he described were undertaken without diagnostic aids other than observation and manipulation, and the patients were mainly old or *in extremis*, it is not surprising that successful outcomes were the exception.[18]

For the first time, the AGM included a trade exhibition of veterinary equipment and medicines. This innovation, indicative of increasing reliance by the practitioner on bought-in products as well as the development of an industry servicing veterinarians, was to become a permanent feature, extremely important in both the drawing power of the meeting and its finances.[19]

The seaside resort of Great Yarmouth hosted the NVA AGM in 1896. President William Bower, in his opening address, referred to a 'want of harmony' between the profession and the Board of Agriculture, which had recently abolished the Veterinary Department, and placed a layman, Major Tennant, in charge of the making and administration of disease control policy. The future veterinary role was simply to diagnose and investigate disease. Bower reported that the matter had been 'rectified' after the president of the RCVS, Professor J. Simpson, had approached the president of the Board of Agriculture 'and the name of the Veterinary Department restored'. He commented, 'By continued and combined pressure [by the RCVS and the NVA] on those in power, appointments pertaining to veterinary matters will be given to members of our profession only.'[20] In fact, he overstated the case. Vets were still 'on tap not on top' within the Board of Agriculture, and were to remain so until 1919, when a veterinary-led Diseases of Animals Division was established.[21] The first clinical session heard a paper on 'Swine fever: its nature and suppression' by Sir John McFadyean. McFadyean, who – one is tempted to say, 'of course' – was a member of the Board of Agriculture's committee on swine fever which was sitting at that time. Its purpose was to review the progress made since control of the disease was centralised in 1893, and 'to supplement that experience by a series of experiments as to its bacteriology and life history'.[22]

After describing case histories and post mortem findings in the disease, McFadyean described the current procedure for dealing with outbreaks, and its shortcomings. He felt that the failure to bring the disease under control was due less to inadequacies in veterinary diagnosis than to difficulties in tracing and containing the spread of disease. He advocated restrictions on the movement of pigs in every district in which swine fever was found.

The audience agreed, and resolved 'That in the opinion of the NVA the enforcement of severe restrictions on the movement of swine in every area in which swine fever is known to exist is absolutely necessary for the eradication of the disease'.[23] This was to bear fruit in the form of new regulations on movement of pigs. Subsequently, swine fever incidence fell, but it was impossible to tell whether these regulations, or improved diagnosis consequent upon the swine fever committee's findings, were responsible.[24]

A presentation with the ambitious title, 'A practical method of gradually, effectively and cheaply reducing bovine tuberculosis to manageable proportions and ultimately stamping it out' by N. Almond proposed the use of tuberculin, then only recently available,[25] to identify cattle reacting to the test which, he said, should be separated from healthy cattle. Calves should be given only milk from non-reactors, or milk which had been boiled. Almond advised that calves should not be reared from cows 'tuberculous to an advanced degree'.[26]

At the 1897 meeting, at Reading, Professor J. F. Simpson presided over an attendance of only eighty-two members and visitors. The sole paper, given by Professor J. R. U. Dewar, was on 'Heredity in its relation to the diseases of animals'. A general review of the subject, it made clear the difference between heritable conditions and those which were congenital. During the lengthy discussion, some views were expressed which inclined to those of Lamarck, that characteristics acquired by an animal in its lifetime may be transmitted to its progeny.[27]

The president went on to urge, as had presidents before him, that meat inspections should be carried out by vets. He castigated the ignorance of local sanitary authorities in appointing 'so-called meat inspectors'. 'In 1896,' he said, 'Battersea had appointed as inspectors four plumbers and three carpenters; Hackney two plumbers, a carpenter, a bricklayer, a florist, a builder, a surveyor and a stonemason.' 'So long as private slaughterhouses are allowed to exist, danger will be incurred by the consumption of tuberculous flesh,' he warned. At the time, London had some 450 private slaughterhouses. It was hoped that the recommendation of the Commission on Tuberculosis in favour of closing all private slaughterhouses would be effective; that was not to be the case.[28]

Of the two clinical sessions, the first discussed a paper by Professor W. Williams, 'Traumatic diseases of the horse's foot'. This dealt with common injuries to the lower limbs and advocated the application of dry iodoform medicated dressings rather than wet dressings, together with the 'strictest asepsis' during surgery on the foot.[29]

The second session, on 'Observations on tuberculin and mallein', by James King, chief veterinary inspector of Manchester, described the use of tuberculin in testing for reactor cows and gave details of its efficiency in identifying tubercular animals. Mallein, a product of the protein fraction of *Brukholderia mallei*, had been found similarly efficient as a test for identifying glanders, he told the meeting. Manchester was progressive in its city veterinary services and King was speaking from extensive and successful experiences of dealing with bovine TB.[30]

In its first visit to the West Country the NVA met at Plymouth in 1899; the president was W. H. Bloy. The papers followed a well worn path. Bovine tuberculosis and its prevention were discussed by Jno. Dunston. He advocated well ventilated, clean and regularly disinfected cow sheds and recommended the establishment of an official laboratory for the production and free distribution of tuberculin as the sole source of that diagnostic agent. He told the meeting that there should be compulsory notification and slaughter of all tuberculous cattle, with government compensation of up to three-quarters of the animal's value. And a comprehensive list of controls designed to avoid the spread of the disease should be put in place.[31]

An extensive and detailed paper on milk fever in cattle, based largely on his own observations and experience, was presented by Cornish veterinary surgeon F. T. Harvey. He suggested that restricting the diet before calving was often effective in preventing the disease and he recommended dosing the animal with tincture of opium following parturition. He disagreed with the practice of bleeding, still apparently popular with some practitioners, as being 'as likely to cause the disease as to prevent it'.[32] Professor Fred Hobday, in his contribution, maintained that ovariotomy in healthy cattle resulted in higher milk yields and increased duration of lactation.

The Dublin meeting, abandoned in 1890, took place eventually in 1900 under the presidency of Matthew Hedley. A proposal that the remuneration of the general secretary (William Hunting, appointed in 1889) should be doubled was put to the meeting and accepted with enthusiasm. However, as the existing amount was 'nil', the increase did not cost the NVA anything. That light-hearted suggestion set the tone for what turned out to be a most successful conference. The *Veterinary Record* commented 'It may safely be said that this year's proceedings have broken the record. In the numbers attending, in the sustained debates, in the interest taken, in the receptions given and in the numbers enjoyed, the Dublin meeting has passed all previous.'[33]

The papers included one on 'crossbreeding telegony in animals'; 'telegony' was the belief held by some at the time that the genetic influence of the sire was carried on in the dam's offspring from subsequent matings by other animals. More conventional topics included 'The parasitic diseases of animals transmissible to man by contact and by food'; and

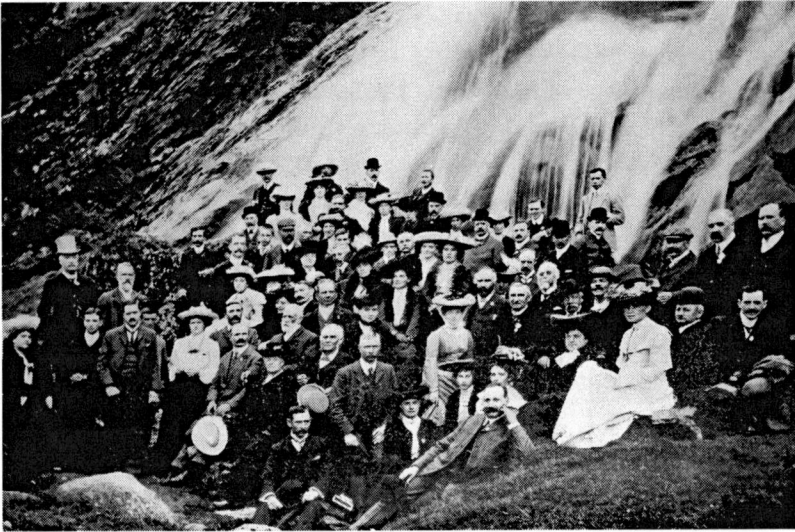

Figure 5. The excursion at the successful Dublin conference in 1904. It established a tradition of photographing all participants to the event.

the 'Medical and surgical nursing of animals'.[34] That was perhaps the earliest reference to the use of paramedical care in veterinary nursing.

The excursion proved to be an enormously enjoyable trip to Glendalough. The AGM proceedings devoted four pages to it. In fact, the whole meeting proved to be so successful that the annual event returned to Dublin only four years later.

Perhaps stimulated by the enthusiasm raised at the 1900 meeting membership had increased to 417 by the 1901 AGM, in Edinburgh, when Professor J. R. U. Dewar was in the chair. That number of members was to be the highest for the next twenty years.

The meeting discussed papers on 'Diseases of young stock, by James Clark; 'Dairy inspection', which included the construction of milking parlours, cleanliness, diseases carried by milk, and disease passed to the milk by the cow, by J. Riddock. 'Meat inspection' by J. McPhail and 'Veterinary inspection at horse and cattle shows' by R. Brydon concluded the clinical programme.[35]

A rare small animal topic was part of the programme at the London AGM in 1902, at which Professor Sir John McFadyean was president. Professor (later Sir) Frederick Hobday of the Royal Veterinary College, a pioneer in the field of small animal practice, said that distemper was 'the greatest scourge in the canine world'. He described unsuccessful trials with vaccines prepared by the microbiologists Phisalix and Copeman. He also demonstrated that calf lymph, which had a popular reputation as a specific, was ineffectual in treating the disease.[36] 'Glanders', by William Hunting (a member of the Board of Agriculture committee on glanders then sitting), and 'Pneumonia', by J. W. Dollar, were the other topics discussed.

The meeting passed a resolution giving NVA support to an RCVS complaint to the War Office about the status of veterinary officers in the Army Veterinary Department. Army veterinary surgeons did not receive an Army commission; they were subservient on certain veterinary matters to non-veterinary superior officers, and received inferior pensions to army medical personnel.[37]

Local man F. W. Garnett was NVA president for the following AGM, which took place in Windermere. Garnett would go on to be president of the RCVS throughout the Great War and to play an important role in the resettlement of ex-army officers thereafter.[38]

MUNICIPAL APPOINTMENTS

A paper by J. S. Lloyd, who was veterinary inspector for Sheffield, described the duties of 'The veterinarian in his relation to state and municipal work'. As well as describing the technical duties involved, Lloyd drew attention to the shortcomings in the structure of the official veterinary services. He told his audience that the government's 'so-called Veterinary Department' was made up of two veterinary surgeons on the staff of the Board of Agriculture and a number of veterinarians 'temporarily appointed as district or travelling veterinary surgeons, mainly to do with swine fever'.

At the municipal level, whole-time appointments were growing, but still 'not far past the teens'. He sought to disabuse his audience of any misconception that the veterinary inspector's life was a comparatively easy one. It was virtually a seven days a week occupation, with work ranging from market inspections to the veterinary management of large local authority stables, dairy inspections under various acts, examination of large groups of animals for the import and export trade and meat inspection. With regard to the latter, he said it was 'remarkable that in England, the veterinary inspector had no power to seize diseased meat'. A not unrelated topic by A. E. Mettam reviewed the 'Duties and liabilities attaching to veterinary surgeons in the exercise of their profession'. 'Anthrax in relation to trade' by Professor J. Wortley Axe and 'Certain septicaemias and other infections of young animals' concluded the clinical sessions.[39]

It was back to Dublin for the 1904 meeting, this time with Dubliner Charles Allen presiding. The papers were: 'Epizootic lymphadenitis (E. E. Martin)', 'Army horses; their collection, selection and purchase', by William Hunting, and 'Haemoglobinurea in bovines' by Professor G. W. Wooldridge of the Royal Veterinary College. G. W. was the uncle of W. R. (Reg) Wooldridge, founder of the Animal Health Trust and a prime mover in the creation of the British Small Animal Veterinary Association.

In a speech at the annual dinner Professor W. O. Williams, a recent president of the RCVS council, introduced a somewhat controversial note by arguing in favour of veterinary students gaining university degrees. Williams had been principal of the Royal (Dick) Veterinary School, which he left in 1873 to establish the New Veterinary College, Edinburgh, taking with him most of the students and staff of the 'Dick'.[40]

He had already provoked controversy within the profession by allowing a young woman, Aileen Cust, to enrol at his college, and supporting her unsuccessful attempt to become a member of RCVS (she was not admitted to membership until 1922). Now he informed assembled members that he had had talks with Liverpool University about transferring his struggling school there. The university had said: 'We will assist you to give university teaching to veterinary students, and we will not interfere with [the Royal College's] sole right and privilege of granting a licence to veterinary surgeons.' Professor Williams had accepted Liverpool's offer and the university's faculty of veterinary medicine and surgery would very shortly grant degrees to the first students who passed the examination of the Royal College of Veterinary Surgeons.

Members of the audience were not impressed with this announcement, nor with Williams' claim that the universities would assist in enabling the profession to know a great deal more than the man in the street. He thought 'without exaggeration' that the 'ordinary man in the street, the horse owner, the horse breeder, the cattle owner and breeder, knew nearly as much as a veterinary surgeon who qualified twenty or thirty years ago'. His listeners responded with 'cries of "Bosh" and "Rubbish" '.[41] In a *Veterinary Record* leader, William Hunting argued: 'All that Liverpool can offer is cheap and perhaps good teaching for class A students, and after that teaching worse than can now be obtained at more than one veterinary school.'[42]

That was the only cloud on what proved to be a very sunny occasion. The dinner concluded in a speech of such hilarity that the *Veterinary Record's* reporter was unable to take an account of what had been said. The speaker's words, he said, had been drowned by gales of laughter (there had also been many toasts drunk during the evening; the *Record's* editor thought his reporter had perhaps over indulged).

A new chief veterinary officer was in place at the 1905 AGM in Buxton. Stewart Stockman, McFadyean's son-in-law, was a man of forceful personality and considerable intellect. Appointed at just thirty-six years of age, he held the post until his premature death in 1926. In his paper 'Preventive inoculation and the serum method' Stockman described the preparation and use of sera to convey short acting (passive) immunity and their use in tetanus and strangles (*Streptoccocus equi* infection) with mixed results. Sometimes, he said, he used serum and vaccines currently administered. He finally described contemporary trials of culture-derived vaccines in a wide range of diseases.

In the treatment of 'Sheep scab and external ovine parasites', a subject about which the Board of Agriculture was currently concerned, R. J. Hicks described the methods of dipping sheep and the formulations used for preventing and curing sheep scab. Arsenic, carbolic acid and tobacco (nicotine) were employed and disinfection of objects and areas frequented by sheep was advocated. The speaker noted that legislation relating to dipping had been in place since 1866, 'and still outbreaks occurred'. As, indeed, they still do. For maggot fly strikes, carbolic oil application was recommended.[43]

A pupilage of 'at least a year' with a competent practitioner in an agricultural district should be insisted upon by the RCVS, said Henry Gray in his paper, 'Veterinary education – ante and postgraduate'. There were, he maintained, many things a veterinary surgeon ought to know which at present could only be learnt in country practice. Gray was also lukewarm about the proposals for university degrees in veterinary science: 'Will it not indicate a place and lower value on our own membership and fellowship degrees?' he asked.[44]

At the AGM at Liverpool in 1906 the Vice Chancellor, Dr Dale, welcomed members on a visit to the university and spoke of his pleasure and enthusiasm for the new veterinary school.

The papers presented at the AGM at Liverpool in 1890 included a discussion on contagious abortion by Professor B. Bang, from Copenhagen, who had recently discovered the bacterium causing the disease, *Brucella abortus*. Bang described, with photographic illustrations, the microbiological investigations of the condition leading to the identification of the organism. 'Animal diseases following war', a subject shortly to have massive significance, 'public health and veterinary science', and 'Insects and ticks in relation to animal disease' concluded the scientific sessions.[45]

The succeeding years saw a preponderance of veterinary medical topics: 'The intestinal parasites of the ox and sheep' by Professor T. W. Cave; 'Actinomycosis and botryomycosis' by Professor G. W. Wooldridge; sterility in mares was discussed by Sidney Slocock. A novelty was an illustrated lecture on 'Dental anomalies and their significance' by Professor O. Charnock Bradley.[46] 'Some skin diseases in the dog', by G. H. Livesey, was another indication of the growing importance of canine topics; but 'Redwater (babesiosis) in cattle', by Stewart Stockman, the new chief veterinary officer, was a regular subject. The prevalence of tuberculosis in livestock was demonstrated by figures presented by John S. Lloyd, who said that in Glasgow (one of the few cities with municipal abattoirs) a total of 3,482 carcasses were condemned in a year because of the disease.[47]

'AMALGAMATION' OF LOCAL DIVISIONS

In 1909, the most important event at the AGM was a special meeting of local division representatives at which Professor Charnock Bradley put forward a draft scheme for the reorganisaton of the NVA 'on a wider basis' to include all the divisional associations.

Orlando Charnock Bradley was a Lancashire man who qualified from the New Veterinary College, Edinburgh, before obtaining medical qualifications. At the time of the Harrogate meeting, he was professor of anatomy at the Royal (Dick) Veterinary College. He would go on to be principal of the college, a long-serving president of the NVA throughout the Great War (1914–1922) and then president of the RCVS.[48]

Charnock Bradley proposed: 'That this conference, approving of the principle of amalgamation [of the local divisions with the NVA], take steps by which a scheme may be formulated and submitted to the various societies for their consideration'. He assured the meeting that there was 'no suggestion of interference with the title or management of any of the existing societies beyond the payment of a subscription for each member to the treasurer of the national society.' The representative of the Central Veterinary Medical Society, Professor J. McQueen, supporting the proposal, said that at the present time the NVA was not fulfilling either its scientific or its professional objectives. 'It has become the occasion of a pleasant outing,' he said. And it was a fact that the Association's only visible activity was the annual meeting. The NVA, he said, should be reconstituted in the face of external economic threats to the veterinary profession such as the introduction of motor traction and in other ways. 'It is necessary that we should combine to fight almost for our very existence.'[49]

The proposal met with general approval – provided it was made clear that there should be no 'interference with the title and management of any existing society' – and carried unanimously.

After further discussion at the AGM the following day, the principle of joining all the local societies under the umbrella of the National Veterinary Association was accepted.[50] Over the next two years, the details were thrashed out by the divisions. Various versions of draft rules for an amalgamation were discussed, with sticking points occurring over subscriptions to the local and national bodies, fears of NVA interference, or even over the title of the Association – whether to add the word 'Medical' to National Veterinary Association. A committee was appointed to work out the details.

In 1910 when Professor McQueen, of the Royal Veterinary College, was president, there was further discussion of the amalgamation – or 'affiliation scheme' as the programme called it. It was reported that the committee appointed at Harrogate the previous year had, 'as far as possible' embodied within the scheme suggestions made by divisions. However, it was decided that they were unable to accept the scheme in its present form: it seems likely there was a lingering suspicion of a loss of sovereignty for the local divisions if they were amalgamated into the national association. In particular, the question of paying subscriptions for the national body to the local division, which would then be responsible for forwarding the money to the national association was a sticking point. The local divisions 'would however, heartily approve of any workable scheme that would place the National Veterinary Association in closer relation with the local societies'. And another committee was appointed to consider the matter further.[51]

Further prolonged discussions were held at the 1911 meeting, the first to be held in Wales, at Caernarvon. It was here that, at last, the proposals for a branch affiliation scheme were finally accepted. Last minute moves to delay the matter for yet another year failed to gain support and the scheme for affiliation of the local societies was accepted. The patience and eloquence of Orlando Charnock Bradley, to become one of the key figures in the Association for the next decade, won the day – almost. The important proposal that local divisions should collect their members' subscriptions for the National was rejected; members remained responsible for payment of their own subscriptions direct to the NVA. The title National Veterinary Association was retained: the addition of 'Medical' would come later.[52]

Charnock Bradley went on to present one of the meeting's main papers. His title, 'Veterinary education in relation to public health' contained the framework for a proposed Diploma in Veterinary Public Health, a concept which came to fruition in 1920. Such diplomas became a recognised qualification. A new departure was a paper on 'Principles of economic feeding of horses and cattle', by H. Taylor. 'Surgical shoeing' of horses by H. Sumner and 'Sclerostomiasis [sic] in equines' by Professor H. E. Annett completed the clinical subjects.

By the AGM in 1912 most of the local societies had become affiliated to the NVA, consolidating the structure by which the main association provided a central organisation based on its constituent divisions. That principle remains in place today. The reluctance of the divisions to accept responsibility for collecting members' NVA subscriptions did nothing to strengthen the Association. In fact, it would have helped weld the divisions together. The risk of fragmentation increased as the number of divisions proliferated over the years. The council structure then put in place meant that individual members, whose subscriptions directly financed the Association, had no direct say in its government. This lay in the hands of a large council whose members were nominated by the divisions. The system was to prove unwieldy and led to problems in the future as the divisions and their nominees proliferated and the number of past presidents (*ex officio* members of council for life) increased year by year.

The AGM in 1912 was at Manchester, with William Woods in the chair. A paper by Lt. Gen. Fred Smith discussed the detailed syllabus of the veterinary undergraduate course in the UK, comparing it unfavourably with some European veterinary schools, and suggested revisions. Arguing the benefits of continued postgraduate education, he said 'the practitioner should not fail to ask himself from time to time, am I honestly satisfied with my results?' The meeting included what was to be the last contribution by William Hunting, on 'Phalangeal ostitis'.[53]

The static state of the membership continued to be of concern and exhortations of one sort or another regularly appeared in the *Veterinary Record.* In January, the journal printed a letter from J. McFarlane, president of the Glasgow and West of Scotland association drawing the attention 'of the profession generally ... to the necessity of becoming members of the National Association, since its reconstitution to embrace all local societies'.[54] The AGM that year reported a membership of 362.

The question of fees for veterinary examinations of animals for insurance purposes was an early example of the NVA's ongoing interest in economic matters. The question of such fees, with allegations of undercutting, was to recur frequently. In 1914, shortly before the outbreak of the 1914–

1918 world war, the Association recommended the following scale, as a minimum for examination and 'report on general health, condition, age, colour, markings and approximate value of animals proposed for insurance':

HORSES AND VALUABLE PEDIGREE CATTLE

(a)	Single animals under the value of £50			5s
	Two animals " " " " "	each		5s
	After the first two	"		2/6
(b)	Single animal valued at £50, under £100	"		10/6
(c)	Single animal " " £100, " £250	"		15s
(d)	Single animal " " £250, " £1000	"		21s

The fee was halved if more than two animals were examined. Mileage charges were made if the vet had to travel more than a mile, at the rate of one shilling for up to three miles, two shillings and sixpence for three to five miles, three shillings and sixpence for five to eight miles, and 'in proportion' for more than that. Post mortem examinations were one guinea (21s.).[55] To put those suggested charges into some sort of context, the national minimum weekly wage for agricultural labourers at that time was 16s. 9d. (The same tables give the yearly salary for 'medical officers, surgeons' as £275; in 1891 the figure had been £475).[56]

William Hunting had been elected president for the 1913 meeting, which was in London. An important paper by G. P. Male discussed the implications for the practicing vet of the new Milk and Dairies Bill – which made it an offence to sell tuberculous milk – and the Tuberculosis Order – which gave local authorities the power to slaughter clinically affected tuberculous cattle, and apply the tuberculin test to suspected cows.[57]

Other papers discussed the foot of the Shire horse (Dr Griffith), gastric and internal diseases in dogs (G. H.

Livesey), and debated the question 'Do we need a new degree?'(Henry Gray).

HUNTING DIES

Only three months after that meeting, Hunting died suddenly. Although he was 77, his death came as a shock; he had just been elected president. With his passing, the Association and the whole profession lost a man whose competence as a practitioner, inquiring mind and foresight had been of immense practical benefit to veterinary medicine and particularly to the NVA.

The contribution made by Hunting to the Association and the whole veterinary world was outstanding. 'If there was any one man of whom it could be said that his personality and literary work were largely responsible for the development of a real unity and sense of corporate responsibility within the veterinary profession, that man was William Hunting,' said an appreciation written fifty years after his death. If the elimination of glanders had been a lifelong passion, his range of involvement in veterinary matters was wide. In the 1870s he had been interested in diseases of the dog; he had experimented with remedial horse-shoeing techniques; and he had demonstrated that treating horses with damaged tendons by 'firing' with hot irons showed no benefit (contrary to widely held belief).As a consultant he had a 'happy knack of putting one at one's ease' in dealing with difficult cases. As a speaker he was 'fluent but not verbose, conversational in delivery'; but on matters of principle 'a determined and fiery conversationalist'. His strong sense of humour could 'create a remark which transformed the whole atmosphere of a meeting'.

Physically, he was said to be 'a handsome man of medium stature', with an auburn beard, and seldom without a cigar. Brilliant in his profession, he was no businessman. 'He was extravagant but had little appreciation of money . . .

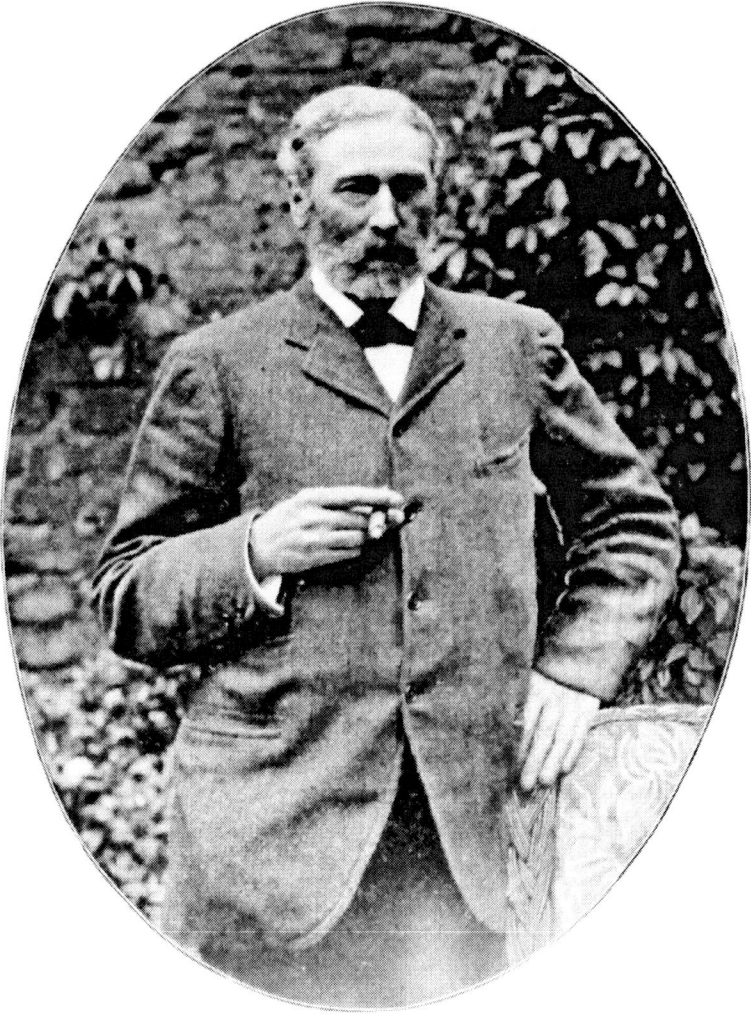

Figure 6. William Hunting, founder and editor of the *Veterinary Record*, in characteristic pose; he was said to be 'the mainspring of the National Veterinary Association' by his contributions to the profession's clinical studies and to the affairs of the Association.

He would buy a box of expensive cigars and then borrow money to buy a train ticket.'

In sum, 'No professional meeting or social function was a real success if William Hunting was absent – he seldom was! It was largely his spirit which animated both the local branches and the National itself . . . He is the mainspring of the National Veterinary Association.'[58]

From the 1920s through the 1950s, the *Veterinary Record's* cover carried the image of its founder. If he had done no more than found and edit the *Record* – critical of the NVA though it was at times – Hunting would have been assured of his place among the early leaders of the profession. An indication of his wider reputation is given by the award to his family of a Civil List pension.

CHAPTER THREE

WAR BREAKS OUT

The outbreak of war on 4 August 1914 meant that meeting the demands of the Army for veterinarians to service its rapidly increasing numbers of horses, and coping with domestic animal health services with the much reduced number of practitioners remaining in civilian practice, became the overriding priority for the profession and, particularly, the NVA. Annual meetings of the Association, and regular meetings of many of its divisions, continued throughout the war, but in a truncated form. The NVA, held together by its wartime president Charnock Bradley, still held its meetings at the premises of the RCVS, 10 Red Lion Square, and the councils of the two bodies continued to overlap in membership. F. W. Garnett was a long serving member of NVA council. NVA president O. Charnock Bradley, also a RCVS councillor, was president of the Association 1914–1922. The chief veterinary officer, Stewart Stockman, was also a member of the councils of both bodies.

The College was soon called upon for assistance by the War Office. On 8 October 1914 it wrote:[1]

Chapter 3

Dear Sir,

There is likely to be a shortage of veterinary surgeons for the new armies which are being formed, and I should be obliged if the Royal College of Veterinary Surgeons could assist in any way to help meet the deficiency.

Yours sincerely,

R. Pringle

Major-General Pringle was director-general of the Army Veterinary Service, and obviously a man of few words. A War Emergency Committee was immediately formed by the College which, included prominent NVA members, the Association's president Charnock Bradley among them.

A notice issued by the Army Veterinary Service offered the following conditions of service to veterinary surgeons joining up:

Conditions of service as relating to temporary commissions

Civil Veterinary Practitioners desirous of serving at home or abroad with the army should communicate with the Director General, Army Veterinary Service, 16 Victoria Street, S.W.

Gentlemen accepted for such service will be granted the temporary rank of Lieutenant in the Army Veterinary Corps and must fulfill the following conditions:

1 They must be members of the Royal College of Veterinary Surgeons

2 They must engage for a period of 12 calendar months or until their services are no longer required, whichever first shall happen

3 Their pay will be that of a lieutenant, Army Veterinary Corps, with allowances as follows:

Pay, yearly	£250	0	0
Field allowance at 3/- per day	54	15	0
Rations at 1/9 per day (approx)	32	0	0
Bonus after 12 months service of 60 days' pay	40	0	0
	£376	15	0

In addition, there was a uniform allowance of £30 and £7 10s. for camp kit. Applicants had to be below fifty and of good character.

When the Army's appeal for recruits was considered at the RCVS council meeting in January, the implications of enlistment for a general practitioner, virtually all of whom were single handed, were discussed. It was agreed that arrangements for cooperation between practitioners should be encouraged, and that 'if a man is to leave his practice, he must have a month or two in which to make his arrangements', said Stewart Stockman, the government's chief veterinary officer. As far as the terms of service were concerned, Sir John McFadyean commented that, while he would be glad to believe that there were no veterinarians in general practice whose income did not exceed £300 a year, he imagined there were considerable numbers who did not make that sum. He felt it would help to induce younger practitioners, whose practices were not large, to accept temporary commissions if some sort of assurance could be given that everything in the council's power would be done to enable them to return to their practices after the war's end. Stockman suggested that 'it might be possible to arrange the matter fairly quickly through the local veterinary societies'.[2]

Accordingly, the College wrote under the heading 'the shortage of veterinary surgeons for the Army', asking NVA divisions to encourage their members to join up. The appeal received much support, with local associations discussing means of 'caretaking' the practices of neighbouring colleagues called to the colours while they were away.

The Midland Counties association (National VMA Northern Branch) saw problems in the proposed caretaking arrangements for the practices of members on war service. It could, one member thought, be difficult to do this without some remuneration in return – some clients might be far afield and involve travelling time. Another member said he 'failed to see how many men could afford to do work for another practitioner without pay'. A third quoted the instance of a practitioner who had joined the Army but declined to allow others to take on his work, saying: 'It would not be just to allow him to do so when he himself was drawing Army pay.' But the division agreed that 'a large

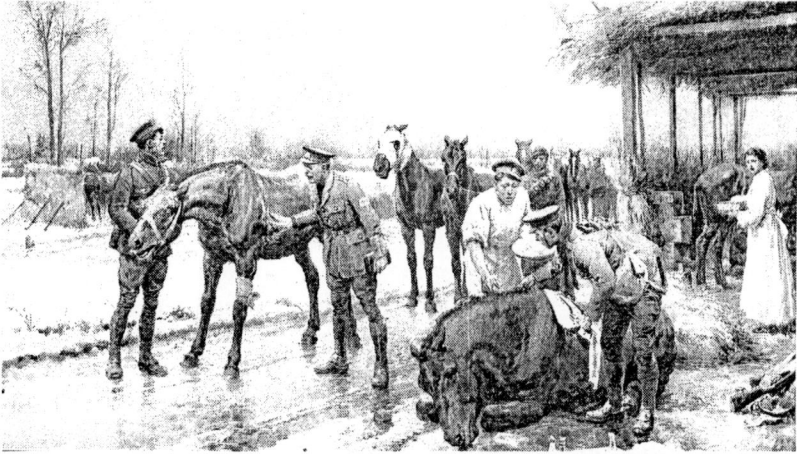

Figure 7. Horses returning from the front in the 1914–1918 war to be treated for wounds at a field veterinary facility run by the Blue Cross organisation. After first-aid, the casualties were drafted to hospital for surgical or medical treatment prior to convalescence.

number of members of this association having joined His Majesty's Forces, all the members pledge themselves to assist in every way they possibly can such practitioners during their absence'. Each case would have to be met on a different basis, it was noted.

The Yorkshire Veterinary Society encouraged members to enlist 'and to entrust their practices to their neighbours. Those in turn are asked to agree not to retain any of the absent man's clients and to pay to his family 20 per cent of any receipts from these clients.'[3] One NVA division after another discussed similar arrangements to assist the war effort. A bone of contention among the profession was that most practising veterinarians who joined up did so as lieutenants, while medical doctors and some vets in government service were given the rank of captain. At a subsequent RCVS council meeting the Midland Counties VMA asked the College to try to establish parity of army rank with veterinary officials of the Board of Agriculture, who were given the rank of captain on joining up, and this argument was pursued (with little result) by the College.[4]

As the war went on, more and more vets were needed for military service. In 1914, the Army had about 25,000 horses (and 80 motor vehicles); by 1917 it was buying 15,000 animals a month. At the end of the war there were some 530,000 horses in military service plus 230,000 mules. There was a total of 2.5 million 'admissions' (casualties or sickness) of which 80 per cent were able to be returned to active service.[5]

In July 1915, Major-General Pringle attended the RCVS council to emphasise in person the urgent need for ever more veterinary officers. The College agreed to pass on his message to all Members of the RCVS who had qualified since 1895.[6]

'Repeated and urgent' appeals from the War Office, with requests to release veterinary students early from colleges for military duties, led to an acute shortage of vets on the home front and fears of continuing shortage in the future. These concerns were not confined to the profession's own organisations. *The Scotsman*, Scotland's leading newpaper, stated that as a result of the number of vets joining the Army 'at the present moment, animal owners in all parts of the kingdom are unable to obtain the normal amount of veterinary service'. It also predicted that, because of a falling number of new entrants to the profession in pre-1914 years and an increase in the number of new public appointments of veterinary officers, the shortage would become worse. 'However acutely the shortage of veterinary surgeons may be felt at the present time, it is clear that in the very near future the shortage will have more serious consequences,' stated *The Scotsman*. It went on: 'Apart from the conservation of the health of the animal – and the incidental protection of the pocket of the owner – the veterinary profession, no less than the medical profession, is essential for the preservation of the health of the public.'[7]

'NEW EPOCH' PREDICTED

As the war continued, practitioners in the local divisions began to have concerns about what the profession would have to face when, eventually, hostilities ended. In an address to the North Midland Veterinary Association in October 1916, Professor J. Share-Jones of the University of Liverpool gave his view of the way in which the veterinary profession might develop. He said the future of the profession hung delicately in the balance. 'Two or three false steps in one direction or the other might make all the difference between our profession taking a permanent place among the ranks of other learned professions and stepping back among those which are still struggling for public recognition as professions.' One of the problems was that there were insufficient entrants to the veterinary profession to maintain the average number on the register. More names were being lost from the register by death than were replaced by new graduates.

One factor not mentioned by Share-Jones was that the expense of a four-year qualifying course, with not particularly profitable career prospects at the end of it, did not make veterinary surgery an attractive option for many young men. The irreversible decline in the horse as a source of motive power as it was replaced by the internal combustion engine meant that that major source of veterinary income, then and for some years to come, was to face serious problems.[8] Share Jones, however, felt there was much potential for expansion of veterinary work. There was a great deal 'that should accrue to the profession that was either not done at all in England or was performed by other people', he argued.

After the war, he predicted, 'there would be a new epoch in the discovery and application of science'. Share Jones said he knew of no branch of science and its application to industry that presented greater possibilities for fruitful results than veterinary medicine and surgery.

One essential opportunity, he suggested, was the routine veterinary inspection and certification of livestock. This, he said, could prove one of the most powerful instruments in preventive medicine. 'What an opportunity it will provide', he said, 'for the veterinary profession to demonstrate its utility!' He made those comments in connection with equine veterinary inspection and certification of soundness for insurance purposes, with reports to the insuring company and the livestock owner. He predicted that such a scheme if widely adopted would be beneficial to production and economic to operate. The content of the veterinary curriculum should make veterinary surgeons 'peculiarly qualified to render signal national service in the development of our milk and meat industries', he concluded. 'The call will be a national one. It is for us, both in numbers and efficiency, to be ready to answer.'[9]

That, of course, was for the future. Meanwhile, the demands of the Army became ever more insistent. The RCVS president, F.W. Garnett, wrote to the War Office in January 1918 – in seeming desperation – pointing out that as many as 1,040 veterinary surgeons out of an estimated 2,460 in active practice were now doing military duty. 'This', he continues, 'represents 42 per cent of the veterinary profession, a far higher proportion than has probably been reached by any other profession'. The official figure was even higher. The RAMC website says there were 364 AVC officers (regular and reserve) at the outbreak of war and a further 1,306 were commissioned, making a total of 1,700 – half the number of active registered vets.

While acknowledging the needs of the Army were urgent, Garnett argued that the needs of the agricultural community were also extremely important. Belatedly, in 1917, the government had recognised the need to intervene actively in food production. To combat milk shortages it laid down generous set prices, while in response to fears about milk quality, it introduced grading and sanitary standards.[10]

These measures can only have increased farmers' demand for – and ability to pay – veterinary surgeons. Garnett was also concerned about post-war shortages, fearing that the numbers of veterinary students coming forward would be too small to replace natural wastage.[11] The War Office reply was unhelpful.

In July, the *Veterinary Record* wrote: 'The endeavours to prevent the calling up of veterinary students have not been successful. ... This is damaging to the profession and mischievous to the prospects of agriculture.' However, some amelioration to the situation on the home front was afforded by a decision not to call up older veterinary surgeons. This 'showed recognition of the fact that the few veterinary surgeons still left in the country have become indispensable for the care of our livestock. ... The experience of recent years has shown us how greatly veterinary science can aid in preserving them.'[12]

MONEY MATTERS

The perennial topic of practitioners' income was taken up once more in a *Record* leader which discussed the factors affecting the economic situation of the practitioner. 'Formerly, many veterinary surgeons profited largely by the sale of medicines. It added: 'There were men, mostly in the country, who were really much more medicine pedlars than practitioners. For various reasons that source of income has declined for many years; and there is no probability that it will ever again approach its old level.' The speculation that sales of animal medicines would decline in importance was very wide of the mark: such sales have continued to be an important part of the business structure of many practices, both rural and urban.

'On the other hand,' noted the *Record*, 'there has been a great increase in such special work as diagnostic and preventive inoculations. ... Veterinary work is now much more strictly professional, requiring the personal attention of the practitioner, than it used to be.' These inoculations included: contagious abortion vaccine, produced by the government veterinary laboratory for extensive field trials; swine fever serum, which the government had introduced in place of the earlier slaughter policy for the purpose of preserving pig life in war-time; and tuberculin, used for diagnosing tuberculosis in cows. However, professional fees, which had never been very high, had not risen much and had not compensated for the loss of income from the sale of medicines. [13]

The National's 1918 AGM at Red Lion Square, London, concentrated on professional fees. With a view to building a stronger profession after the war ended, a paper was presented by veterinarian Peter Wilson which put forward a proposal for 'an organised (i.e., by the NVS [*sic*]) attempt to improve the present fees'.

The three classes of fee he considered were insurance fees (for examining an animal for insurance purposes), fees for local authority work (meat and market inspections, etc., and private fees – those for practice clients). Wilson acknowledged the complexity of his proposal and the difficulties it would present. The urgency of the need to increase fees was acknowledged and a subcommittee was appointed to consider the matter. Meanwhile, the AGM agreed the following resolutions;

PROFESSIONAL FEES

That we send forward to the branches for comment and criticism certain recommendations respecting night calls, percentage increase on existing fees; fees for insurance, examination of horses for soundness, and castration; and the payment for the use of the veterinary surgeon's car.

The recommendations are as follows:

1 That there be a general increase on prewar fees of 'not less than 25%'.
2 That double fees be charged for night work, commencing at 6 pm in winter and 8 pm in summer.
3 That the minimum fees for examination for soundness should be one guinea; and for castration 10/6.
4 That the scale of fees previously recommended for insurance companies be not reduced, but increased 25%.
5 That government offices and public bodies shall be requested to pay to veterinary surgeons using their own car or trap the same fees as they would have paid to the garage or livery stable car for trap hire.[14]

Branches were asked to consider the resolutions and submit comments for discussion at the next meeting of the NVA

Chapter 3

The following year the following scale of minimum fees was proposed:

Town visits 3/6 Mileage 1/3 per mile

Foaling or calving 1 to 2 gns; removing placenta 10/6 mare, 7/6 cow; inflation of udder , (Milk fever) 5/-

Medicines. Draughts, cows and horses 2/6; drenches, cows, cleansing, etc 2/-; Lotions, 8oz 2/6; Liniments, 8oz; Blister 2/6 to 5/- according to size; Powders, horses and cows, 8/- per doz; Balls 1/6 each; Pessaries 1/- to 2/- each

Dog medicines. Pills 1/6 per doz; Medicine 2oz 1/6, 6oz 2/6; Worm capsules 1/- each; Whelping 10/6 to 21/-; Castration with chloroform 21/-; Board and Treatment at Infirmary 2/- per diem [indicates that many vets also ran boarding establishments for dogs].

Operations. Horses. Etc. –
Castration horses, Single 21/-, Two15/-, Three or more 10/6 each; Docking 5/-.
Castration, calves 2/6 each; Bulls 1 year and over 10/6 each

Ringing Bull 5/- (ring extra)

Intratracheal injection (used to treat livestock for lung worms), 5, 3/6 each; up to 10, 2/6 each; above 10, 2/- each

Tuberculin test, Single 21/-; Next two 10/6 each; after first three, 5/- each

Antitetanin [*sic*] Injection 7/6 each

Raising and slinging horse 10/6; hire of slings 2/6 per week[15]

Some comparisons with fees charged around 1870 – half a century earlier – show not a great deal of change: visits and examinations were then between 1s 6d and 2s 6d; castrating a colt, 5s; medicines, between 1s 6d and 2s 6d.[16] 'Inflation of the udder' – 'pumping up' the teats – was practiced to treat milk fever as a pragmatic treatment; it was later discovered that the pressure prevented the loss of calcium by the cow which caused the condition. Antitetanus serum was used following injury to a horse; tetanus was an important and not infrequent condition in working horses.

The scale was circulated to all divisions and also to MRCVSs who were not members, pointing out the benefit to be derived 'from associating with members of the Association'. Divisions discussed the proposed scale, generally with approval; how widely they were adopted is not known. The adoption of a uniform scale of fees throughout the country was 'a more than doubtful proposition. . . .The difficulties of establishing such a scale are great.'[17] And so it proved; complaints about low fees did not stop.

The list gives an illuminating picture of the common practice procedures at the time. Medicines were then, and remained, an important part of the veterinary practitioner's income. The great majority of the medicines and lotions dispensed would be made up at the practice; the dominance of proprietary products manufactured by the pharmaceutical industry would await the therapeutic revolution in medicine during the 1950s and 1960s.

ARMISTICE

Four months after that 1918 meeting, the need to meet the insatiable demands of the battlefields was overtaken by events. The armistice of 11 November meant that the priority became resettlement of those returning from the war.

Discussing the forthcoming demobilisation of those members of the profession who had been away on active service, the *Record* comments: 'It will be no light matter to arrange for the resettlement of these members in civil life.' There would be problems with resettling those returning from war service in the practices they had 'loaned' out to neighbours. Some clients will not want to go back to their former veterinary surgeon, and obviously cannot be compelled to do so. Further, 'practically none' of those who had graduated since June 1914 had seen much of civilian practice. The *Record* suggested that 'younger members holding temporary commissions, if offered a permanent one, would do well to think before refusing a permanent commission'. Acceptance of a permanent commission would mean 'a settled career, with a fair pension assured after its termination', while 'the present prospects of civil practice are much more dubious',[18] warned the article.

In its last issue of 1919, the *Veterinary Record* published a leader which looked at the situation in which the profession found itself, and was cautiously optimistic about its future in peacetime. It said, 'This year has not been satisfactory for the nation [it had been a period of unemployment and industrial unrest] but it can hardly be called unsatisfactory for the profession. Veterinary surgeons, confronted with much the same difficulties as other men, are dealing with them more successfully than are many classes. Vets were urged to support the NVA, and the College: 'Future progress depended on consistent and patient development of our resources.'[19]

The fact, however, was that the NVA was in fairly low water. Membership and finances were not yet recovered from the exigencies of wartime. One of the reasons why only a small proportion of the veterinary population were members of the Association had been raised earlier in the year by a correspondent to the *Record*. 'Strong Unionist' wrote: 'The principal reason the Association is not representative of the professional generally is that members have no money to spend to enable them to attend meetings, having to pay locums if they are desirous of doing so. When veterinary fees and charges are more uniform the membership of the National will be greatly increased, I am certain: and the sooner the better.'[20] That opinion was at odds with the rather more favourable economic view from the *Record*.

The Association remained optimistic: a post-war revival of its affairs was heralded by the journal: 'One of the most hopeful signs of the changing conditions at the present time is the resumption by the NVA of its normal functions, which have necessarily been in abeyance during the absence of so large a proportion of its members.'

And it was clear that the war, with all its problems, had not been without benefit to the veterinary profession, largely in relation to its heroic efforts in caring for the army's horses (the Army Veterinary Corps was made the Royal Army Veterinary Corp in November 1918) but also for the work it had done in maintaining civilian veterinary services when most of its members were away on active service. The Yorkshire Veterinary Society president, S. Sampson, said in August 1919, after referring to the difficulties endured by those vets who had 'kept the home fire burning' that the profession had 'more than acquitted themselves well' during the war. Veterinary surgeons, he said, 'had gained during the last four and a half years that which would have taken us a quarter of a century to achieve under our pre-war conditions'.[21] While he did not specify what those gains were, Sampson must have had in mind the fact that the heroic war efforts of both civil and military branches of the profession in striving to maintain the health of the nation's livestock had brought veterinary matters into the eye of the public, and appreciation of its services to government.

THE *VETERINARY RECORD* ACQUIRED

The Association's general meeting for 1919 – held in October because that planned for July had to be cancelled due to a railway strike – had heard that the NVA's finances were in a poor state. The treasurer, Professor G. W. Wooldridge, did not present the accounts: 'The auditor's fee is five guineas (£5 5s) and the total receipts for the year only £11,' he told his colleagues.

Nevertheless, it was agreed that the time had come when the Association needed to appoint a paid secretary 'at the earliest possible moment' to deal with the increasing amount of business. That moment was not just yet, however, and the proposal was not acted upon.[22]

Chapter 3

The most important decision taken, and one which had a profound and beneficial effect on the future of the Association, was the adoption of a proposal 'that the National Veterinary Association proceed to the establishment of a journal of the Association and that if possible the *Veterinary Record* should be acquired, and that with this object in view a committee be formed.'

It was also decided to change the name of the Association to the National Veterinary Medical Association of Great Britain and Ireland and to incorporate it as a registered company to facilitate the running of the *Record*, when it was acquired, as a business while limiting the liability of members in the event of its failure.

Col. J. W. Brittlebank, the general secretary (and Manchester's chief veterinary officer), moving that resolution, said that while there were some 2000 practising members of the veterinary profession in the British Isles, membership of the Association was 'somewhere under 350'; so that it was rather difficult to justify the claim that they were a national association and had the right to speak on behalf of the profession. He asked how they were to increase membership and suggested that their own journal was the only choice. He said 'propaganda' – he presumably meant publicity – 'is essential. Without propaganda this Association may continue for very many years as an association having for one of its prime objects, meeting every year for social intercourse. If we are content with that, well and good; but I think that you will find that during this period of reconstruction the profession is not content to remain where it has been. . . .The profession cannot stand still; it must go ahead.' The proposal, perhaps not surprisingly in view of the NVA's parlous financial state, met with considerable opposition. Sir John McFadyean suggested that they needed to know much more about the finances of the *Veterinary Record* before seeking to acquire it. They should not be hasty in the matter. A number of members made similar points. However, when the matter came to a vote the proposal was accepted and a committee was formed to decide whether or not to recommend that the

Association should go ahead with the acquisition of the journal.[23]

Twelve months later, in July 1920, one of the most important events in the development of the Association occurred. The NVA became the NVMA and purchased the *Veterinary Record.*

The acquisition of the *Veterinary Record*, when the reserves of the NVMA were very low, was a brave step. Although the price paid, a modest £500, was low it meant that the Association was left with virtually no working capital. The recommendation to make the purchase was accepted at the AGM on 28 July 1920. In spite of the opposition expressed at the previous year's meeting, 'the resolution ... was passed very unostentatiously. ... The decision might have been one of little consequence and not the origin of a new departure of fundamental importance.'[24]

'It is hoped that by the management, publication, and the issue of this paper the Association will accomplish a deep and far reaching effect on our progress and well-being, and that by appropriate organised propaganda the need for the education of the public with regard to the special fitness of trained veterinarians for public works as, for example, dairy inspection and meat inspection will be generally recognised and acted upon.' This emphasis of the 'public' role of the veterinarian was to be a recurring theme of the Association. And while the benefits of the acquisition in both the long and short term would be enormous, following the 'public works' role was to prove a pretty hard path.[25]

The author of those optimistic comments was John Malcolm, a former general secretary and innovative veterinary inspector to Birmingham, who helped to reform the milk supply in that city by inspecting cows for tuberculosis.[26] Although appointed editor to the *Record*, he was never to take up the post or to see his hopes fulfilled: he died before his comments were in print.

As it had been for many years the expressed wish of the NVMA to publish its own journal, why did the Association not acquire the *Veterinary Record* before this? After the sudden death of William Hunting in 1913, while he was president of the NVA, the question does not seem to have arisen. Although that would appear to have been an appropriate opportunity to take over the journal, for whatever reason no action was taken at the time. The outbreak of war in 1914 meant that other events assumed precedence and the ownership of the *Record* passed to W. R. Brown, the representative of the journal's printer.

Brown's enthusiastic involvement kept the journal afloat during the war years. He had acted as sub-editor during Hunting's editorship while Hunting was engaged in his own professional work and as general secretary of the Association. After his death Brown assumed the role of editor with the technical advice of a small editorial committee of the NVA. Most of the editorial comments had been written by W. Roger Clarke, a member of council.

In a valedictory message in the last issue published under his proprietorship, 25 December 25, 1920, Brown writes that when he took over the *Record* he had already decided that the NVA should have first refusal of the journal. Had it not been for the outbreak of war 'it is probable that the NVA would have possessed a journal of their own five years ago'.[27]

The achievements of the veterinary profession in caring for the huge equine population during the war, which 'appears to have wrought a remarkable development of confidence among the veterinary profession',[28] plus the post-war surge of general optimism, no doubt gave the Association the confidence finally to take the plunge into publishing.

In the first edition of the *Record* published under the Association's ownership, the NVMA's president, still Orlando Charnock Bradley, reiterated the Association's rationale for taking over the journal: to learn from each others' views, enable council to act more effectively and influence other bodies, and be representative of its members. Importantly, it had to be able to speak for the profession as a whole. 'If the Association and its journal are to fulfil expectations it must be possible to assert that those members of the profession who are not members of the Association are numerically and professionally negligible.

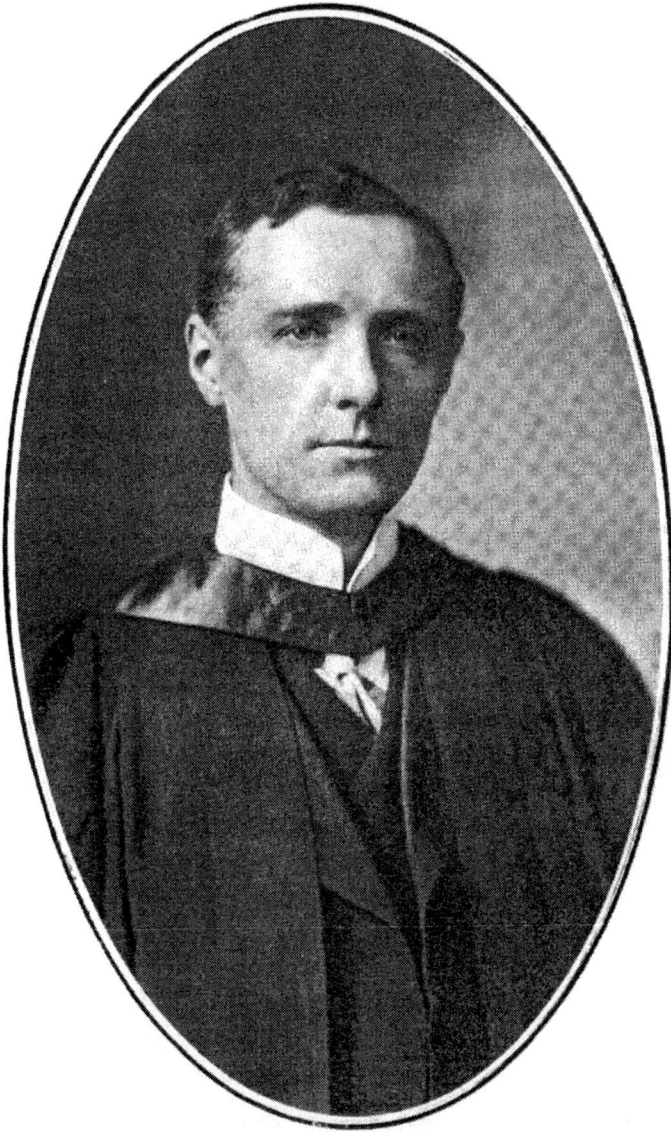

Figure 8. Orlando Charnock Bradley, principal of the Royal (Dick) Veterinary College, who headed the National Veterinary Association throughout the 1914–1918 war and on to 1922. He was a firm advocate of amalgamation of the Association's divisions into a cohesive body.

Unless this can be done ... its full power cannot be exerted or its full value realised.'[29] In other words, the journal must be a powerful reason for furthering the profession's ends – and, specifically, those of the NVMA.

The same theme was emphasised by Basil Buxton, in an address to the Southern Counties Veterinary Association. He said that 'since the National is nothing more or less than the profession, it is quite obvious that it depends on the profession for its existence. Its function is to coordinate the views of the individual members of the profession, to collect and to condense the numerous rays of individual opinion, and to focus them in such a manner that the concentrated beam shall have greater force.' Buxton said he wanted each member of the profession 'to realise that the well-being of the whole profession, that all hope of the future advancement of the body as a whole, depends entirely upon the support of the individual'.[30]

That 'coordination' did not go so far as to make the NMVA into a union; although the Association would come to provide many of the mediation and representation services customary in unions, it was never unionised.[31]

Bringing the *Record* into the Association's ownership had the immediate effect of both increasing the number of members and the NVMA's revenue. When the Association bought the *Record*, it had fewer than 400 members. On becoming the proprietor, the membership subscription, which had been fixed at 10s. 6d. since its foundation, was raised to £2 2s. a year, to include the journal. A year later, membership exceeded 1,000: the 1921 AGM at Chester saw the membership at 1,205 and there were some 300 additional subscribers. At a stroke, therefore, a major advance had been made towards the Association's target of being truly representative of the veterinary profession. There was still some way to go, however, as the membership of the RCVS was about 3,400. Nevertheless, having a third of all qualified vets in membership and a readership among veterinary surgeons very much greater, gave the Association strong support for its claim to be able to speak for the whole of the veterinary profession.

While the acquisition of the *Record* brought an immediate increase in the revenue flowing into the Association finances of the journal were, however, tight. A page cost £2 to print, while advertisers paid only £3 for a full display page. There was still some way to go before the NVMA acquired the financial stability needed to back up its ambition to be the profession's only significant voice.

The lack of substantial funds did not dampen the enthusiasm that followed the acquisition of the Association's own journal. Office premises, consisting of two rooms in Buckingham Palace Road, London, were rented and a secretary and office boy hired, the extra staff made necessary to deal with the additional business of running the *Veterinary Record.*

Apart from a modest redesign, the journal itself underwent no radical changes under its new ownership. A typical issue would contain reports, normally verbatim, of Association and RCVS councils and NVA territorial division meetings with discussions, clinical reports and general correspondence from readers on matters of the day. The leading article would comment on current political and professional issues and there would be notes and news on events of veterinary interest at home and abroad. In spite of the aspiration of the founder, in those early days there were few scientific papers; there was little research being done. Reports of the papers presented at the annual congress provided the main information of advances being made in techniques and medicaments. Occasional clinical and scientific papers were published, but for many years the scientific content was small. Few practitioners, although frequently asked to do so, submitted anything other than correspondence. Even fewer vets were involved in research; and for those, there was not the requirement to publish that exists today.

Management of the editorial content was in the hands of an editorial committee of variable composition, the comment usually being written by one of its number (often the general secretary) who was the nominal editor. Supervising the content of a weekly publication was no light responsibility for the part-time volunteers, all with responsible professional or academic appointments, who undertook the task. Greater attention was paid to obtaining advertising, with one of the editorial group being nominated to undertake that responsibility. Sub-editing, layout, general production and seeing through the press was in the hands of William Brown, a young journalist who had qualified as a vet but devoted his career to the journal. Although he was not formally designated editor until 1945, Brown was the virtually anonymous figure who managed the publication, subedited the contents, and saw it through the press every week for almost thirty-five years. Almost single-handedly he was responsible for all aspects of the *Record* except those relating to editorial policy, which were decided by a committee whose composition and effectiveness varied over the years. Shortly before he was due to retire in 1954, Brown died suddenly. There were many tributes to him, as a person and as an editor, from past and present officers and contributors. His long-time colleague, the general secretary Fred Knight, wrote 'Those who receive the *Veterinary Record* each week do perhaps not always realise the amount of work involved in dealing with material received for publication, getting clinical articles approved, editorial decided upon,. abstracts ready on time, large advertisements fitted in and small ones collected, editorial [committee] meetings arranged and endless correspondence carried on.'[32]

But because there was no single guiding hand the editorial policies of the journal and some of its procedures 'seem to have been haphazard, to say the least. There was no proper panel of scrutineers without whom it is virtually impossible to maintain standards. Congress papers good or less good were published automatically.'

Editorial articles were contributed by a variety of hands, sometimes that of the general secretary of the day – at other times by the president or a member of the editorial committee. Clinical papers were hard to come by and the *Record* was more like a house journal than the production of a scientifically orientated profession; 'Its reputation outside the profession was less high than could be wished,' according to his successor, Charles Mitchell.

Over the years of Brown's tenure, some presidents and editorial committee members took a keener interest in the Association's journal than others. J. T. Edwards worked to raise the quality and variety of papers published. W. R. Wooldridge did the same and also contributed effective leading articles A. W. Stableforth, director of the Central Veterinary Laboratory, encouraged his staff to contribute material and so did W. S. Gordon, director of the Institute for Research into Animal Diseases, Compton.

The correspondence columns were sometimes rather sparse, but always received a boost when matters affecting the status and education of the profession arose. Events such as the Loveday reports on the profession and the ending of the so-called single portal system of entry and its replacement by university degrees, or establishment of the Supplementary Veterinary Register would always fill the letter pages.

When Brown died, the editorial committee, chaired by Professor D. L. Hughes, decided that the time was right for a change in the *Record's* affairs. They proposed that a professional journalist, not a veterinary surgeon, be appointed editor, with proper editorial authority over the journal. The proposal was not at first welcomed by council. A compromise advertisement was placed stating that a veterinary surgeon would be preferred for the post, but the office was not exclusive to members of the profession. Apparently, no vet with journalistic experience applied: perhaps the salary was not attractive.

The person appointed to succeed Brown was Charles Mitchell, a journalist of the old school (a former essayist for the *News Chronicle*) who had been the Association's press officer since January 1954. Mitchell, on appointment, said that, as new editor, he was faced with a daunting task. He was, he said, expected to help put a somewhat ailing publication on its feet in all matters: scientific, literary, professional and financial, with a staff of one. The total income was less than £20,000 a year; there was no advertisement manager; there were few papers submitted and little correspondence. There were no leading articles, few serious readers and an abundance of serious critics.

He indicated that 'the new editor [i.e. himself] should be expected to accept considerably greater responsibility than had been the case in the past'.[33] In other words, he expected to be able to exercise appropriate editorial authority over the running of the journal. As part of the changed role it was agreed to reduce the size of the editorial committee from fifteen members to six; the editor would deal directly with the panel of scrutineers of clinical papers, consulting the committee only in cases of 'uncertainty or doubt'. Finally, leading articles would be written by the editor, (a change from the longstanding custom) but 'submitted to the officers if matters of policy were concerned'.[34]

His first priority was to increase the publication's revenue. He set out to improve the attractiveness of the journal to readers, contributors and advertisers. The finance committee was persuaded reluctantly to provide an additional member of staff – a typist – to help with the advertising. This young lady proved to have a flair for selling space and dealing with advertising agents. The journal's income increased rapidly and part of the increase was ploughed back with 'gratifying results'. To encourage the submission of papers, Mitchell visited veterinary schools and research institutes, invited constructive criticism, and began to commission papers on specific subjects. He was helped in his efforts by the now more effective editorial committee whose members gave him enthusiastic support.

When Mitchell took over, there were few leading articles published because of what was always referred to as the 'Yarmouth resolution'. This was a decision made at the annual general meeting in 1939 that any leading article touching on a sensitive or controversial subject should be approved by council before publication. This meant that there were hardly any leading articles published, it being totally impractical to get prompt approval for a proposed leader on a subject of topical interest from over 100 individuals. In effect, the journal had lost its voice. The more sensible policy of submitting leaders before publication to the president, or another officer if the president was not available, was adopted.[35]

The *Record* was still the only English veterinary journal published weekly and the major contributor to the Association's finances. In 1955 it showed a profit of £6,700 on an income of £21,439; the Association's subscription income was £15,128.[36]

However, not everyone was happy with the more scientific articles whose submission Mitchell had encouraged, or the rejection of more anecdotal articles. They gave rise to the comment that the *Record* had become 'very highbrow'. J. H. Wilkins, major commandant of the RAVC, suggested that a BVA journal of veterinary research would be the answer to such criticisms.[37] Other correspondents complained about the rejection of their contributions. D. C. Lancaster maintained that the editor – a layman – had no right to refuse letters and articles from members of the profession.[38] Joan Joshua, member and former chairman of the editorial committee, and not one to mince her words, defended the editorial policy of the *Record*. She pointed out that only a small proportion of the material submitted for publication was rejected, but 'were some of the tripe and drivel submitted in this small proportion published, not only the *Record* but the authors would be the laughing stock of the veterinary world'.[39]

G. N. Henderson, in the same issue, also defended the journal. He said that recent innovations (including more modern typography and layout) indicated that it might not be a bad thing that in choosing the new editor the BVA had paid more heed to experience in journalism and professional writing than in academic knowledge of veterinary science. 'The standard of veterinary skill in this country is second to none. I feel that our journal is, however slowly, beginning to reflect that standard as well,' said Henderson.

The suggestion of a purely scientific journal was pursued by Mitchell and eventually agreed to by council.[40] The title was to be *Research in Veterinary Science*. An editorial board of eminent veterinary scientists was appointed and Mitchell acted as executive editor. It was decided to appoint an outside publisher to handle printing and distribution due to pressure of work in the editorial department. Among those who tendered for the job was Captain Robert Maxwell, of the Pergamon Press (long before he achieved notoriety as a national newspaper publisher); he attended a meeting of the editorial board and, according to the minutes of that meeting, made a favourable impression.[41] Blackwells was appointed publisher; the Association's editorial department brought the journal in house in 1973.

The *Record* thrived under Mitchell's editorship; by the time he retired in 1971, its revenue had grown to £105,000, more than 60 per cent of BVA revenue. His successor, Peter Wood, who had joined the staff about a year before with a view to the succession, had rather different ideas on how the journal should be run. If Mitchell had found the *Record* somewhat old-fashioned when he took over seventeen years previously the same applied to Wood.

Among his innovations, he printed articles featuring particular practices; when these were owned by vets whose methods were considered a little too commercial, some members were not happy. When he made arrangements to change printers from the long established H. R. Grubb but neglected to involve the editorial committee, the proposal was quashed. Wood did not believe that there should be a leading article in every issue. And in the issue of the *Veterinary Record* dated 1 April 1972, he printed an article 'Some observations on the diseases of *Brunus edwardii*', a witty spoof by the veterinary scientist D. K. Blackmore and colleagues, which some thought *infra dig*. In a little under two years his appointment was terminated. If his tenure was brief, that article is his lasting memorial: it is still in print as a booklet.

In the six month interval between Wood's departure in April and the arrival of the new editor, the journal was produced by a caretaker regime consisting of a young assistant editor, with oversight by the secretary, Pat Turner, and the former editor, Charles Mitchell – with production left to the printer.

The new editor, Edward Boden (the author of the present volume) joined the *Record* from *The Pharmaceutical Journal*. The first thing he discovered on taking up his post in October 1973 was that his duties included that of executive editor of *Research in Veterinary Science*, a fact that had not been mentioned at his interview. The second was that his office, a pleasant room on the first floor of 7 Mansfield Street, contained only two reference books: the 1928 edition of Black's Veterinary Dictionary and an even earlier edition of the Shorter Oxford Dictionary. He also found that the staff, two assistant editors (one for the research journal), a manuscript secretary and the editorial secretary, were helpful and efficient, and that the system for scrutinising manuscripts was excellent.

The new editor introduced some changes; the typographic layout was modernised and the cover redesigned with the intention of presenting a more easily readable appearance. The cover had been a rather drab green and black and the text pages looked flat. The first reaction to the changes came when the then deputy chief veterinary officer came in to the editor's office and said; 'I just want to tell you that I hate everything you're doing to my *Veterinary Record*.' Which taught the new incumbent two things: that the members have a strong proprietorial interest in their journal; and that they tend to be rather conservative in their attitude to change.

The Association's reliance on the revenue-earning function of the *Record* that had been encouraged by its virtual monopoly in the field of veterinary periodicals began to be questioned as more journals, in various formats, some distributed free to the profession, entered the field (some of the officers thought any vet who was involved with such upstarts was something of a traitor!).

Revenue was earned from two types of advertisement: display and classified. The former required active selling; the latter efficient administration involving many small accounts. Josephine Francis, then and for many years after, was the efficient display sales manager; the management of classified sales fell to the lot of the tiny and overburdened accounts staff; this was in addition to handling all the other financial transactions of the BVA, from membership subscriptions to staff salaries. They were frequently hard pushed to keep their invoicing up to date. Clearly, changes were necessary.

It was decided that all advertising for the *Record* should be put in the hands of a specialist advertisement management company who would take on board all the administration and sales functions, bear all the expenses involved and deliver the proceeds, net of their commission, to the BVA. Mrs Francis joined that company, T. G. Scott & Son, taking her expertise with her, and the accounts department no longer had to struggle with the classified ads. The association with Scotts proved satisfactory to both parties and was to last for over thirty years. The close link between the two was illustrated by the fact that Derek Williams, Scott's former managing director, was eventually elected chairman of the BVA's board of management.

Another long overdue change was to arrange a contract with the Post Office by which the despatch of the journal was charged by bulk weight, rather than being charged by the fee for a single copy multiplied by the total number sent out. And every copy was franked individually. This had meant that on occasion, when an issue fell slightly over the weight for a particular price band, all the copies would be trimmed to avoid the higher fee. That is why some bound volumes of the *Record* in the 1960s and early '70s have very tight margins.

It soon became clear that Wood had been correct in his wish to change printers, countermanded by the officers. H. R. Grubb had been printing the Record since 1930. The same antiquated equipment was still used – operated, in some instances, by the same staff; this was taking tradition too far. But it would be 1978 before the officers could be persuaded to agree to a change.

The third journal launched by the Association was *In Practice*. The 1970s saw a proliferation of medical journals, many of which were devoted to practice educational topics, following the new requirement for keeping professionals up to date with a faster rate of change in medical practice: continuing professional development (CPD). Similar influences were to be found in veterinary practice. It was decided that a journal consisting mainly of articles on topics of immediate practical interest, specially commissioned as 'opinionated review articles' from veterinary surgeons with specialist knowledge, would be welcomed by members in practice.

An editorial board was appointed, and *In Practice* launched in 1979 as a six-times-a-year supplement to the *Veterinary Record.* Introducing the new journal, the *Record* said it was 'specifically intended as a contribution to continuing postgraduate education for the veterinary profession. The presentation of the material is designed to combine technical soundness with an easily assimilable format. Each issue will cover subjects usually of seasonal or other topical interest in a form which encourages the reader to update their knowledge.'[42] At the first council meeting after the launch of *In Practice* it was reported that members were enthusiastic in their reaction to the new publication.[43]

The editorial board consisted of a mix of academics and experienced practitioners. The first chairman was Professor (later Sir) James Armour, of Glasgow University veterinary school. It was Jimmy Armour's brilliant chairmanship, combining a vast breadth of knowledge of the profession with an apparently easy-going affability, that put the stamp on the new journal's success. He was the catalyst by which ideas tossed around the board table were able to take tangible form. Armour could put his finger on subjects needing coverage and help identify authors either from the board or elsewhere. The meetings were quite short, but productive.

The liberal use of colour in illustrations and layout – unusual for its day, more like a magazine than a learned journal – assisted the attractiveness of presentation and the number of issues per annum soon rose from six to ten, the present frequency.

The BVA produced the *Equine Veterinary Journal* on behalf of the British Equine Veterinary Association in 1980, the *Journal of Small Animal Practice* for the British Small Animal Veterinary Association in 1987, and the *Veterinary Nursing Journal* for the British Veterinary Nursing Association in 1990. They also produced the *SPVS Bulletin,* the *Journal of the Association of Veterinary Students,* and a range of occasional books and informational publications. Over time, it was decided to concentrate on the core publications; *Research in Veterinary Science* (which enjoyed a healthy circulation among scientists, but hardly any among BVA members), was sold to another publisher and the other publications taken back in house by the divisions to which they belonged.

One of Boden's final projects at the BVA was a collaborative exercise with the Royal Pharmaceutical Society; publication in 1991 of the first edition of an important standard text: the *Veterinary Formulary*, the authoritative compendium of information on animal medicines and their uses.

On his retirement as editor in 1990 Martin Alder was appointed editor. Alder, a Cambridge science graduate, brought to the post a wide experience of medical and scientific publications; his journalistic career had actually begun as a subeditor on the *Record* a dozen years earlier. Under his leadership the publications continued to develop; a particular strength was the weekly editorial article, many of which were adopted as BVA policy statements.

A new chapter in the history of BVA publishing was opened in 2009, when production was outsourced to BMJ Group, the publishing arm of the British Medical Association. The BVA and BMA have, of course, many overlapping interests and the BVA felt the larger organisation had the infrastructure and technological expertise to help its journals' growth.[44] The editorial staff moved en bloc the short distance from Mansfield Street to BMA House, Tavistock Square.

CHAPTER FOUR

A TROUBLED DECADE

The 1920s was a troubled decade for Britain. There was economic depression and industrial unrest, including a general strike in 1926. Problems in the agricultural community included the catastrophic series of FMD outbreaks which brought serious criticism of the veterinary profession for the way the disease had been handled. Country practice in general remained a hard option for the veterinary surgeon. The depressed state of agriculture; the fall in the value of farm animals together with a steady increase in whole time municipal and Ministry of Agriculture and Fisheries (MAF) veterinary officers (taking over TB testing and inspections under the Diseases of Animal Acts and Milk and Dairies Act); and a dearth of part-time employment were eroding the incomes of many general veterinary practitioners' districts and rendering their practices almost valueless. A country vet commented: 'A practitioner turning over £600 a year has to work hard and has practically nothing left after expenses have been paid; it is a dog's life. Farmers grumble at their bills and expect the veterinary surgeon to be at their beck and call at all hours. They frequently paid their veterinary surgeons' bills after three or four years.'[1]

Yet at the end of the decade the NVMA was stronger than it had ever been; its membership quadrupled over the ten years, its finances were sound and it had developed the basis of a political and administrative structure that would serve it for years to come.

Leading vets then, as today, were frequently preoccupied with speculation about the future. Indeed, 'a concern with the nature and implications of change can be viewed as one of the few constants in the profession's history'.[2]

At the 1921 AGM in Chester, Henry Gray, a prominent London veterinary surgeon who established the London Infirmary for Animals, gave his view of 'the future of the profession'. He said that veterinary practice should be devoted more to the prevention of diseases of animals than to curing them. It would, for example, be much more economical to prevent tuberculosis than to allow it to exist and to endanger the health of animals and man. But the elimination of tuberculosis would occupy the time of veterinary surgeons for a long period, he predicted.

Gray drew a pessimistic picture of the professional future for the general practitioner. He pointed out that 'the most profitable patient of the veterinary practitioner' – the horse – had declined since the advent of the motorcar. It was a plain fact that the equine population of the country had fallen dramatically since the start of the century. From the estimated 3 million or so horses in 1901 there were fewer than 2 million by 1924.[3] The rate of decline would accelerate rapidly thereafter. Canine and feline work was also on the decline, according to Gray; that prediction was to prove wildly inaccurate, as will be shown. And 'If it were not for the increased value of cattle, sheep and pigs, occasioned by the war, the number of practitioners in country districts would also have dwindled appreciably,' he said. That increase in value, and the relative prosperity it brought, were not to last. Gray was speaking before the great betrayal of agriculture by the government's repeal of the Agriculture Act in 1921 left the rural economy in deep depression, leaving many practising vets struggling to make a living wage.[4]

He also felt that better education for the farmer would mean that many of the minor veterinary tasks would be done by the farmer himself. While, over time, he foresaw a great reduction in the total number of veterinary surgeons, he said, much better veterinary education would mean that what was lost in quantity should be made up in quality. He felt that a sufficient number of highly trained veterinarians should be maintained so as to be available when 'rapidly spreading epizootic diseases made their appearance'.

However, the increasing expense of training for a veterinary qualification meant that veterinary surgery was 'not a profession congenial for the great majority of men' with money and intellect, Gray believed. The 'social position, leisure and emoluments' were too limited. 'Unless the state was prepared to subsidise veterinary education and perhaps to give grants for maintenance of students there will, I have no doubt, be a scarcity of veterinary surgeons.'

The bulk of the future veterinary surgeon's education, he argued, should be concentrated not on the horse but on the detection and prevention or elimination of contagious parasitic, enzootic and nutritional diseases of food animals including sheep, pigs, fowl, and rabbit; and on those diseases of the dog and cat transferable to man and to food animals.

Gray felt that the greatest drawback to the progress of veterinary medicine and of its recognition of esteem by the general public was professional snobbery within its ranks. Before motors came along, 'one encountered practitioners who confined their attention to the horse, who looked down sneeringly upon the practitioner who attended cattle, sheep and pigs and even contemptuously on those who treated cats, dogs or poultry'.[5] And some horse vets who themselves used cars to travel to clients were embarrassed to own up to the fact and left their motor out of sight. The account of Gray's paper and the discussion that followed took up a dozen pages of the *Veterinary Record*. Much of the debate was dominated by those who maintained, in the face of the facts, that the advent of motor traction in agriculture would never replace the horse to any great extent. Others accepted that the day of the horse as a major source of motive power in both the rural and the urban environments had gone, but saw great potential for well trained veterinary surgeons in the fields of preventive medicine, farm livestock, and small animal practice.[6]

Although Gray was not quite right in some of his predictions of the way the profession would develop, it was in many ways a perceptive analysis of the situation as it was at the time and might develop in the future. And his pessimism was no doubt influenced by the depressed state of the UK's economy. As the decade moved to the 1930s, unemployment was around 1 million, with a further 600,000 workers on short time (the country's population at the time was around 35 million).[7] Prices for agricultural produce fell by 34 per cent between 1929 and 1933, bringing them to the same level as before the first world war.[8]

AIMS AND OBJECTS

The objects of the NVMA, as promulgated in 1922 (see panel overleaf), are a testament of its aims. The document, expanded in the Articles of Association that are revised periodically, set out the core of the activities encapsulated in its first sentence: The promotion and advancement of veterinary and allied sciences and the maintenance of the honour and interests of the veterinary profession.

It is thus primarily concerned to look after the interests of its members in the exercise of their professional activities. Those activities, of course, include the financial interests involved in earning a living. That is the fundamental difference from the RCVS, whose prime consideration is the public interest. The difference is quite plain; nevertheless, the roles of the two bodies, and their purpose, are often confused by the general public and not infrequently by veterinarians. This is not surprising, because the interests can overlap; for example in education, relations with official bodies (particularly government), and standards of professional practice.

The third of the stated objects, To support the claims of members of the profession to legitimate veterinary appoint-ments, has − as evidenced in this book − been frequently

Objects of the Association, 1922

The promotion and advancement of veterinary and allied sciences and the maintenance of the honour and interests of the veterinary profession.

To hold meetings of members of the Association for the branches and divisions from time to time in various parts of the country for the discussion of veterinary topics and kindred subjects, and to publish the proceedings of the said meetings.

To support the claims of members of the profession to legitimate veterinary appointments.

To collect and disseminate news and information.

To publish periodicals or books connected with operating on subjects relating to veterinary science and medicine or kindred subjects or professional matters.

To obtain the money for the objects of the Association in any lawful manner and deal with the same in such manner as may be considered most desirable for effecting such objects.

Should the finances of the Association permit, to grant sums of money out of the funds, or otherwise assist branches or divisions in the provision of scientific demonstrations and lectures for investigating animal diseases, or in other manner promoting the veterinary science, and to make grants to institutions and individuals to enable them to make research into and investigate animal disease and the causes thereof, and other matters in furtherance of veterinary science and medicine, and to bring out instruments for veterinary work, and to publish books and pamphlets dealing with veterinary science or medicine or kindred subjects.

To apply, petition for, or promote any act of Parliament, Royal Charter, or other authority with a view to the attainment of the above objects or any of them.

To do all such other lawful things that are incidental or conducive to the attainment of any of the above objects.

called upon, particularly where terms and conditions of state and municipal officers and official veterinary surgeons were concerned The Association had from its early days made much of its claim to speak on such matters for the whole profession. Yet the Association is not a trade union, although it acts in some ways like one. Its calls for action in disputes could never be supported by legal sanctions, although measures in support of the Association's case, such as representations to ministers and the media, may be vigorously pursued.

One reason why it has never sought unionisation (although that has been sometimes suggested) is that the majority of its members are, traditionally, a diverse group of highly individual self-employed professionals (some employed vets may, of course, be members of the organisations employing them).

The commercial activities covered by the objects – sales from publications, conferences, etc. – have grown in importance as the organisation has grown in size: a board of directors has oversight of the Association's financial affairs.

Holding meetings remains a major activity, one that has changed greatly over the years. In its early days, the annual meeting, or congress, was uniquely important as if was the sole public activity. The long-established regional meetings were strongly supported, matching the Association itself in size and influence. Specialist divisions representing animal species or special technical interests did not (apart from the Society of Practising Veterinary Surgeons) develop until the 1950s.

That situation changed radically: now, the largest veterinary meeting in the UK is that of the BVA's largest division, the British Small Animal Veterinary Association. Other specialist associations thrive strongly. The area divisions, for so long the mainstay of the profession, while still active, struggle in some areas to attract members against the competition of the special interest divisions.

One important omission from the 1922 objects is any mention of animal welfare or ethical treatment. That is a major concern of the BVA, which founded the BVA Animal Welfare Foundation in the 1983, and has ethical treatment of animals as on ongoing organisational involvement.

ADMINISTERING THE ASSOCIATION

In 1922 council, no doubt as a result of the increased membership (now standing at 1,256), enhanced financial prospects, and the need to make the Association's influence felt more widely, decided to meet four times a year instead of holding one major meeting with occasional extra meetings called as necessary.

A formal committee structure was set up so that the widening range of activities of the Association could be dealt with more effectively.(an Executive Committee consisting of the president, treasurer and secretary had already been set up in 1919).[9] The committees were: Finance and Advisory; Biological Products; Appointments; Articles of Association; Editorial; and Veterinary Inspectors and Public Health. This last took over the administrative aspects of the National Association of Veterinary Inspectors, which had been disbanded and incorporated as a division of the NVMA – the first specialist division, in fact.

Not all the committees were intended to be permanent. The biological products committee was established because of concerns about the distribution and standardisation of tuberculin. The availability of tuberculin to anyone who wished to buy it had led to an 'extensive and far reaching system of fraud' which cast doubt on the accuracy of the test and the honesty of the veterinary surgeon applying it.[10] The articles of association committee was set up to consider new articles and a change of title; new articles were approved but it was decided to retain the title National Veterinary Medical Association of Great Britain and Ireland.

To cater for the greater activity produced by increased committee meetings and the expanding work of the *Veterinary Record*, more spacious offices were acquired at 10 Grays Inn Road, London, and a junior clerk appointed at a salary of 30 shillings a week. And three years later it was decided that, at last, the NVMA could afford to pay its general secretary and editor (G. H. Livesey, a practitioner, held both posts) a salary. The sum agreed was £500.

The year 1921 saw the end of the long reign of Orlando Charnock Bradley. He had been head of the Association since 1914, throughout the difficult years of the war, and played a large part in both ensuring the survival of the NVA and its post-war resurgence as a much stronger and potentially more influential organisation.[11] In his valedictory address at the 1922 AGM, Charnock Bradley paid tribute to the 'loyalty, self-sacrifice, devotion and labours of the executive officials of the Association' who had kept the NVA going. He mentioned three factors, among many, that had engaged the attention of council during his final year of office: salaries attached to public appointments, veterinary education, and research. He said that while the Association might draft a scale of salaries, it was another matter to try to enforce it, particularly as veterinary surgeons continued to apply for posts offering remuneration considered too low for the responsibilities involved.

That problem was to be a continuing one. Although, 'taking all in, veterinary education had advanced as fast as any reasonable person would demand', Charnock Bradley complained that public money for the encouragement of veterinary education and research was being 'doled out in an astonishingly niggardly fashion'.

There were only two established sites in England for the pursuit of research into animal diseases: the state veterinary department's laboratory at Weybridge, overseen by Stewart Stockman, and his father-in-law John McFadyean's lab at the RVC. In Scotland, recent initiatives by a group of farmers had led to the foundation of the Animal Diseases Research Association (ADRA, the forerunner of the Moredun institute), which funded investigations at Glasgow and later Edinburgh veterinary schools.[12]

The recommendation made by the government's post-war development commission for the maintenance of veterinary research amounted to no more than about £9000. That miserly provision was made in spite of the fact that the commission's own advisory committee had drawn attention to the very large losses arising from disease in livestock, and also noted that the facilities for research in the five veterinary schools, barely those of the school science classroom, 'constituted a national disgrace'.[13]

Concluding on an optimistic note, however, Charnock Bradley said 'I am more than ever confident that, in the Association, the veterinary profession has the germ of a powerful instrument such as it never had before.'[14]

THE NVMA AND ITS DIVISIONS

The question of the nature of the relationship between the local veterinary societies and the NVMA, ever a delicate subject, was raised at a meeting of the Central Veterinary Society in March 1926. Professor Bernard Gorton said that when the local veterinary societies had become divisions of the National Veterinary Association some of their members did not join it; that remained the case. On the other hand, a veterinary surgeon might be a member of the NVMA and yet not a member of a local society. And again, there were people who were members of more than one society. This created the situation in which members were either not represented on council at all or, as it were, were represented two or three times as each division sent representatives to council in proportion to its own numbers. Professor Gorton suggested that the subscription (two guineas) to the National Association should include the subscription to a local society. He pointed out that such a scheme would mean that the local societies would have to 'sink their identities'. But he was sure that the results would be worth such a sacrifice. A long, inconclusive, discussion followed.[15] Seventeen years earlier, Charnock Bradley had argued for a similar proposal, again without success.

In a comment on the discussion, the *Veterinary Record* said that during all the 'tedious and wearisome' negotiations that led to the reorganisation of the Association 'it was clearly seen that an essential condition for harmonious cooperation between the divisions and the main organisation was the preservation of the autonomy of the individual societies'. If the Association had created its own divisions absolutely from scratch, that would have been different. But to ask existing societies to become divisions, which is what had been done, was simpler and far more expedient.[16]

The president at the 1926 annual meeting, held once again in Dublin, was a most distinguished veterinary scientist, Professor J. Basil Buxton. A member of the RCVS council since 1920 and a former general secretary of the NVMA (1920-1922), Buxton was the first veterinary surgeon to be appointed to the Wellcome physiological laboratories and the first veterinary surgeon on the scientific staff of the Medical Research Council. He had recently been appointed as the first director of the Institute of Animal Pathology at Cambridge, a post he held from 1923 to 1936. He was able to report success in the adoption by 'several counties' of the Association's recommended minimum fees for work done in certifying attested cattle under the Tuberculosis Order.

Buxton was succeeded as president by Professor George H. Wooldridge. As a student at the Royal Veterinary College he had swept the board by winning medals in every subject of the course; on graduating in 1899 he was appointed a tutor at the college, followed almost immediately by his appointment as professor of veterinary science and bacteriology at the Royal Agricultural College. Then he was appointed to the chair of medicine at the Royal Veterinary College of Ireland, followed only five years later by his appointment in 1908 as professor of *materia medica* at the Royal Veterinary College. He was also the author of veterinary text books and holder of a wide range of appointments to veterinary and medical bodies. Wooldridge had been treasurer of the Association for sixteen years and concurrently honorary secretary throughout the Great War.

An innovation among the subjects discussed at the 1927 congress over which he presided was electrotherapy. High-frequency application, it was said, had 'a wonderfully bracing effect on the whole system'; ionic medication could localise the application of soluble medicaments in topical therapy; 'fulguration' (electrocautery), and ultraviolet treatment were also considered by the author, E. Middleton Perry.[17]

Among the papers presented at the congress at Newcastle on Tyne in 1928 was a discussion on lamb dysentery and its prevention by Thomas (later Sir Thomas) Dalling. He had researched the disease at Glasgow veterinary school on behalf of the Animal Diseases Research Association, before moving in 1923 to the drug company, Burroughs Wellcome, to help develop a vaccine. Dalling was later to become chief veterinary officer (1948–1952) before joining the United Nations Food and Agriculture Organisation.

Sir John Moore, in a paper entitled 'the horse as a national economic factor', presented a spirited case for 'the urgent necessity for the maintenance of due regard and interest by the public in the horse and in horse production'. Sir John wished 'to ensure the continuance of the horse as an indispensable factor in the defence of the realm, the agricultural industry and the considerable element of sporting pleasures'. Sir John (1864–1940) was himself something of an old war horse – he had seen service in the Boer War and had been the general officer commanding the Army Veterinary Corps, 1914–1918. Moore produced figures to support his argument that a strong economic case could be made for the continuing wide use of the horse for both industrial and pleasure purposes.[18]

Financial matters during the year had included, yet again, concern over inadequate salaries for veterinary surgeons in public appointments. The Association had also failed to gain the support of the RCVS in its attempts to secure parity of fees paid to veterinary surgeons acting as professional witnesses in court with those payable to members of the medical and legal professions. The College had said that the question of securing adequate fees was 'a matter for negotiation by the individuals concerned'.[19] The College, of course, had always maintained that such matters were the business of the Association, as in the 1914 war.

If the Association itself was modestly thriving, with a full-time paid secretary and larger offices at 2 Verulam Buildings, Grays Inn, many of its members, particularly those in rural areas, were having a hard time. They were not alone. The whole country was in deep economic crisis exacerbated by a return to the gold standard. Unemployment was running close to 3 million out of a population of under 40 million; real poverty was widespread.

In 1925 Arthur Gofton had called in his presidential address for the establishment of a national veterinary public health service. There was in the profession a continuing conflict of opinion about the relative roles of salaried municipal and county veterinary officers – full time or part time – and private practitioners on a more uncertain and variable income. The need for some source of income which was regular and independent of the vagaries of practice had long been recognised. Vets had never had recourse to income from 'poor law, club, or friendly society practice' as had the medical profession. In 1920 a practitioner had written to the *Veterinary Record* calling for 'the adoption of the panel system as is used for the insured patients of the medical profession'. He complained of an awkward situation arising where, for example, two vets operated practices in a neighbouring area. If one of them held a licence and the other did not, the licensed vet might be asked to test animals belonging to his unlicensed neighbour. That would put him in an invidious position.[20] The diseases of animals branch of the Ministry of Agriculture employed in the early 1920s only forty full-time veterinary inspectors and 239 local veterinary inspectors engaged mainly in TB testing. Fewer than fifty veterinary surgeons were employed by local authorities, mainly on TB testing, meat hygiene, and inspection of livestock markets. 'For a profession with some 3,300 members' there were 'meagre pickings' in part-time employment.[21]

The sense of financial insecurity lay behind much of the veterinary desire for a state service and shaped the profession's conception of how the service should be staffed and run. It was little wonder that veterinary surgeons looked wistfully towards the National Health Insurance scheme and the panel practice that had secured the incomes of medical men and raised their social status.[22]

But if the veterinary surgeon in the country was having a hard time, his colleague in the town was not much better off. G. P. Male, making those points in his presidential address in 1930, commented: 'It may be that a state system of veterinary practice will be evolved with panel patients, as in the human medical practice.'[23] He was echoing the point made ten years previously by a correspondent to the *Veterinary Record*.[24] In fact, such sentiments seem to have been widespread. In an address the following year to the Western Counties division the division's president, H. W. Townson, complained that agriculture was 'at a very low ebb and we are told that worse is to come'.

At the same time, sales of 'quack' remedies to farmers to treat their own animals were thriving. 'What a boon the panel must be to the medical man,' he said. 'When a government really tries to help the farmer we may have one, too, some day.'[25]

While many vets in general practice were struggling financially, officers employed by boroughs or counties also felt their services were undervalued. The Association was continuing its efforts to have salaries of such employees brought into conformity with a national scale. The following scale was proposed: Chief veterinary officer, from £700 to £1,200 per year; veterinary officer – for an officer working alone, where only one veterinary officer is required – .commencing salary £600 a year upwards; senior assistant veterinary officers, £500 a year upwards; assistant veterinary officers, £400 a year upwards. It was expected that increases commensurate with the duties performed would be made. The Association strongly recommended the provision of a contributory superannuation scheme for all veterinary officers.

A 'tentative' minimum scale for veterinary research workers was drawn up after consultation with the Agricultural Research Council: grade 3 £320–£380 a year; grade 2 £425 a year with annual increments of £20 to a maximum of £625; grade 1, £630 a year with annual increments of £25 up to £830; for a director, £1,000–£1,200 a year.[26]

Copies of the scale were sent to all the appropriate county council and local government bodies. Although the recommended salaries could only be taken as guidance, the scale did have the effect of providing a benchmark. The Association recommended that its members should not apply for any post advertised at a lower salary than that proposed in the scale. Somerset County Council and the Animal Diseases Research Association (ADRA) were among the non-complying organisations. In spite of that recommendation, members continued to apply for such posts; jobs were in short supply and there was unemployment in the profession.

Although members had been advised not to apply for the post of head of the Animal Diseases Research Association, Moredun, because of the low salary attached to it, the distinguished veterinary scientist Professor J. Russell Greig, an NVMA member, applied for the position and was appointed.[27] And as the problem continued, it was decided to remove from membership a number of members who had taken posts advertised by local authorities at salaries below the Association's recommended scale for whole time veterinary officers.

The Association's salary recommendations for veterinary surgeons in public appointments appeared to have had some effect. Two years later, it was 'gratifying to report the salaries of most full time appointments by local authorities conformed to the NVMA scale'. However, efforts to bring about improvements in the commencing salaries at the lower end of the scale were 'unfortunately nullified by the action of certain members and others in accepting posts at salaries advertised in the lay press'.[28]

An attempt to improve the situation for private practitioners by gaining an increase in fees paid for the examination of animals for insurance purposes was rebuffed. The insurance companies refused the request because of the 'continuous and considerable fall in the value of animals and the consequent reduction in premiums'.[29] The NVMA also failed in its attempt to require that all applications to license a bull intended for breeding purposes, a requirement of the Improvement of Livestock (Licensing of Bulls) Act 1931, should be accompanied by a certificate of health from a practising veterinary surgeon. The reason given was that 'it would impose a charge on the owners of bulls for which there was not sufficient justification'.[30] The Act had been introduced to prevent the use of substandard animals for breeding; with artificial insemination increasingly common, a single substandard bull's defective genes could be passed to numerous progeny.[31]

Increasing dissatisfaction with their situation was exacerbated in 1933 by the availability of free advice given to farmers by veterinary advisory officers from the government's Veterinary Investigation Service. This had a long tradition, dating back to 1922 with the regional laboratories established in the agricultural colleges. Their dissatisfaction led practitioners, inspired by a group in Wales ('the wild men of North Wales')[32] to form the Veterinary Practitioners League, which became the Society of Practising Veterinary Surgeons. The need for such a body, according to the joint secretaries, H. Llewellyn Jones and Leonard Jones, was that 'official and comparatively sheltered members of the profession' had long had their own organisations of veterinary inspectors and municipal officers associations; but general practitioners, 'by far the largest party in the profession, had never been organised as such'.[33]

The Association made some modest steps in supporting the practitioner economically by the introduction of a pension and family provision scheme in conjunction with an insurance company.[34] Certificates for recording the results of tuberculin tests, which were designed to meet the requirements of auctioneers at cattle sales, were made available. And the Association also approved a scheme by which commission on motor insurance arranged on special terms for members should be paid to the NVMA for donation to veterinary benevolent funds.[35] They had limited success.

Competition from unqualified salesmen added to the qualified vets' financial problems. While they were not allowed to advertise their services in newspapers and magazines, no such restrictions applied to unqualified persons who purported to offer veterinary service, or indeed to the animal charities. The urban vet was facing increasing competition from the animal charities offering free treatment for the pets of the indigent.[36] The Association responded by placing 'counter adverts' in the newspapers concerned and also submitted articles to the press advising the public how to distinguish a veterinary surgeon from a 'quack'. A request to the RCVS that it should allow 'dignified advertising by members of the veterinary profession, and methods of combating the quackery' was, however, rejected.[37] The College's staunch resistance to advertising was to last until pressure to accept a modest degree of commercial enterprise was forced on it in the 1960s.

The poor economic situation for the veterinary surgeon did improve somewhat after 1927 with the gradual expansion of veterinarians contracted to provide local authority public health services, in response to concern about bovine tuberculosis and the risk of human infection from tuberculous milk. At first, however, when the system came into operation, those local practitioners not contracted to provide municipal services often found their work reduced because local authority services such as TB testing were offered free or at comparatively low cost.

CHAPTER FIVE

FOOT-AND-MOUTH DISEASE: THE FIRST MAJOR OUTBREAK

The overriding animal health concern in 1924 was foot-and-mouth disease. A series of outbreaks had begun in 1922 and early undetected outbreaks spread widely. They took eight months to clear up and necessitated the slaughter of 56,000 livestock caught up in the 1,440 outbreaks; compensation payments amounted to £1.25 million. Further outbreaks, beginning in August 1923, were even more devastating. The county of Cheshire bore the brunt of the diseases and between the start of the outbreaks and May 1924 some 300,000 livestock were slaughtered in 2,691 outbreaks, 1,700 of which were in Cheshire. The county lost one third of its dairy cattle and in some areas as many as 60 per cent of farms were cleared of livestock. The compensation costs of those further outbreaks amounted to £3.3 million, an enormous sum of money in those days. The events of this epidemic call into mind those of the 2001 epidemic of FMD in Britain, which devastated rural Britain.

The government policy of eradication by slaughter was called into question as the numbers of livestock destroyed escalated. The long serving chief veterinary officer, (now Sir) Stewart Stockman, was put under great public pressure by those alarmed at the consequences of the 'slaughter and compensation' policy. That policy, and the veterinary surgeons who supported it, were severely criticised in the national press and by the medical profession, many of whom felt they knew more about the control of infectious diseases than did veterinary surgeons.[1]

The *Veterinary Record* commented: 'At no time during the life of the present generation has our profession stood in a more difficult position than it does now, and at no time has suffered more from adverse criticism.' The journal complained about the 'flood of abuse and ill-conceived comment' in the lay press. Even worse were the letters and articles from medical men, whose 'extraordinary lack of knowledge' was 'really remarkable'. 'Many of the suggestions made to effect isolation or to prevent the spread of infection would shame a first-year student.'[2]

Despite a barrage of opposition, Stockman stuck to his guns. In an address to the council of the NVMA in January, at the height of the outbreak, the chief veterinary officer said that the Cheshire outbreak was entirely different from any other outbreak he had ever tackled before. Up until 1922 all the initial outbreaks were confined to a definite area. In the present instance he felt there was a possibility of birds being a carrier of infection to the UK: a large number of outbreaks had taken place on farms where there had been no outside contact.

Stockman had published a paper which discussed the possible role of bird migration in the introduction of FMD to the country. It included a series of maps showing the route of migration both in the UK and from the continent and plotting outbreaks of foot and mouth disease connected with the migration routes. He gave the credit for the work involved to his co-author, Miss M. Garnett.[3] He also speculated that imported foodstuffs from the Argentine, 'where there had been an enormous spread of FMD', might have been the cause. It had also been alleged that there had been a malicious spread of the disease although there was no evidence for that.

'What happened in this case', said Stockman, 'was that we had all of a sudden something like twenty outbreaks miles from each other all at or about the same time.' All the ministry's staff had been involved and outside veterinary

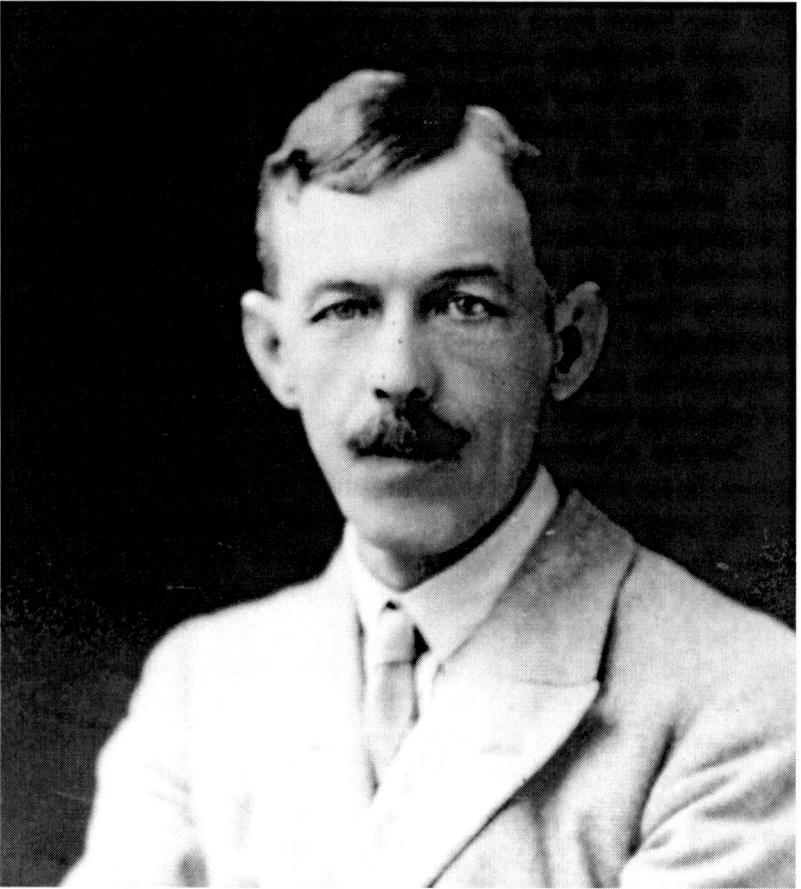

Figure 9. Sir Stewart Stockman, the government's chief veterinary officer in the foot-and-mouth disease outbreaks of the 1920s and a staunch advocate of the 'slaughter and eradicate' policy adopted.

surgeons (temporary veterinary inspectors) had been recruited in 'large numbers'. 'They had done exceedingly fine work – but, of course they had to be put through a large amount of training' before they could be deployed.

In the Cheshire outbreak, he said, a number of animals at Fleetwood on the Lancashire coast which had completed their quarantine had been visited by a veterinary surgeon who had previously visited an outbreak of FMD near Blackpool. Also in the Fleetwood dock were 1,000 sheep which were then distributed all over the country, including to Cheshire, with some going to Crewe market.

Unfortunately the local authority's veterinary inspector did not publish an order restricting local movement in the area and livestock was sold on, spreading the disease.

Another factor in the spread of the disease was that a general election was taking place at the same time and all the police, who should have helped to control livestock movement, were on other duties; and there was a great deal of traffic in and out of farms.

The outbreak had also bought into prominence the question of research into FMD and the possible production of a vaccine. Opinion in the medical profession was that this was the course that should be followed and one of Stockman's concerns was that any research institutes to be established would be dominated by doctors and not vets; another was the risk of virus escaping from the laboratory. In the event, the slaughter and eradication policy was confirmed and remained in place as the method of control for subsequent outbreaks. While effective in the UK's island environment, and with the relatively small herds customary in the nineteenth and early twentieth centuries, the policy became increasingly difficult to justify as effective vaccines were developed and modern methods of livestock production made the spread of infection devastatingly rapid. By the time of the horrendous outbreaks in 2001, the scale, social impact and expense of the destruction involved brought the policy into question and many thought the slaughter/eradication policy no longer sustainable.

In spite of Stockman's misgivings, the government decided to initiate research into FMD, under the aegis of an FMD research committee, populated by vets and doctors. Several institutions were involved, including the MAF laboratory run by Stockman, the National Institute for Medical Research (later the Medical Research Council). In addition, a field station was set up at Pirbright. The bulk of the committee's early work focused on the epidemiology of the disease: finding out how it entered Britain and by what means it spread. Vaccines research only began in earnest as the second world war approached, and their use in the UK was not authorised until over sixty years later with the advent of the Animal Health Act 2002.

FMD RETURNS

In 1951, on 14 November, FMD returned to the UK. It had spread from the Continent where there had been an epidemic originating in Germany, then spreading through Denmark, Belgium and France. It was believed that migrant birds had been responsible for transmitting the disease to the eastern counties of the UK. The traditional remedy of eradication by slaughter and a standstill on the movement of animals was applied. On this occasion, however, there was widespread controversy about that long-standing policy. There was debate in the press and parliament in which the supposed advantages of vaccination, rather than slaughter, were advocated.[4]

The Association stayed firmly on the side of the existing policy that argued against vaccination on three grounds: cost, the need for regular revaccination, and the risk of some vaccinated animals acting as symptomless carriers of the disease. It was pointed out that in Germany an outbreak in 1937–1938 was estimated to have cost £83 million while in the UK during the ten-year period 1940–1950 inclusive the cost was approximately £222,000 a year. And in the 1951 outbreaks, of which there were 116, the total compensation paid for slaughter was £310,000. By the end of the following year FMD outbreaks had risen to some 600, with the slaughter of 85,000 livestock costing about £3 million. But, argued the Association, 'if this recurring threat to our livestock is to be reduced or removed it seems the problem of the control of FMD and other contagious animal diseases must be tackled on a wider basis than at present. Control must be exercised not only on a national but on an international scale.'[5]

After the outbreak had subsided, MAF appointed a departmental committee under the chairmanship of Sir Ernest Gowers to look into the most recent epidemics. The committee was instructed to focus its attention on the vaccination question. The BVA appointed its own committee to prepare and submit evidence to Gowers. The Association had been asked to deal with the question of slaughter policy and possible alternatives, and whether there were any relevant points which the Association felt the committee should investigate. The BVA was also asked whether it had any criticism or suggestions to make in connection with MAF's procedure in dealing with outbreaks of foot-and-mouth disease.

Largely the work of Dr R. F. Montgomerie, director of veterinary research at Burroughs Wellcome & Co., the Association's evidence came down firmly in favour of the existing system.

Its conclusions were summarised as follows:

1 It is contended that Great Britain must remain a country in which foot-and-mouth disease is not endemic.

2 The present policy of the Minister of Agriculture, the so-called slaughter policy, is the only line at present available which will surely maintain this position.

3 The success of the slaughter policy is largely dependent on early notification and immediate action. To these ends an improved procedure for dissemination of information to the veterinary profession is essential. Stockowners must be made more conscious of their obligation to seek professional advice when any unusual condition appears among their livestock and to report immediately any suspicion of foot-and-mouth disease.

4 The evidence at present available indicates that there is no good case for the use of improved foot- and-mouth vaccines or specific serum in Great Britain.

5 It is suggested that Great Britain should collaborate with the appropriate international authority to devise a scheme of vaccination which will limit the spread of foot-and-mouth disease on the continent of Europe and create a barrier area there, to reduce the risk of introduction of the virus into Britain.[6]

So, although solidly against the use of vaccines in the UK, the Association appreciated that in the countries where

FMD was endemic they might well have a place, and could potentially reduce the risk of transfer of infection to the UK.

When the Gowers committee report was published in 1954 it was rather more equivocal than MAF, or the Association, had anticipated. By that time, however, public interest in the outbreak, and how FMD should be controlled, had dissipated. The report's findings received relatively little attention. Those findings were that 'in the circumstances of today, and of the immediate future, any idea that it would be possible to do away with stamping out by making the whole susceptible animal population – or even cattle – immune by vaccination is in the realms of fantasy. In present circumstances stamping out must continue to be the policy in Great Britain.' However, the report went on to say that if advances in vaccine technology were achieved in future, vaccination could eventually replace slaughter as the preferred method of controlling FMD in Britain.[7] That rider was played down in MAF publicity about the Gowers Committee's conclusions.

ANOTHER OUTBREAK

When foot-and-mouth disease (FMD) hit the country once more, in October 1967, there was little warning that the outbreak would be even worse than that in 1924. But a month later, eighty cases a day were being diagnosed. Soon the whole country was declared a 'restricted area'. Minister of Agriculture, T. F. (Fred) Peart, in a statement to the House of Commons on 20 November 1967, said 'this is one of the gravest epidemics of foot-and- mouth disease which has occurred this century, not only because of the number of outbreaks, the number of animals slaughtered or the cost of this, but also because of the virulence of the virus type 1, the speed with which symptoms have appeared in infected animals and the speed with which the disease is spread has been unprecedented. The number of outbreaks so far this year is 639; the number of animals slaughtered approximately 57,500 cattle 26,500 sheep and 31,000 pigs.

There have been 291 outbreaks in Cheshire, 223 in Shropshire, 44 in Flintshire, 37 in Denbighshire; and others in Montgomeryshire, Staffordshire, Lancashire, Derbyshire, Worcestershire, Westmorland, and Gloucestershire.[8]

By the time the epidemic was over, in June 1968, some 450,000 cattle had been slaughtered and £27 million paid in compensation; the ancillary losses suffered by farmers and rural businesses more than trebled that amount.

As it happened, the BVA president that traumatic year was Mary Brancker, the first woman to be elected to that office; she rose magnificently to the occasion. Fred Peart was unusual for a minister of agriculture: he knew the veterinary profession extremely well, having previously been a Privy Council appointed member of RCVS council for eleven years. Opening the BVA congress in September, Peart (by now Lord Privy Seal) spoke of the great help given by the profession during the outbreaks. He paid particular tribute to Mary Brancker 'for your cooperation when we were in great difficulty'.[9] Lord Peart was made an honorary member of the Association in 1977.

The method used to deal with this latest FMD epidemic was the traditional one: slaughter and eradication. The BVA was involved both through the active participation of its members and, behind the scenes, with liaison with MAFF.

Although publicly supporting the slaughter policy, fears that the epidemic might run wild and out of control had forced the Minister of Agriculture to consider resorting to vaccination. Five million doses of FMD vaccine were imported and the chief veterinary officer, John Reid, consulted the BVA president on planning a vaccination campaign. Mary Brancker later recalled: 'We calculated the number of animals to be vaccinated, the number that could be vaccinated and examined in an hour, and the number of daylight hours available in December. These calculations gave us the number of veterinary surgeons required ... finally we agreed the rate of pay for them.'

BVA members had given wholehearted support to the FMD campaign, often neglecting their own practices to do so; but they felt the Association had not made the public at large aware of their contribution. Members complained of the poor public relations effort in presenting the profession's point of view during the FMD outbreak.[10] Council member Henry Carter's comment was typical: he said the Association's public relations had been a total disaster for the profession. Misinformation by lay persons had been published in the newspapers without a word of rebuttal from the BVA. There had been no mention of the large number of veterinary surgeons who had temporarily left their practices to assist the Animal Health Division. 'In the matter of public relations it was time that, like the medical profession, we too dragged our Association kicking and screaming into the twentieth century.'[11]

And support for the slaughter policy was by no means universal. J. K. Brown opposed it on 'practical, economic, humane, scientific and moral grounds'. Among the points he made was that the elimination of the virus by slaughter was only logical if fresh imports of virus from the importation of meat could be prevented[12] (the chief veterinary officer's report on the origin of the outbreaks concluded that frozen lamb imported from the Argentine was the cause of the initial outbreak).

However, the worst was over and the disease began to abate. Once again, the slaughter policy had survived – just. But the repercussions of the outbreak on the important international trade in meat, particularly with Argentina, were serious.

FMD'S MOST SERIOUS OUTBREAK

All other Association matters were put on one side in February 2001 when foot-and –mouth disease was confirmed at an abattoir in Essex. The first major outbreak since 1968, it was unprecedented in its scale and devastating effect. MAFF's long-standing contingency plans were inadequate to cope with the size and range of the epidemic. The plan had been based on the supposition that there would not be more than ten infected premises at any one time: in fact, 'At least fifty-seven premises were infected before the original diagnosis was made.'[13]

The resources of the State Veterinary Service were quickly overwhelmed. As in previous outbreaks, licensed veterinary inspectors' (LVI) services were mobilised and other practitioners were called on for their help as temporary veterinary inspectors. An appeal for 'many more' veterinarians to come forward to help was made in a letter to the *Record* from BVA president, David Tyson. On 24 March 2001, he wrote that there was an enormous backlog of tracings of foot-and-mouth disease to be dealt with and a great need for extra veterinary input 'right now'. The Association appealed to all types of practice to offer help. The BVA had also agreed to encourage the use of students in support roles. Cumbria was a priority area but vets were desperately needed all over the country.[14]

In March, the *Record* said that 'five weeks into foot and mouth disease there can now be no doubt that things will get worse before situation improves'. In the space of five weeks the number of animals slaughtered in an attempt to control the disease had already exceeded the total slaughtered during the six months of the 1967/68 outbreak. The current outbreak differed markedly from that one in the speed and geographical scale of the spread of infection as infected animals (mainly sheep and cattle) were traded in markets across the country. The problems involved in controlling the outbreaks remained formidable; MAFF sought organisational assistance from the army to help free veterinary surgeons' time so that they could devote themselves to tasks for which they were better suited.[15]

BVA headquarters acted as a kind of sorting office for information on the outbreak, giving over 1000 media briefings and liaising with MAFF and the National Farmers Union, giving advice to members and dealing with practical matters such as remuneration and recruitment of temporary veterinary officers.[16]

There were complaints from vets who wished to join in the fight against the disease that MAFF refused to employ anyone over sixty-five years old. Past president Don Haxby was one of a number; he said 'those of us even in our seventies are capable of executing the duties required. Any vet over sixty had experienced foot and mouth disease in the 1967/68 epidemic.'[17] Other letters noted that, although many practices' income had been hit badly by the FMD outbreak, vets were willingly helping in its control. The need for veterinary manpower was so great that, among the more than 2,500 temporary veterinary inspectors engaged, 704 were from overseas; in addition, over 650 veterinary and technical staff from foreign governments were called in to help.[18] The situation had not been helped by cuts in State Veterinary Service (SVS) resources: between 1979 and 2001 the number of field veterinary officers had been more than halved, from 597 to 286, and the number of SVS divisional offices was down to twenty-three from a 1969 figure of seventy.

Policies of wholesale slaughter of suspected FMD cases, as well as confirmed ones, with many vets being inexperienced in dealing with farm animals, plus a policy of slaughtering all (healthy) stock on contiguous premises, added to the carnage. Pedigree herds and flocks built up over years were killed and burnt; the effect on the farmers who owned them, and on the vets who had to supervise the slaughter was very traumatic. The welfare of animals held on farms while they awaited slaughter raised serious concern.[19] Strong doubts were being expressed by vets about the effectiveness of the 'slaughter and burn' policy still being employed,[20] and the mathematical model on which it was based.

After six months the epidemic was at last defeated. The financial damage, coming immediately after the astronomical sums spent on dealing with bovine spongiform encephalopathy (BSE), was staggering: direct costs to the public sector were estimated at £3 billion, while private sector costs would be even higher, about £5 billion, much of it from lost tourist revenue.[21]

The aftermath of the FMD outbreak brought a rash of retrospection. Inquiries and reports came from a Parliamentary select committee, the Royal Society and its

Edinburgh counterpart, and the Farm Animal Welfare Council. The major investigation was a 'Lessons to be learnt' inquiry commissioned by the government, with Dr Ian Anderson as chairman, to which all those affected were invited to submit evidence

Veterinary evidence came from the RCVS and the BVA. The College concentrated on criticising the way the outbreak had been handled: inadequate contingency planning, poor management of resources, and deficiencies in the MAFF – which had now become the Department of the Environments, Food and Rural Affairs (DEFRA) – command structure.[22] The Association, rather than dwelling on shortcomings in dealing with the unprecedented epidemic, focused on how to prevent such a disaster recurring. It called for rigorous controls on import of animals, to prevent disease entering the country, and improved veterinary surveillance to detect any disease that did occur. Pointing to the part that movements of animal from one area to another area had played in the rapid spread of disease, it called for better systems of identifying and tracing animals, particularly through markets; and improved biosecurity, medicines use and traceability of feed. To ensure that sufficient veterinary manpower was available to deal with any outbreak, BVA advocated a 'Territorial Army-style' reserve of private practitioners.[23]

One of the very few welcome side effects of the FMD disaster was a promise from the government of an extra £25 million over five years in funding for the veterinary schools.[24]

CHAPTER SIX

STATE VETERINARY SERVICE PROPOSED

The 1927 congress at Torquay included a special section on veterinary state medicine which discussed the role of the veterinary surgeon in meat inspection, and diseases of the cow in relation to milk legislation; further progress was stalled, however, for seven years. That might have been because there was little enthusiasm for the idea among the Association's council at the time.

Then, in pursuit of its aims for a more formally recognised system of veterinary involvement in meat inspection, and in particular in the control of tuberculosis spread by milk from infected cows, the Association decided in 1934 to support the establishment of a State Veterinary Service. This recommendation was no doubt made in anticipation of the forthcoming report of the committee on cattle diseases and milk production by the Economic Advisory Council chaired by Sir Frederick Gowland Hopkins. In January council passed, not without dissent, the following resolution:

> That there should be a State Veterinary Service under one central government department of animal health in which shall be invested the duties of appointing staff and controlling the whole of the veterinary services of the country, to include veterinary duties under the Diseases of Animals Acts and Orders, the Milk and Dairies Acts and Orders (including the

housing of animals), meat inspection and the Veterinary Advisory Scheme.

That the veterinary practitioner shall be incorporated in the service as well as the whole time veterinary officer.[1]

The insistence on the participation of the private veterinarian was fundamental to the improvement of the practitioner's financial health.

Seeking the wider opinion of the whole profession, the following year the Association sent a questionnaire to every MRCVS in the UK to establish details of the animal health services offered by official bodies and by private practitioners. Of 2,366 questionnaires mailed out, only 284 were returned, mostly from veterinary surgeons in private practice. A lengthy analysis of the findings was published two years later shortly before the announcement of plans for a centralised service.[2]

As is typical in such surveys, respondents were mainly those with a particular axe to grind. A wide divergence of opinion was revealed. Practitioners who had seen their practices affected by the free services offered by municipal or county veterinary officers, and feared further official services, looked to the establishment of a panel model in which they could be involved. A second group of practitioners, who were already holding part-time official posts and had no wish to lose income from that source, were content with things as they were. Finally, there was the small group of full-time municipal and county and government employees who were naturally insistent that the system was best run by full-time veterinary officers.

The fact that the survey took so long to report its results was perhaps because its authors, disappointed with the scant response and equivocal outcome, hoped that everyone would have forgotten about it by the time it was published.

The 1934 resolution in favour of a State Veterinary Service can have had no effect on the Hopkins committee which had by that time virtually completed its deliberations. Their report, published later in that year, recommended an expansion of local authority veterinary services, on a full time basis, under the Ministry of Agriculture. It was estimated that some 300 full time veterinary surgeons would be needed and, while that establishment was created, part-time appointments of practitioners would be continued *as a temporary measure.*

That proposal, which would have had the effect of virtually eliminating part-time official work for the practitioner, was greeted with consternation. 'For the veterinary politicians of the NVMA, who were committed both to a unified profession and to the welfare of individual members of the profession which alone would make such unity possible, this proposal was little short of disastrous.'[3]

The report, according to H. W. Steele-Bodger, by then secretary of SPVS, 'bristles with many misstatements and contradictions'. The committee, he alleged, had ignored the view of veterinary witnesses who had urged that the appointment of a full-time staff of veterinary surgeons would be detrimental to the interests of veterinary practitioners generally. But 'We do not accept this view', Gowland Hopkins stated, 'as the advice given [free] by veterinary surgeons in the public service, by directing the attention of the farmer to incidents of disease . . . tends to make him call in his own veterinary surgeon more freely for the purpose of treatment.' Steele-Bodger doubted whether that opinion would be supported by a single veterinary surgeon.[4]

The Association, too, while commenting, diplomatically, that it was 'in marked sympathy with the bulk of the recommendations made by the Hopkins committee' for the control of diseases in cattle, was unable to support the recommendations made on the organisation of the profession itself. The NVMA argued that any effective scheme had to have the support of a united veterinary profession; which would not be given if the committee's recommendations were implemented as they stood.[5] It will be seen that the establishment of a united veterinary profession was, like nirvana, not to be attained.

The Association published its own recommendations in response to those made in the report. These urged the establishment of a Department of Animal Health under the control of a principal veterinary officer 'whose status should be equivalent to that of the chief medical officer'. The country would be divided into four or five areas each supervised by an area officer directly responsible to the principal veterinary officer. County and municipal officers would regularise standards throughout the country and coordinate the work of panels of private veterinary practitioners. These part time appointments, which would consist of 'as many veterinary practitioners as can be employed for the purpose', would be established on a permanent basis to carry out routine work under the supervision of county veterinary officers. Finally, it was recommended that each area should have a laboratory run by veterinary officers.[6]

Those proposals, which attempted to satisfy the aspirations of salaried veterinary officers as well as private practitioners, did not of course quite achieve that aim. There were complaints from members in municipal service that not only did the scheme appear to be designed for the benefit of veterinary general practitioners, but also that it was directed only towards the control of animal diseases and failed to take account of the interdependence of animal disease control with the public health functions integral to the work currently undertaken by the local authorities.[7]

One veterinary officer complained about the lack of attention given to meat inspection and public health in the discussions on the Agriculture Bill. He commented: 'In a very few years it will be realised that acting under the stimulus of the Society of Veterinary Practitioners (SPV) [the future Society of Practising Veterinary Surgeons] the NVMA has thrown away all hope of progress for the profession.' He predicted that the provisions for veterinary service in the Agriculture Bill would lead to the abandonment of all claims to public health and the ruin of their municipal veterinary service: not only that, but the general practitioners would find they have no place whatever in the public veterinary service[8] (not surprisingly, H. W. Steele-Bodger, on behalf of the Society of Veterinary Practitioners, strongly refuted those assertions).

A dichotomy between veterinary care mainly concerned with the live animal and the public health and meat hygiene aspects of professional work would grow; the eventual creation of the Meat Hygiene Service in 1995 was its logical outcome.

Nevertheless, the Association continued to press its case with the government and when, in 1937, the outline proposals for a centralised veterinary service went before Parliament as part of the Agriculture Bill, they appeared to be very similar to the Association's own proposals. The only cavil was that the meat inspection services would be left in their 'present unsatisfactory and disorganised position'.[9]

In a leader, commenting on that year's NVMA congress, the *Record* was able to say, 'with the passage of the recent Agriculture Act it may truly be said that the veterinary profession in this country has embarked upon a new era.' The Minister of Agriculture, W. S. Morrison, spoke at the congress of the government's 'great enterprise, which involves a centralised State Veterinary Service, to commence an attack upon the problem of animal diseases on a scale and on a front of the magnitude which has not yet been imagined'. And that could not succeed without the profession's cooperation, he said.[10] The mention of the profession's 'cooperation' was significant.

A consultative committee of the NVMA was set up to work with the Ministry of Agriculture with the intention of coordinating, as far as possible, government and Association policies. All seemed set fair for a satisfactory outcome. However, the euphoria evident at the August congress was short lived. Disillusion set in when on 12 December 1937, the trade journal *Farmers Weekly* published details of the proposed new service – before the Association had been given the information. Britain was to be divided into seventy-eight divisions, each in charge of a divisional inspector; the divisions would be grouped in areas, each headed by a superintending inspector. The service would at first employ between 300 and 350 full-time officers and it was contemplated that eventually a staff of 500 would be needed. Laboratories would be provided in each division for the examination of milk samples, and provision would also be made for area laboratory facilities.

It was proposed that staff to be appointed at the commencement of the service on 1 April 1938, would be assisted by panels of part-time veterinary surgeons which would be reduced as the number of permanent staff was increased. The Association's consultative committee had been committed to confidentiality and had kept to that agreement; the source of the leak was not discovered. The fact that the information had surfaced in a farming journal and not through the profession itself added insult to injury.[11]

The *Veterinary Record* commented: 'Unfortunately the counsel of the profession has not truly been sought, its consultative committee has been presented with defined schemes in which it has been expected to acquiesce almost at once. A policy of secrecy, the spirit suggestive of dictatorship and an apparent assumption of omniscience have prevailed. The goodwill of the profession has been shocked and dissipated, for on no material point has its wishes been met. Its county men are to be absorbed by the State, smarting under petty injustices, the municipal officer is to be left in large measure to work the broken system of duties concerning public health, while the practitioner is expected to welcome temporary inclusion within the service. Such intentions are widely different from those which the profession had been led to expect and have not unnaturally annihilated its confidence.'

GOVERNMENT PROPOSALS 'A TRAVESTY'

The scheme, said the *Record*, was 'a travesty of all that is meant by a coordinated attack upon the diseases of livestock'. It had little, if any, hope of success.[12] The bad feeling caused led to difficult relations between the ministry and the Association.

A special meeting of council in December received a report from the Association's consultative committee on the confidential negotiations held with the Ministry of

Agriculture. Dissatisfied with the proposed scale of salaries, the committee had submitted its own proposals, similar to the scale NVMA had recommended in 1934 (see above). These the minister, W. S. Morrison, had turned down flat. The committee requested a personal interview with the minister to press its case for a review of the scale, which request was also refused. Presumably realising that the government held all the cards, and was well aware that the Association had found itself powerless to stop its members accepting what it regarded as unsuitable salaries for veterinary officer posts, the committee reluctantly accepted the salary scale on offer.

In response to criticism from some members of NVMA that the case for the transfer of meat inspection to the new central service had not been pushed as hard as it might, the committee responded that it had made the point throughout its discussions; it submitted to council the resolution: 'The Association deplores the omission of powers to include the entire public health veterinary services within the new centralised service and pledges itself to press the necessity for such change.' It also intended to seek a further interview with the minister to discuss points about transfer to the state service of those already in municipal or county veterinary posts, and their superannuation and salaries.

Very serious issue was taken with a ministry statement that the employment of part-time veterinarians as local officers would be only a temporary measure, contrary to the undertaking contained in a MAF memorandum which indicated that 'even after a full complement of full-time veterinary inspectors has been completed . . . there will still be considerable scope for the employment of part-time men'. The NVMA president, Donald Campbell, wrote on 9 December 1937 expressing the concerns of the veterinary profession, complaining that each time the ministry had met the profession's representatives it had been faced with a *fait accompli*. He proposed a date the following week for such a meeting. An exchange of correspondence between the president and the minister's private secretary followed.

The president's rather straightforward style of argument was no match for the literary diplomacy of a senior civil service mandarin. A lengthy final letter from the ministry dismissed each of Campbell's points in turn and concluded that the minister 'does not feel that any useful purpose would be served by his receiving a further deputation from your association on the matters dealt with in this letter to which he has given the most careful consideration'. He concluded that the minister 'cannot believe that, if the members of the veterinary profession are fully apprised of the steps which have been taken and are being taken to create a State Veterinary Service which will offer congenial work and an attractive career to a large body of veterinary surgeons in this country, there could be any reason whatever for the dissipation of goodwill to which he alludes'.[13]

Notwithstanding this rebuff, the Association decided to ask once again for an interview with the minister. The letter making the request set out principles which the Association considered essential for the success of the new service. These were:

1 Permanent inclusion of private practitioners in the service;

2 Freedom of choice by the stock owner of the practitioner to be employed [for examination and testing];

3 An invitation for existing full-time officers employed by local authorities to accept appointment in the service;

4 An arbitration board to deal with any question arising between the ministry and veterinary officers employed.

When on 5 January 1938 the president called on the minister's representative, Donald Vandepeer and the chief veterinary officer, Sir John Kelland, and invited Mr Vandepeer to address the Association's council on the minister's proposals, the invitation was emphatically declined. Vandepeer described some of the recent articles in the *Veterinary Record* as scurrilous and showing a lack of experience of negotiation. Further, acceptance 'would not accord with the dignity of the Ministry'. Both Vandepeer and Kelland appeared to resent the Association's 'going over their heads' by writing direct to the minister. It was also pointed out that, by appealing direct to the minister, negotiations automatically stopped pending his reply. The *Record*, in a comment headed 'A specious plea of dignity' considered that its expressions of views were in the public interest and should not have offended 'so delicate a departmental dignity'.[14]

On 10 January, the president wrote to Vandepeer asking for a comprehensive statement of the ministry's scheme for a State Veterinary Service 'as a whole', as hitherto its proposals had had to be dealt with piecemeal.

The minister replied on 12 January to both the earlier and the last letter. He brushed aside the four basic principles which the Association had spelt out and indicated that he saw no useful purpose in a further interview. If the Association wished to discuss detailed proposals that were being formulated, it should do so through the medium of the consultative committee and the ministry's representatives, he intimated.

NEGOTIATIONS RESUMED

Although the minister himself refused to meet a deputation, his permanent secretary, Sir Ronald Fergusson, offered to meet representatives of the Association and to resume negotiations with the consultative committee, but only on the basis of complete confidentiality (which had, in fact, been the basis of negotiations throughout and which the NVMA's team had scrupulously observed). No report of the progress of the meeting was to be published unless by mutual agreement.[15]

Clearly, the minister and his advisers must of necessity have become perplexed as to how to deal with 'these troublesome people'. Parliament had decreed that the State Veterinary Service was to be established and the minister was under an obligation to set it up; already the appointed day had been changed from 1 January to 1 April (April Fool's day, as it happened) and the role of part-time officers had barely been touched upon in the negotiations to date. There were also many loose ends concerning the transfer of the local authority officers yet to be resolved. It must have seemed imperative that the cooperation and goodwill of the profession be regained, as without it the scheme must founder.[16]

In early February 1938, following these further negotiations, the structure of the new service was finally revealed. The service would remain under MAF; it would be headed by the chief veterinary officer, Sir John Kelland, two deputy CVOs and a chief superintendent inspector. As had originally been published in the *Farmers Weekly*, the country was divided into seventy-eight divisions each in charge of a divisional inspector; these were grouped into twenty-two areas, each under the control of a superintendent inspector. Of those twenty-two areas, thirteen were in England, two in Wales and seven in Scotland. Ninety-one full-time veterinary officers would be employed on duties in the field. A further twenty-nine would be employed on headquarters duties at the Ministry in London and in Edinburgh; on port duties; and at the Pirbright experimental station and the London quarantine station. The whole-time strength of the new service, when it commenced operations on 1 April, was thus 120 veterinary surgeons. The county and municipal veterinary services would be dismantled and their employees, or the very great majority of them, absorbed into the centralised service.

As for the part-time officers (veterinary surgeons in private practice) they would be divided into two panels. Panel A would deal (only) with notifiable diseases and market inspections. A specific area would be allotted to each part-time officer in consultation with the officers concerned at a conference with the superintendent and divisional officers. Panel B would deal with 'eradication duties' which would include tuberculin testing and taking blood samples under a proposed scheme for controlling contagious abortion. Those duties would normally be carried out by the appointed practitioners within their existing practices.

However, practitioners appointed to panel A would also be eligible to undertake the designated 'eradication duties' among their own clients.[17]

So practitioners had, at last, got a 'panel' system, something they, or some of them, had long desired. Whether the system they were landed with was the one they wanted, was a different matter.

The Association hoped that this scheme, which removed the provision by which the 'panel' veterinary officer appointments (local veterinary inspectors) would be temporary ones lasting only until the state service had achieved its full complement of full-time officers, would be welcomed by the profession in general. The scheme it hoped, 'should secure both efficiency and harmony'. It was a vain hope. Within three months of the scheme coming into operation on 1 April, sharp dissenting voices were being raised by practitioners aggrieved at the financial losses they would suffer by failure to be appointed to panel A. Eventually, however, the dust settled and a kind of tacit moratorium seems to have been declared while the system found its working order.[18]

A year later, opinions as to how the scheme was settling down differed. The Association, speaking through the *Veterinary Record*, commented that the large-scale schemes introduced under the 1937 Agriculture Act would take a considerable time to develop (already there were 670 Panel A vets – local veterinary inspectors). Although it acknowledged that 'serious harm' had been done to meat inspection by the closure of local authority services it hoped that the shortcomings would be quickly rectified. It was also aware of 'this difficult time in international affairs'.[19] The 'difficult time' referred to was the international crisis leading to the outbreak of the 1939–1945 war in September.

That doyen of the profession, Sir Frederick Hobday, took a much less emollient line, international crisis or no. The new arrangements were disappointing; he was outraged at the dismantling of the local authority services, which had 'embraced many aspects of public health'. He particularly resented the way in which the meat inspection service had been omitted from the new system and 'left to die'. 'We must demand a fair deal for our veterinary services and, above all, that meat inspection shall remain one of the essentials of a municipal or state veterinary service.'[20]

Hobday had a valid point. Local arrangements for veterinary meat inspection and the monitoring of milk quality were significantly disrupted by the transfer of veterinary staff to the centralised service. Even the distractions of war did not long obscure the reality that the ideal of a unified public health veterinary service had been undermined by the 1937 legislation. 'The paths of human and animal health diverged in Britain once more. .... If the financial security of the ordinary members of the profession was the price of greater political unity, then the price must be paid. The ideal of a public health veterinary service was an aspiration abandoned [by the NVMA] in the act of achieving a State Veterinary Service,' he argued.[21]

Throughout the long and difficult negotiations, the Association's president, Donald Campbell, and the secretary, Fred Knight, played a major part. They and other representatives of the NVMA, veterinary surgeons with full-time jobs, thrust into an unfamiliar role, had put up a creditable performance against senior civil servants. The fact that the State Veterinary Service remit completely ignored meat inspection and veterinary public health was due not to any shortcomings in the case presented by the Association's negotiators but to the fact that it was never an option included under the Agriculture Act. And one important point had been firmly re-established: the National Veterinary Medical Association was truly the representative body in negotiations between government and the veterinary profession.

In spite of the difficult negotiations, relations between the Ministry of Agriculture and the Association had so much improved by 1939 that the new chief veterinary officer (CVO), Daniel Cabot, opened the 1939 congress. The *Veterinary Record,* in a comment on the CVO's address, welcomed his announcement that contagious abortion of cattle and diseases of poultry would soon be brought within the activities of the service. Looking at the wide range of diseases and other conditions which are included in the term 'animal health', said the comment, it was apparent that there was no branch of veterinary science outside the ambit of the state services. The author wondered whether it was now possible to foresee the day when 'every practising veterinary surgeon will be a unit of the service',[22] adding that many would view that prospect with alarm. But, the *Record* continued, each extension of official measures should increase the recognition of the general practitioner as, in the chief veterinary officer's words, a 'part of a large team'.

The CVO's speech was welcomed with 'loud applause'. But the hope that 'every practising veterinary surgeon would be a unit' of the State Veterinary Service proved to be very wide of the mark.

A NEW PRESIDENT AND ANOTHER WAR

At that same congress Harry Steele-Bodger was elected president; at 38, he was the youngest man to hold that office; he had already proved his mettle as secretary and guiding light of SPVS.

Steele-Bodger is an unusual name: he was an unusual man. It is said that he inherited a love of animals from farming antecedents on the Bodger side, an aptitude for medicine from the Steeles of his mother's side and his flair for politics from his ancestor Sir Richard Steele. Even before he qualified as a vet (a term he hated − it was always 'veterinary surgeon') he had had a colourful life. Too young for Army service in 1914, he had volunteered for an ambulance corps attached to the French army; he then joined the Royal Engineers and became a shoeing smith before gaining a commission as an instructor in horsemastership. In France he was wounded and gassed. On recovery, while training raw horses, he was kicked in the face and reported killed. The eye lost in that accident was the reason for the monocle he sported.[23]

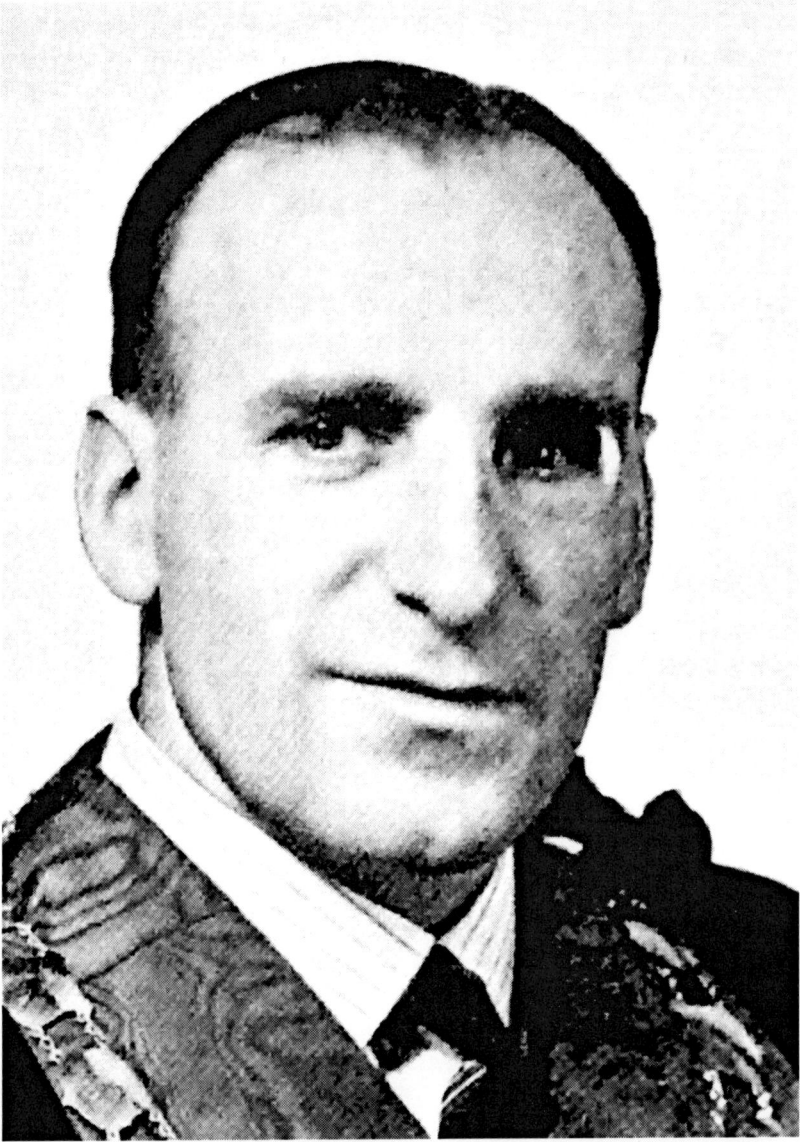

Figure 10. Harry Steele-Bodger, activist in both clinical and veterinary political matters, as a leader of the Society of Practising Veterinary Surgeons and the youngest president of the NVMA.

On 4 September, only a few weeks after his induction as president, war was declared. Steele-Bodger wrote in the first issue of the *Veterinary Record* after that date: 'When my biographer referred to me as the first post-war graduate to be president of the NVMA he did not imagine that within a month we should be at war again. ... It would seem inevitable that many of the schemes which I had hoped to have seen brought to fruition during my term of office will have to be postponed, but members may rest assured that we shall do our best under the circumstances.'[24]

Those 'circumstances' would soon prove difficult for the Association. Bombing in and around 36 Gordon Square, which it had acquired in 1937, meant that its offices had to be evacuated. The home of the general secretary, Fred Knight, received a direct hit and was totally destroyed. Fortunately Knight and his family were unharmed. The editorial office was removed to Welwyn Garden City, and Association's headquarters moved to the premises of the president, Steele-Bodger, in Lichfield.[25]

The situation of the veterinary profession in the Second World War was, however, very different from what it had been in 1914. There was no longer a demand for a huge number of Army horses to be looked after. The demand, rather, was to secure the country's food supplies by increasing livestock productivity on the home front. It was to this end that the efforts of the veterinary profession would be directed. Members of the profession, however, were classified as belonging to a reserved occupation because there were fears that Germany might utilise animal diseases as weapons in biological warfare.

One of the first wartime initiatives of the Association was its involvement in the National Air Raid Precautions for Animals Committee (NARPAC). This body, to which Steele-Bodger had been appointed as the NVMA's liaison officer, was formed mainly of representatives of various animal charities. Its role was to organise the prompt treatment, or slaughter when treatment was not practicable, of animals injured in air raids. Steele-Bodger, in an early report of the committee's activities, spoke of the difficulty of 'welding together a heterogeneous mass of workers into a coherent whole'.[26]

Perhaps that is not surprising in view of the Association's poor relationships with some of the animal charities involved and the reluctance of some vets to work with such colleagues. In 1942, a Farm Livestock Emergency Service was set up with MAF backing to cater for any air raid activity affecting animals in rural areas, rather than relying on the town-centred NARPAC, which was left to cater for pet animals. A joint NVMA/RCVS committee was set up with the aim of coordinating efforts to persuade the government to utilise the services of the veterinary profession more fully in the national interest. On the South Coast, the evacuation of towns had led to the euthanasia of many pets, with the virtual elimination of veterinary practices in those areas, exacerbating an already serious employment situation in the profession.

WARTIME ANIMAL HEALTH SCHEMES

Driven by Steele-Bodger's enthusiasm to win the cooperation of the farming industry, a joint committee was formed with the National Farmers Union to help promote the Association's animal health proposals. These proposals were initiated with a series of technical leaflets for veterinary surgeons setting out schemes for the prevention and control of many of the common diseases in livestock and the more effective use of veterinary medicines. Steele-Bodger believed that 'if one could only capitalise on waste in this country due to preventable disease, the sum of money involved would be staggering – it would subsidise any scheme of disease control or eradication'. His supporters in, and major contributors to, these early animal health schemes, the survey schemes as they became known, were Professor Tom Dalling, Professor W. C. Millar and Dr W. R. Wooldridge.[27]

On an immediately practical level, improvements in cattle fertility were sought to raise standards of milk and meat production; the government backed an NVMA scheme to tackle infertility. The first step in any attempt to improve rates of conception was early diagnosis of whether cows that had been served were pregnant so that, if not, they could be got back in calf quickly. Back then, there were relatively few veterinary surgeons skilled in the appropriate techniques; with the encouragement of the Ministry of Agriculture, three fertility experts toured the country instructing colleagues in the necessary procedures. Steele-Bodger, Sam Hignett (a lecturer in the agriculture department at Leeds University shortly to become director of veterinary research for Burroughs Wellcome & Co) and George Gould, a West Country practitioner, were those selected.

The survey committee did a remarkable job. With the backing of MAF from 1942, which pressured an initially reluctant NFU into cooperation, it introduced a preventive medicine scheme (also called the 'panel scheme') by which, for a flat fee paid by the farmer, his vet would visit and advise at least four times a year. The conditions intended to be covered by the scheme were infertility, contagious abortion, mastitis and Johne's disease.

By 1941, the demand for milk, encouraged by government promotion of its merits as a food, was increasing. Feedstuffs for livestock were at a premium so the need to maximise production per animal was paramount. By highlighting the contribution that the veterinary surgeon could make to milk supplies by showing farmers how to improve conception rates for cows, the NVMA initiative was well timed. MAF accepted the case for veterinary intervention and agreed to support the scheme. Incidental benefits which accrued were improved relations with farmers, greater expertise among veterinary surgeons – and the removal of the unemployment which existed in the early days of the war.

The work of the survey scheme pioneers was to receive the gratitude of wartime Minister of Agriculture R. A. Hudson who, speaking at the 1942 congress, paid tribute to 'the few veterinary surgeons experienced in that field [infertility] who devoted time to train their colleagues and were prepared to sacrifice their practices and their leisure in order to do this'.[28]

Mary Brancker, a young colleague in the Steele-Bodger practice at the time, recalls that there were considerable periods when the staff did not see the principal from Monday morning until Friday evening and were on duty for 24 hours a day during that period. Steele-Bodger himself was a workaholic; if, after an exhausting period without a break an assistant asked for a day off, he would respond, in some surprise, 'what for?'[29] Mary Brancker also recalled that during the time the Association's headquarters were based at the Steele-Bodger practice, when close liaison between the ministry and the profession was a regular practice, she would drive to the station to collect Professor Dalling, then attached to the Ministry of Agriculture, and deliver him to the Lichfield meetings of the survey committee.

In 1944, the introduction of the official calfhood vaccination scheme using S19 brucellosis vaccine, brought further success to the fertility scheme. However, after 1945 the NVMA scheme, according to MAF, lost much of its attraction; it was eventually terminated in 1950.[30] An indication of how farmers had come to value the regular veterinary input brought by the scheme is that when it was closed the main critic of that decision was the NFU.[31]

The activities of the survey scheme and the technical information committee's publications represented the first structured attempts at continuing professional development (CPD) for the veterinary profession: the NVMA was the trailblazer in that field. The production of technical information leaflets by the Association continued throughout the war and, indeed, to the 1970s when they were superseded by other CPD activities. But the widespread adoption of preventive medicine techniques was much longer delayed, until the widespread adoption of intensive livestock production.

Steele-Bodger was followed as president of the Association by Dr W. R. (Reg) Wooldridge, eminent academician and research scientist. Wooldridge was the brilliant nephew of another notable past president, G. H. Wooldridge. Following qualification at the Royal Veterinary College, gaining a BSc in chemistry along the way, he went up to Cambridge on a Ministry of Agriculture scholarship and after a short stay at the Institute of Animal Pathology worked as a researcher under Sir Frederick Gowland Hopkins, specialising in the effect of bacterial toxins on mammalian tissue. He was appointed lecturer in biochemistry at the London School of Hygiene and Tropical Medicine in 1931, since when he had been active in the affairs of NVMA, proving an extremely efficient committee chairman and negotiator in the Association's service; he had been honorary secretary for four years before succeeding to the presidency.

When he gave his presidential address in 1942 the country was in desperate need of home-produced food. He surveyed the task of the veterinary profession in regard to the health and welfare of the nation's livestock and advocated the setting up of a comprehensive veterinary service. In considering the type of personnel needed to operate such a service, he argued that some of the work of the veterinary surgeon could usefully be done by lay assistants, provided they had sufficient training 'to appreciate the value of the work they were doing'. But, he emphasised, it was essential that those lay assistants received veterinary supervision and direction, particularly in so far as giving advice was concerned. This proposal, of the use of trained lay assistants, was to return over the years, often to face opposition from private veterinary surgeons.

Wooldridge's idea was that a comprehensive service dealing with the health of all animals should incorporate all branches of the profession. Such an efficient and progressive organisation, he considered, could only satisfactorily be developed on the lines of an official body, but one untrammelled by ordinary civil service restrictions.

He envisaged the formation of a corporation, with governors appointed by the state and a veterinary surgeon as its chief executive, similar in structure to the BBC. The control and inspection of human foods of animal origin would be an integral part of the organisation.[32]

Wooldridge's successor in office, R. G. C. Hancock, had views on the future of veterinary practice that were even

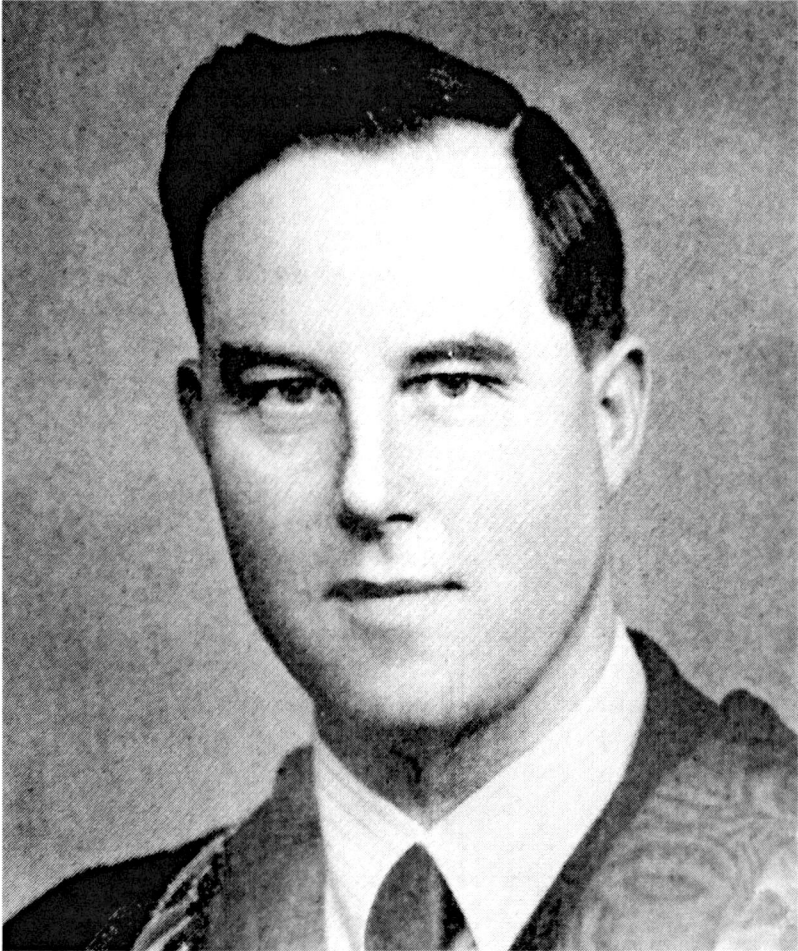

Figure 11. Dr W. R. 'Reg' Wooldridge, Association president with radical ideas; he went on to become founder and head of the Animal Health Trust.

more radical. He suggested that 'when opportunity arose' private practices should be bought by the state. Private practitioners would run such practices as their own; they would be paid a basic salary for veterinary inspector duties, but would be allowed to earn fees from private practice in addition.[33] Neither of those proposed schemes came to anything; they may possibly have been intended as no more than Aunt Sallys. Wooldridge's advocacy of what would have

121

been a wholly state-incorporated profession, certainly was not likely to gain support from many practitioners.

However, the stresses of life in a country preoccupied with fighting for its very survival, and the fact that most veterinary surgeons were involved to an increasing degree in MAF-generated or sponsored duties, presumably made such suggestions of increasing state involvement in practice less indigestible than might formerly have been the case. Hancock had prefaced his remarks by the comment that 'even now, it has become impossible for the majority of country veterinary surgeons to be sure of earning a decent living unless they were willing to take part in the local activities of the Animal Health Division'.[34]

This period, when very many activities were subject to one form or another of official control, was also the time when the Beveridge proposals for a National Health Service were being discussed.[35] The Beveridge plan's recommendations for cooperation between the state and individuals, and radical changes in the organisation of medical services, revolutionary at the time, would have had resonances for the veterinary profession. Consideration by its leaders of ideas to regularise some of the uncertainties of veterinary existence were not surprising.

VETERINARY EDUCATION PLANS

What had become increasingly clear during the war was that existing facilities for veterinary education were inadequate to produce practitioners who could service the needs of an efficient, productive agricultural industry. The fact that the Minister of Agriculture in his address to the 1942 congress had spoken of the need for special training for veterinary practitioners so that they were competent to implement the animal health measures brought in by the dairy cattle diseases control scheme, served to draw attention to the shortcomings in the knowledge of the average veterinary surgeon. Wooldridge's intention in setting up a veterinary education trust (the Animal Health Trust [AHT]), which he also announced at the 1942 congress, was specifically to provide better facilities for veterinary postgraduate education.[36] The AHT was to develop into one of the world's foremost veterinary research establishments – particularly in the equine field and that of canine ophthalmology.

The need for a thorough overhaul of veterinary education had, of course, been recognised for some time and the Loveday committee (the interdepartmental committee on veterinary education) had been set up before the war to look at the whole system of veterinary education and training. Consideration of the committee's recommendations, published in 1938, had added to the workload of the Association's officers during 1938 and 1939. They culminated in a detailed presentation by NVMA council officers and members, led by president Robert Simpson, to the RCVS council, with the aim of ensuring a united front by the profession in its approach to the proposals; in fact, the Association was in broad agreement with the main thrust of Loveday's report and there were no major differences on the report between the two bodies.[37]

Implementation of the recommendations of the Loveday committee had largely (if not entirely) been overtaken by the outbreak of war in 1939. In 1943 'in the light of the altered circumstances arising from the war' it had been recalled and asked to review its earlier recommendations. The recalled committee based its considerations on MAF's revised estimates of the number of veterinary surgeons that would be required in the changed circumstances since 1938; it was now estimated that there would be a need for some 220 veterinarians annually for a period of about ten years, with a possible reduction to 150 annually thereafter. The committee did not consider the estimate of 220 was excessive and had framed its recommendations accordingly. It added that it could see no reason to believe that the demand would fall to 150 after a decade.

The Association welcomed the reconvening of the committee and the fact that it had been asked, again, to give evidence. The Association's council, broadly in favour of supporting Loveday's 1938 recommendations, agreed that 'degrees granted by the universities should be accepted by the RCVS as qualifying for registration and membership of the College provided that safeguards as to minimal educational standards can be devised and agreed to. The RCVS would then retain all its disciplinary powers, including license to practise.'

The 1943 annual general meeting, however, was against any change to the existing 'one portal' system of entry to the profession; that is, qualifying after passing the examination of the RCVS. A motion to the effect that such a change would be a 'threat to the existence of the Association and the integrity of the profession' was passed by 120 votes to 33.[38]

The BVA council had, in fact, misunderstood what Loveday intended: it did not propose to change the principle of the 'one portal' system of qualification. What seems to have caused the misunderstanding, which persisted for some time, was the objection taken to the principle of accepting a university degree as the academic qualification recognised by the College; it would remain the case that the RCVS diploma, granted on the basis of an acceptable degree, was the registerable qualification.

When the Loveday committee issued its second report in 1944 its recommendations confirmed, and expanded upon, those made in 1938: that two new veterinary schools should be established, and that all future veterinary surgeons should qualify after taking a degree awarded by a university; those degrees should be registerable qualifications. The College would be given powers similar to those of the General Medical Council in relation to the standard of the training given by the schools and would have power to inspect the schools, and make recommendations, as it found necessary. The RCVS council would be reinforced by the appointment of 12 representatives from the six schools; four representatives would be appointed by the Crown. The remaining seventeen members would be elected by the membership. The recommendations maintained the principle that licence to practise should be restricted to those graduates registered by the College. It was emphasised that membership of the RCVS would remain the sole means of entry to the profession.

Other recommendations related to the provision of improved teaching facilities for students, with each school to have a field station which included a large animal hospital. Specific funding for research ('an essential function of the teaching institution') was recommended and the provision made that all students should undergo a period of at least six months with a veterinary surgeon in practice during his or her course.

Loveday also recommended that bursaries should be available for students so that no one should be precluded from training because they could not afford it. Finally, the existing schools should be incorporated with the appropriate universities and the two new schools established at Bristol and Cambridge.

A vocal minority of members continued their protests against any change to the existing system of entry after sitting examination by the College. Throughout 1944 the *Record* published more than forty letters commenting one way or the other, but mainly supporting the existing 'one portal' system; they were pushing at an open door. One correspondent who went against the tide by praising the advantages that would follow the adoption of the Loveday recommendations, was a young veterinarian who would herself go on to be an important contributor to the veterinary profession: her name was Olga Uvarov.[39]

Eventually Wooldridge, both a leader of the Association and, as a member of the Loveday committee a signatory of the report, sought to correct 'various misunderstandings that some are trying to engender concerning the committee's second report'. Foremost among those misunderstandings, he wrote, was the misapprehension that the recommendations of the report would result in the abolition of the single portal entry to the profession. Wooldridge pointed out that the council of the RCVS would remain the body concerned with maintaining a minimum standard of all examinations, university as well as College. He emphasised that the College council remained as the supreme professional body over its own affairs and that no new General Veterinary Council was recommended.[40] That remained the case until after 2010.

CHAPTER SEVEN

AFTER HOSTILITIES

The war had brought about a revival of agriculture and a better appreciation of the veterinary profession, what it stood for, and the vital part they could play in conquering diseases.[1]

The end of hostilities found 'a diminished number of overworked practitioners manfully dealing with the increasing demands of an enlightened agriculture'.[2] But by 1945, the veterinary profession had, at last, weathered the sea change from being largely devoted to horses to a more broadly based practice serving the needs of livestock, companion animals and mixed practice generally.

The profession had acquitted itself well, as it had done in the First World War, but in a different way. The mechanisation of the armed forces in the inter-war period had diminished the need for veterinary surgeons to provide and maintain transport animals for the army, as they had. That does not mean to say that the Royal Army Veterinary Corps had not played its part. As well as training military dogs, providing horses and mules for transport in Italy, India and Burma proved to be increasingly vital as the war progressed; the strength of the RAVC grew from 190 in 1939 to 4,500 in 1945, and the need for Army veterinary surgeons increased to the extent that the reserved status had been removed from younger vets.[3]

However this role was complemented by the profession's increasingly important activities on the home front, in maintaining the productivity and health of livestock to feed the whole population.

Such activities remained vital after the war, due to the ongoing global shortage of food. The introduction by the government of guaranteed prices for livestock, measures to expand food production by encouraging the use of artificial fertilisers, draining land and grubbing out hedgerows to increase arable acreage[4], all maintained the prosperity of farmers. The robust financial situation thus ensured that farmers had the wherewithal to pay their veterinarians' bills. In their turn, vets found more demand for their services for routine vaccinations, piglet castration and cow dehorning as well as for the traditional 'fire brigade' treatment for sick animals.[5] As a corollary, the shortage of veterinary surgeons to cater for an increased demand continued. So did the need for improved veterinary education, recognised by the reports of Loveday and others.

Those shortages were among the matters on the agenda of the first post-war congress of the Association, in September 1945, in London, little more than a month after the surrender of Japan. It saw, as the *Record* put it, 'the social functions happily restored' after truncated meetings in wartime. The main social function was the congress luncheon; the list of guests indicates their status: they included Earl De La Warr, chairman of the Agricultural Research Council; the Duke of Norfolk, lately Parliamentary Secretary, Minister of Agriculture; Sir Henry Dale, president of The Royal Society; Dr Thomas Loveday, chairman of the Committee on Veterinary Education; Sir Walter Monckton, recently solicitor-general; the president, Dr H. S. Soutar, and secretary, Dr Charles Hill, of the British Medical Association; the editor-in-chief of the Press Association; and senior officers of the National Farmers Union and of the BBC – to name, as they say, only a few.[6]

In his speech, Earl De La Warr commented that the livestock industry comprised over 70 per cent of the output of the farming industry, and the losses from animal diseases amounting to £20 million indicated the 'absolutely vital part which veterinary surgeons can contribute to the future of agriculture – still our largest industry'. He went on to refer to the shortage of veterinary surgeons in the UK and said that, although the Loveday report had been issued eighteen months previously, they were not one single step nearer an increase in educational facilities for the veterinary profession (the Loveday report recommended an increase both in numbers and the breadth of training of veterinary students). 'Unless your leaders and universities are able in the near future to come to some agreement, there would be very wide support in parliament if the Minister of Agriculture eventually decided to overrule whoever might be responsible for the hold-up,' he said, adding that 'the present impasse cannot be allowed to continue'.[7]

The impasse to which Earl De La Warr referred was the row over 'single portal' entry to the profession which had been simmering since 1943. The hiatus, as we have seen, had been caused by the entrenched opinion of that section of the profession which was opposed to any change in the existing regulations. It continued to disagree that a university degree should be the qualification for granting membership of the Royal College of Veterinary Surgeons rather than the College's own examination. The NVMA president, Professor W. C. Miller, in his response acknowledged the need for urgency to come to a decision on the Loveday report's recommendation: the parties concerned were still jockeying for position and in the meantime 'the milk is lost, calves die and production remains less than it might be', he said.

Before this matter could be settled, however, the long running, indeed perennial, complaint by the Association about the salary scale of state veterinary officers broke out again. Negotiations with the ministry continued throughout Miller's presidency and into those of his successors, G. N. Gould and Guy Anderson. Gould was an outstanding practitioner from a long-standing veterinary family whose grandfather had been veterinary surgeon to Queen Victoria. He had built up an extensive practice based on the principle that veterinary services should not be limited to the treatment of individual animals but should be concerned with herd health as a whole, including feeding, pasture management, breeding and herd management. He was also experienced in the wider world of veterinary organisations, as well as that of his local community.[8]

Anderson, a younger vet with experience in Canada as well as Britain, was a forceful advocate when arguing the Association's case in the later stages of the Veterinary Surgeons Bill, which would replace the old Veterinary Surgeons Act 1881

The Association felt that the low salary scale for state veterinary officers was discouraging recruitment. The numerical strength of the service had fallen to a danger level, increasing vulnerability of the country to diseases such as foot-and-mouth disease and an increased risk of more widespread epidemics following modern means of transport, of animals and animal products. Recruitment to the public sector was not helped by the growing opportunities and wages in private practice, which reflected the resurgence of the agricultural industry.

However, the minister maintained that the salary of the chief veterinary officer must remain at the ceiling of £2,000 a year as opposed to the £3,000 recommended by the Association. NVMA council was told that meetings with the minister and his representatives had been fruitless and further representations in writing, backed by the National Farmers Union and the Parliamentary and Scientific Committee, had invoked the response from the minister that '£2,000 a year was the most that can be justified'.

The NVMA argued that 'the difference of £1,000 a year between the salary of the chief veterinary officer, Ministry of Agriculture, and that of the chief medical officer ... has a most injurious effect on the status not only of the government service but that of the profession as a whole'. Council resolved to refuse advertisements for the ministry's veterinary staff for insertion in the *Veterinary Record* at the existing scale of salaries. Veterinary surgeons wishing to apply for appointments advertised elsewhere would be

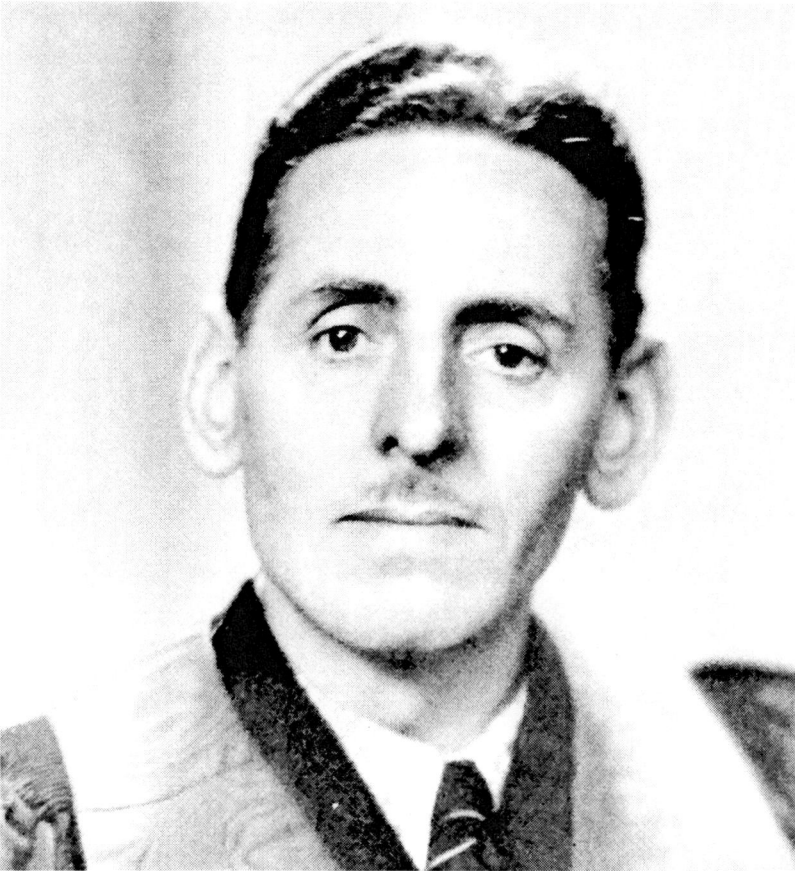

Figure 12. George Gould, scion of a Victorian veterinary family and pioneer of herd health schemes, who clashed with government over State vets' remuneration.

asked to contact the Association's general secretary before applying for any post.[9]

Later that year, 1946, Tom Williams, the Minister of Agriculture, was scheduled to propose the health of the Association at the annual congress banquet. At a very late stage – a matter of hours – the minister said he could not do so because of the continuing differences over salaries for veterinarians employed by the state service.[10] This left the president, George Gould, in a very difficult situation but fortunately he was able to persuade his friend Sir John Boyd Orr to step into the breach at the very last moment.

Gould read out the letter he had received from the minister:

Dear Mr Gould

Sir Donald Vandepeer [Parliamentary Private Secretary, with whom the NVMA had had dealings when the State Veterinary Service was being set up in 1937] has reported to me the result of the discussions between representatives of the Ministry and of your Association on the policy of 'active non-cooperation' recently adopted by the NVMA to express their dissatisfaction with the revised salary scales which have been fixed for the National veterinary service. I have also seen the terms of the resolution passed at the special meeting of the Council of the Association held yesterday morning to consider the serious situation which had arisen as a result of last Friday's talks in which the council reaffirmed their decision to refuse to allow advertisements for vacancies in that service to appear in the *Veterinary Record* and to advise members of the Association not to apply for such vacancies.

I am myself quite satisfied that the salary scales as now revised are appropriate and adequate. Your Association clearly does not share that view. We are both entitled to our opinions, and if that were the only issue we could agree to differ on that subject and continue to cooperate on the other; but the deliberate policy adopted by the Association to further its aims makes – as it is expressly intended to make – cooperation between the Ministry and the Association impossible.

In these circumstances I have decided, with very great regret, that for me to attend your Association's dinner on Thursday evening and propose a toast to the Association would imply that continuance of the relationship which unfortunately has been terminated by the action of your Association. I am sorry to have to reach this decision at this late hour but I am afraid it has become inevitable.

Yours sincerely,

T. Williams[11]

Gould told the gathering that the discussions with the minister had been going on since 1937 when a salary scale for state veterinary officers was imposed to which the Association could not agree. Negotiations had been proceeding, albeit slowly, until recently when the situation arose which made it necessary for the Association to protest strongly at the imposition of a status that would not allow the development of the animal health services in a way which the nation urgently required. The Association thus found itself faced with an ultimatum to accept an unsatisfactory salary scale, to withdraw the ban on advertisements and to refrain from giving advice to members of the National Veterinary Medical Association about the conditions of service within the ministry's animal health division. He continued: 'This ultimatum was one that a democratic association such as ours, representing about 90 per cent of the active members in this country, could not accept – and this is what is described as "active non-cooperation" in the letter.'

Nevertheless, continued the president, the position the two sides were in was not unusual in the course of a dispute; and with goodwill on both sides – 'and I think that goodwill still exists' – the solution should not be difficult to reach. He concluded: 'I am still hopeful, and failure will not be for want of effort on my part or on the part of the council of the NVMA.'[12]

That 'solution', however, proved harder to achieve than Gould's optimistic hopes imagined.

In June, 1947, the *Record* returned to the subject of Ministry of Agriculture pay for its veterinary personnel in a leader headed 'A lamentable impasse'. It refers to the salary scale imposed by the ministry the previous year as one that 'simply perpetuates a running sore'. The disparity between the pay of medical and veterinary officers (which had existed since before the 1914 war) still rankled. The pay and prospects for a young vet joining the service at age twenty-five at the initial basic salary of £420 year plus bonus and increments might appear superficially attractive. But that veterinary officer would be forty-two years old by the time he was on the maximum scale for the veterinary investigation officer, £840 a year. Most of his bonus payments would have been swallowed up by the cost of having to remain completely mobile and by inadequate allowances for car mileage and subsistence. If he 'plods his weary way to higher salary grades' he could have a salary of £1,050 after twenty-five years' service and by the time he was fifty-four he would have attained the 'munificent' figure of £1,300 a year. If there was any prospect of stepping into the shoes of the deputy CVO (£1,700) and later CVO (£2,000) the attainment of the maximum salary grade would virtually coincide with the eve of his retirement on superannuation.

By comparison, it was pointed out, a young assistant in a practice could expect a starting wage of £500 a year, often with a house and car provided; and according to advertisements in the *Record,* there were three times as many situations vacant as there were applicants for a post.

Those figures, said the *Record,* explained the discontent rife among the staff of the ministry's animal health service and why the NVMA was bound to warn its members that the rewards of the civil service career could have no attraction for the 'zealous young veterinarian who is sincerely desirous of playing a worthy part in the great battle for animal welfare'. The article concluded: 'It would be lamentable if nothing could be done to remove the impasse until the ministry is convinced that inadequate salaries explain the dearth of applicants for ministry appointments.'[13]

The urgency of the ministry's veterinary staff situation may be gauged by the fact that of a total complement of some 450 full-time professional personnel, 140 vacancies were being advertised, although about half were filled by temporary appointments.[14]

Nevertheless, perhaps in an attempt to prove that the ministry's salary scales would not attract applicants, the *Record* agreed the following month to publish an advertisement from the ministry seeking to recruit staff. The same issue also carried a double page feature carrying messages from divisions supporting the Association's stance on the matter and a prominent statement from the NVMA once again setting out the Association's position, stating that the council of the NVMA expected the full support of all members of the profession, at home and overseas, 'in this fight for the profession's status. They rely upon members not to apply for posts within the animal health division until a scale of salaries satisfactory to the Association has been formulated and agreed.'[15]

Further exchanges of letters followed. The president, by then L. Guy Anderson, assured the minister that 'we all share your desire that nothing should be done to aggravate a difficult situation'; but he denied the minister's allegation that the Association had misrepresented the facts in material respects.

The ministry provided a lengthy explanation of civil service staff structure and salaries and concluded that 'the salaries of the veterinary staff were fixed after a careful review of the salary scales for comparable civil servants. . . . The comparisons illustrate that the salaries of the veterinary inspectorate are not out of line with other civil service salaries.'

The Association responded with its own interpretation of the salary situation, also denying any suggestion that the Association had ever adopted a policy of non-cooperation with the ministry. It reserved its 'democratic right to freedom of expression of its views and its right to *advise* [NVMA italics] its members according to its interpretation of the known facts'.

That particular exchange was concluded by Anderson's offer to refrain from any public comment on the dispute if the minister would be prepared to consider 'our present differences'. He felt that this did in effect produce the conditions required by the minister for reopening negotiations. Anderson repeated his request that Williams should receive a delegation from the Association to reopen discussions.

Eventually, the ministry did receive a deputation, on 17 March 1948. At that meeting the Association representatives pressed their case 'most forcefully'. The result was a negative one, perhaps not unexpectedly given the dire state of the UK economy at the time. The pound had been devalued and the war-damaged economy was suffering badly.[16] The response from the permanent secretary, Sir Donald Vandepeer, that 'without entering further into the merits of the case, on which our respective views are I think well known on both sides, I must, I am afraid, tell you that the circumstances described in the White Paper on personal income [which imposed a virtual standstill on salaries in the public sector] completely preclude any revisions of the present time of the scales fixed at the end of 1946 and now in operation'. Vandepeer threw out a crumb of comfort. He ended his letter by assuring the NVMA that the ministry was well aware of the Association's position and realised that 'you will feel bound to renew your claims when times are more propitious'.

The reply to a question in Parliament on 21 June drew a line under the matter as far as the ministry was concerned. Asked whether the Minister of Agriculture was aware that the dispute about the unsatisfactory scale of salaries for the veterinary staff of his ministry was still unsettled, the minister, Tom Williams, replied 'I do not agree that the scale is unsatisfactory. Taken as a whole it is at least as favourable as the scale of the scientific officer class.' He reiterated that the White Paper on personal incomes precluded any revision at present.[17]

The Association made one final attempt to obtain some amelioration of the salary position of state veterinary officers. It asked if it would be possible to amend the way in which existing staff had been assimilated into the salary scale – this being one of the greatest reasons for dissatisfaction within the service. The answer was that the ministry 'could not hold out any hope of any further concession in this matter'.

Conceding defeat, council on 2 July decided that 'having considered the facts appertaining to the dispute with the Ministry of Agriculture on the status and salary of its veterinary officers, is reluctantly compelled to accept the fact that no further action can usefully be taken in this matter at the present time'. However, the Association's 'deep dissatisfaction with the existing scale and its determination to see the state veterinary service given the status and salary which the interest of agriculture and the profession demanded' were reaffirmed.

No further action would be taken which would impede recruitment to the animal health division, it was decided.[18]

VETS AND THE ANIMAL CHARITIES

Despite the prominence and length of the discussions over state veterinary salaries, in the eyes of the general membership of the Association the dominating event at the time was the intention of the government to introduce a new Veterinary Surgeons Bill. The Bill was proposed at the instigation of the People's Dispensary for Sick Animals (PDSA) to regularise the position of unqualified practitioners who were engaged in the treatment of animals. The PDSA was the main charity offering free treatment for the pets of the poor. There were some 500 men, many of them employed by the PDSA, who would have to be accommodated, one way or another, within the provisions of the Bill.

The provision of charitable, or *pro bono,* veterinary treatment for the animals of the deserving poor had long been accepted informally by veterinarians. The subject had grown in significance with the increasing importance of small animals and of the charitable organisations offering free treatment for them. Over the years, the NVMA had had occasional discussions with the RSPCA on arrangements for the treatment of the animals of those who could not afford to pay – and also of strays. On the whole, it had tended to leave to their own discretion the involvement of practitioners with such organisations. And as the animals concerned were mainly dogs and cats, species with which many vets had been little involved, the matter had not been of major importance to its members. By the mid to late 1940s, however, the importance of small animal practice to the typical vet was growing rapidly and the number of animal charities was increasing. So were the services they were offering free or at nominal charge.

The Royal Society for the Prevention of Cruelty to Animals (RSPCA), founded in 1824, operated a system of local branches, some of which ran clinics. No doubt prompted by the initiative of the PDSA described below, it began in 1926 a scheme by which its clinics issued vouchers to those applying to have their animals treated; the voucher entitled the person concerned to have free treatment from a veterinarian who agreed to participate in the scheme. The vet worked in an honorary (but not necessarily unpaid) capacity and the RSPCA met the cost of the medicines, dressings, etc.[19]

The PDSA was a different proposition. Formed in 1917 by Maria Dickin, it had become under her formidable leadership a major international organisation and 'a large thorn in the side of the private veterinary profession'.[20] It did not employ veterinarians; it operated its own clinics, many of them in mobile caravans, staffed by technicians who although not qualified as veterinarians, were not untrained. The PDSA enjoyed royal patronage, advertised widely and received substantial funds.

This funding enabled it to build in 1926 a very sophisticated facility on a thirty acre site at Ilford, London. The Sanatorium, as it was called, offered the latest equipment, including X-ray equipment, operating theatres, stabling, kennels, lecture rooms and outpatient facilities. The Sanatorium also ran a training school, in charge of a veterinarian, for its technical staff, with a three- to five-year course; a pharmacist supervised medical supplies. 'The Sanatorium was looking very much like a rival veterinary college, issuing its own internally-generated licence to practise.'[21] The opening of this impressive undertaking received widespread publicity and proved very popular.

The RCVS saw this development as a threat; any certificate issued to its technicians by the PDSA, and carrying the stamp of royal patronage, was seen as a 'bogus qualification' frustrating the provisions of the Veterinary Surgeons Act 1881. The College launched its own press campaign, writing to newspapers and journals complaining of the PDSA using such terms as 'fully qualified' in relation to veterinary work when applied to unqualified people. The NVMA was equally concerned about competition from the charity's free services and issued 'counter advertisements' highlighting the services that were available only from a registered veterinary surgeon.

The Association was not, and had never been, opposed in general to charitable treatment of their animals on behalf of the indigent owner. Following the modest provision made in 1931, it agreed to the suggestion by Sir John McFadyean, RCVS president, that NVMA divisions should hold meetings to see how veterinary surgeons might best involve themselves in treating the animals of the poor by cooperating with the existing RSPCA/Association's scheme. Because of a Royal College ban on publicising veterinary surgeons' services, that scheme was not well known.

At a joint meeting between the two bodies in 1933, the NVMA president, P. J. Simpson, promoted the scheme.[22] As well as centralised clinics attended by a veterinary surgeon, in other areas voucher treatment could be given by private veterinary surgeons. An effort to improve publicity for veterinary practices was made by issuing press advertisements indicating that veterinary surgeons could always be identified by the letters MRCVS or FRCVS after their names. The joint scheme progressed; by 1937 the RSPCA was able to report that from a few thousand at its outset, it had treated 238,320 in that year.[23]

Meanwhile, the RCVS had been holding discussions with the PDSA in the late 1930s and had come close to an agreement about regularising the status of PDSA-trained technicians engaged in veterinary services and coming to some accommodation about the future status of the veterinary personnel it employed. Those discussions ceased on the outbreak of war.[24]

There matters stood, with the PDSA, the RSPCA and the profession maintaining their respective stances, until it became apparent that a Bill to replace the outdated provisions of the 1881 Veterinary Surgeons Act was in the offing. This new Act was being promoted on behalf of the PDSA to regulate their unqualified technicians as 'veterinary practitioners' and consolidate the position of that body as a provider of veterinary services. This prompted the

Association to reconsider its own situation in relation to the animal charities.

In December 1947, a special meeting of NVMA council was called to discuss 'unqualified practitioners and veterinary attendance of sick animals of the poor'. A report on the subject had been prepared for council with the aim of ascertaining 'the extent and nature of unqualified practice in the UK and the number types and locations of clinics run for the treatment of sick animals of the poor'.

It was accepted that the profession was not 'at present' able to organise and provide such services itself; there was a continuing shortage of veterinarians, a fact that strengthened the arm of the animal charities. It was therefore felt desirable to collaborate with 'such animal welfare societies as will adopt an ethical policy acceptable to us in every way'. Council felt it was regrettable that an 'atmosphere of suspicion and distrust' existed in some quarters regarding the activities of the charities. The Association had to recognise that, in the main, animal welfare societies were doing work which the profession had to support. If close liaison existed between the societies and the Association at all levels, much good could accrue to all parties concerned, especially to the sick animals of the poor, it was argued. The Association recommended very strongly that the veterinary profession should reconsider its attitude to the animal welfare societies. The president (Guy Anderson) commented 'the only way to control societies who employed unqualified practitioners was to control unqualified practitioners'. Although not welcomed by veterinarians, that control would, in due course, be achieved by the establishment of the proposed Supplementary Veterinary Register.

The following conclusions were arrived at with regard to future relations between the major welfare societies and the profession:

Peoples Dispensary for Sick Animals As the PDSA did not accept the principle that clinical work should be done by vets, close collaboration was unlikely to be achieved at present. The PDSA employed 'a very small number of vets' with about 230 'technical officers' who had received at least four and a half years' training.

Royal Society for the Prevention of Cruelty to Animals This society had shown greater willingness to work with the profession and a large number of veterinary surgeons acted as officers. Differences have occasionally risen but existing machinery proved adequate to resolve them.

National Canine Defence League The NCDL employed 'two or three' vets and a number of lay practitioners. It had not been possible for the Association to achieve agreement with the NCDL on free treatments. [The NCDL became the Dogs Trust in 2003]

Our Dumb Friends League Veterinary surgeons were employed in its clinics.

It was believed that the two latter societies might be persuaded to work in closer cooperation with the profession if definite proposals were put on this.[25]

A year later, a special meeting of council was convened to consider the opinions of the divisions on the 'the future of small animal practice in relation to the agreement between the RSPCA and the NVMA'. After a long discussion, mainly about fees to be paid by patients and those to be paid to vets working in the charities' clinics, no concrete decisions were made. Council merely noted the opinions of the divisions.[26]

The matter of admitting unqualified individuals to the Supplementary Veterinary Register, via Section 7 of the Act, was still causing problems. There was a backlog of PDSA trainees whose licenses had not been issued; there were others scheduled to complete their training, and who the PDSA had expected to be licensed, whose status remained uncertain. The charity felt that MAF, encouraged by the RCVS, was dragging its feet.

In an attempt to sort things out, the Minister of Agriculture appointed in 1950 a committee 'to examine and advise upon the problems raised by applications for licences under Section 7 of the Veterinary Surgeons Act 1948 with particular reference to intentions that have been expressed for the immediate future'.[27] The Champion committee (named after its chairman, A. J. Champion) whose five members did not contain any veterinarians, recommended that the PDSA should liaise with the BVA (the NVMA changed its name in 1952 – see panel) on conditions of service for its veterinary- qualified employees; that part-time as well as full-time veterinary surgeons could be employed by PDSA, and that no more licences would be granted after the end of 1953 unless the minister was satisfied that neither part-time nor full-time vets could be recruited. And the PDSA should put in place a stricter system for examining the status of those seeking charitable services (almoning) for their pets' treatment.

The report was accepted, and the outstanding applications for admission to the Supplementary Veterinary Register were granted.

An important inclusion in the Champion report was its reference to the potential for delegation of 'activities which were not necessarily carried out by qualified veterinary surgeons, such as wound dressing, general nursing, castration of young animals, first aid and painless destruction'. This was another step towards recognition for the role (and eventual professional status) of veterinary nursing.[28] The Association, too, was beginning to accept that nurses should have some recognition of their role in veterinary care. Referring to proposals made in 1955 by the RCVS, BVA president Professor Alexander Robertson said the Association had been approached by the College for 'cooperation and advice' in relation to a scheme for the recruitment and training of animal nurses. It was felt that the 'creation of a body of properly trained and certificated lay people, controlled by a code of ethics, could prove a useful adjunct to the profession'.[29] Twenty years earlier, in 1936, the Association had disagreed with the College's opinion that 'it is desirable that canine nurses should be registered after having undergone a proper course of training and a proper examination'. It felt 'the time is not opportune' for action.[30]

FROM NVMA TO BVA

It was as long ago as 1932 that the then president, P. J. Simpson, had called an extraordinary general meeting of the Association to discuss certain proposed changes to the Articles of Association. Only one of the proposed changes gave rise to discussion: that was the president's own resolution 'That the name of the Association be altered from "The National Veterinary Medical Association of Great Britain and Ireland" to "The British Veterinary Association" '. There were immediate objections by and on behalf of Irish members. The Irish Free State had just been established, and the new state was in political turmoil. P J Howard, from County Clare, proposed an amendment that the matter be deferred for twelve months 'until a more opportune moment'. His amendment was carried.[31]

The matter resurfaced regularly over the years until the AGM in 1947 resolved 'That the name of the Association be changed to the British Veterinary Association with effect from January 1, 1952. Presumably, the opponents of the change thought that something that had been put off for five years might not happen.

When the postponed resolution came up at the 1951 annual meeting there were objections, as had happened at every previous occasion that it had been discussed. On this occasion the council of the Veterinary Medical Association of Ireland had asked the Association not to implement the change and instead suggested the title 'British and Irish Veterinary Association'. However, the NVMA council pointed out that there was no reason why, if the resolution was implemented, the Irish Association should not be associated with the BVA if it so desired. The Irish association had replied stating that while no difficulty was visualised for individual members, it was the position of the Irish association itself which would be difficult. After discussion, during which comments were made that all the arguments about the Irish members had been made before, 'the only thing to do now was to make the decision'.

The resolution to change the name to British Veterinary Association on 2 January 1952 was carried, with two voting against.[32]

There was still unhappiness of the part of practitioners about competition from the charities' clinics. They objected to the 'constraints on publicity suffered by the professional'; clinics scored over 'freedom of advertising, as well as freedom to use drugs without the meticulous regard to cost'; not only that, but the clinics could often offer a better service, wrote one typically disgruntled vet. He considered the present unsatisfactory position had been reached by a lack of public relations.[33] The Royal College was called upon to allow a 'decorous increase' in the signs they were allowed to exhibit.[34] The growing amount of work that was being generated by small animal work was noted; one vet thought there was a danger that the welfare societies might completely take over the treatment of small animals.[35]

Former BVA president, L. Guy Anderson, tried to argue the case for the private practitioner. He said the charitable clinics could not offer a seven day a week, twenty-four hours a day service; that few had facilities for major surgical work or hospitalisation. 'Was a crowded waiting room a suitable place for an animal with an infectious of contagious disease?' he asked. The clinics, he said, were left with minor cases. Were the clinics run 'for the relief of suffering or for propaganda for the societies that run them'?[36] The practitioners' concern about the activities of the clinics continued: in 1955, Professor Robertson, expressed concern about the 'encroachment' of the animal charities on to private practice.[37]

UNREGISTERED PRACTICE AND THE 1948 ACT

Progress on the Veterinary Surgeons Bill had continued while the vets argued back and forth about the activities of the charities' clinics. The government's preferred choice of title for unqualified individuals who would be entitled to registration by the College was 'veterinary practitioner'. That suggestion drew howls of protest, led by members of the Society of Veterinary Practitioners whose membership was, of course, restricted to properly qualified and registered veterinary surgeons. But resentment was widespread among the profession. Both the Royal College and the Association made formal protests.

The Association wrote to all MPs stating its strong objection to the title 'veterinary practitioner' being conferred on unqualified practitioners included in the proposed Supplementary Veterinary Register. The president, L. Guy Anderson, said the title veterinary practitioner was protected (which was not, in fact, the case) and to the general public would always denote a person qualified by education and examination to practise the art and science of veterinary medicine and surgery. It was important to them and the public, he said, that the brass plate of a man [no mention, even at that date, of women] qualified by five years' scientific training should not be confused with that of a man who lacked this scientific grounding.[38]

This supported a similar message from the Royal College, which had written on 3 June 1948 – the day before the second reading of the Bill – stating that, while the RCVS had by a majority vote agreed to withdraw its opposition to the title 'veterinary practitioner', it had done so reluctantly and only because the College had been informed that such opposition would seriously hamper the passage of the Bill through Parliament. In spite of the fact that it had formally withdrawn its opposition, the RCVS, and the NVMA reiterated their unanimous objection to the title on the grounds that the terms 'veterinary surgeon' and 'veterinary practitioner' were synonymous.[39]

The *Record* noted that, while 'at no time had the Royal College agreed to sacrifice the title', it had to be appreciated that the Bill was a government measure which was supported in both Houses of Parliament. It had been made quite clear that in spite of the objections inherent in the question of title, the College had been unable to secure any concession on that point.

The agitation over the matter was even greater than it had been over the perceived loss of the 'single portal' entry to the profession. Letters to the *Veterinary Record* illustrated concerns felt by some members. 'I am deeply concerned at the prospect of having a motley collection of quacks foisted upon us under the title veterinary practitioner. ... It is obvious that the government is purely concerned with the welfare of the quacks,' wrote J. F. Kinghorn.[40] 'The Bill is an insult to the profession and public alike. Our leaders have meekly bowed down and cowered before dictatorship. Had this Bill been presented to the profession first it would have been hurled into the refuse bin where it belongs,' was the opinion of R. F. Townson.[41] 'To those of us who are proud to call ourselves professional men this is indeed a bitter pill – to become associated directly or indirectly with a body of quacks,' said W. Scott.[42]

There were more reasoned voices. T. A. R. Chipperfield pointed out that once a government department had made up its mind to introduce legislation, sectional interests such as those of the veterinary profession were of no moment.[43] G. N. Gould, a past president of the Association and a member of the Royal College council who had reluctantly voted in favour of accepting the disputed title, commented that 'the lack of serious criticism by the profession of the bulk of the provisions within the Bill may be taken to indicate the success achieved by the College council in their negotiation. Even those sixteen, among whom I am numbered, who voted for the reluctant withdrawal of the opposition to the title, did so after making it quite clear that it was just as objectionable to them as to those who voted against. But careful consideration had led them to believe that that action was justified in the best and proper interests of education and practice.'[44]

Another member, relating a similar situation that had occurred in New Zealand, recounted that when the Veterinary Surgeons Act had been passed in that country in 1926, the very same question, the title of the practitioner, had been a serious bone of contention. Since then the greater number of 'those practical men' had retired or died. 'It will not be long before the term "veterinary practitioner" will be extinct.'[45] Some thirty other individuals voiced their opinions one way or the other in the correspondence pages of the journal.

Meanwhile, the Bill continued its progress through parliament. The professional objection to the term 'veterinary practitioner' was not without its supporters in the Commons.

Moving the second reading of the Bill, the minister (Tom Williams) reminded the House of Commons that the main object was to provide the means of filling the urgent need for more veterinary surgeons. Its provisions also meant that, following the recommendations of the Loveday report, veterinary studies would be given university status and the appropriate degree would entitle graduates to qualify for registration as a veterinary surgeon and to have their name printed in the register of veterinary surgeons maintained by the Royal College. For its part, the College would have oversight of the quality and standard of the courses and examinations held at the universities for registerable degrees.

The one point where some difference of opinion still existed, continued the minister, was in regard to the title 'veterinary practitioner'. That title had hitherto been reserved for those who are qualified as a veterinary surgeon by examination. He noted that alternatives such as 'registered animal practitioner' and other titles had been suggested (the Chancellor committee, set up to consider the question of unqualified veterinary practice, had recommended the term 'animal practitioner' for such practitioners).[46] However, after a very long discussion the government had been driven to the conclusion that the right thing to do was to allow those given a licence to practice under Section 7 of the Bill and registered by the College (in the supplementary register) to use the title 'veterinary practitioner' leaving the title veterinary surgeon to those who qualified by examination.

In discussion, the MP for Ripon argued that the Royal College had made it abundantly clear that, although they had reluctantly voted in favour of accepting the compromise, they were unanimously against the use of the words veterinary practitioner for unqualified men as they were 'thoroughly misleading to the public'. He also pointed out that the Chancellor report had recommended that unqualified men 'should not be permitted to use the description veterinary practitioner or any name reasonably calculated to suggest that he was a member of Royal College of Veterinary Surgeons. It was also a fact that there was a body of veterinary surgeons called the Society of Veterinary Practitioners and many veterinary surgeons had the inscription on the brass plate of their surgeries – "Mr So-and-So, veterinary practitioner" ' This argument was supported by other speakers.

The debate was replied to by the Parliamentary Undersecretary for Agriculture, George Brown. He noted that the only academically unqualified people with limited qualifications placed on the supplementary register would be those who were at least twenty-eight years of age, were of good repute and had made their living as a practising veterinarian for at least seven of the previous ten years.

Further, the size of the problem was not as great as some members seemed to think; it was not likely to be much more than 500 compared with 4,000 qualified people on the main register. There was another point: they would all be brought under professional discipline. And if they subjected the unqualified to the obligation to accept professional discipline, then they had to give them professional status. He noted that not so long ago men 'with a little knowledge' (and no formal qualification) had been permitted to call themselves veterinary surgeons. The government had considered very carefully what term to use. He thought the term in the Bill, veterinary practitioner, was 'a sufficiently good one'.[47]

During the committee stage of the Bill on 24 June, the minister, returning to the subject of the title of 'veterinary practitioner' said that over the past seventy years Parliament had passed a number of Acts [affecting professions] which established a clear pattern for the treatment of existing unqualified practitioners. The pattern had always been that statutory protection was given to the profession and titles always provided for the unqualified practitioners. The existing unqualified persons had been admitted to a register and had been given a professional title. That had made them subject to control.[48]

The Bill was read for a third time and passed on 8 July 1948. The Under Secretary, George Brown, said 'for good or ill they had embarked on a course which everybody agreed would ultimately be in the interests of the profession. How much, it would be dependent on them and the outside world.'[49]

The Association reluctantly accepted the fact that the Supplementary Veterinary Register would be a reality and that all persons claiming to have been earning their living from veterinary practice for at least seven out of the previous ten years could apply to be included on it. It advised its members to accept the inevitable with good grace. 'No persons can be more fully aware whether an unqualified practitioner meets those requirements than the veterinary surgeons practising in his area,' it noted. 'It is therefore incumbent on every member of the profession to lay before the RCVS council any evidence or information which will enable the council to reach a just decision on the merits of each application'.

That applied not only to unfavourable evidence, but also to evidence which was favourable to an applicant. 'There are unqualified practitioners well-known to veterinary surgeons who by a length of practice of the nature of their work are fully entitled to registration in the Supplementary Veterinary Register. . . . So long as the Supplement Veterinary Register endures it will be necessary for all the members of the profession to treat with courtesy and dignified cooperation persons entered on the register.'[50]

And no doubt to signify that that particular battle between the Minister of Agriculture and the veterinary profession was over, the president of the RCVS, H. W. Dawes, gave a small and informal luncheon party for the minister, Tom Williams. 'There were no formal speeches but the minister replied to his address of welcome briefly but in a happily phrased speech. The cordial atmosphere of the small gathering was felt by the veterinary representatives and was endorsed by the minister's good wishes for the future of the veterinary profession,' it was recorded.[51]

For its part, the Association praised the 'enormous amount of well-balanced charitable work carried out by societies like the RSPCA in conjunction with the profession'. The experience thus gained had to be applied to the solution of present problems, it maintained. 'If we go forward willingly in cooperation with the societies we should settle this, the last of our serious outstanding problems, and bring unqualified practice . . . to an end for all time.'[52]

However, relations with the PDSA continued to be unsatisfactory. Eventually, following a series of private meetings in 1955 between the PDSA and BVA officer H. F. Hebeler, formal meetings under the chairmanship of George Brown, Parliamentary Secretary, Ministry of Agriculture, at the House of Commons between the PDSA, the BVA and the RCVS were held. These established the basis for a proper working relationship with the charity in regard to the employment of veterinary surgeons at its clinics and which led to the gradual ending of the services of unqualified veterinary practitioners.[53]

Some individuals, however, carried on the fight after the war was lost. Harry Steele-Bodger – that stalwart of the Society of Veterinary Practitioners, which would have to change its name as a result of the Act – resigned from the RCVS council, mainly over the way the council had handled negotiations over the Veterinary Surgeons Act 1948 in respect of the title of veterinary practitioner.[54] In the event, Steele-Bodger was not long away from RCVS council; he offered himself for re-election in that year's council election and regained his seat[55] (in the 1970s, when the present author was editor of the *Record*, one had to be careful not to refer to a 'proper' veterinary surgeon as a 'veterinary practitioner').

Steele-Bodger's publicised resignation was to be almost the last political gesture by one of the Association's, and the profession's, great men. He died in January 1952.[56] The travelling scholarship for young veterinary surgeons established in his name serves as a lasting memorial; and he was made, posthumously, an honorary member of the Association.

Legislation affecting the professions does tend to be subject to modification over time, however. And the battle lines were reopened in 1965 when a new Veterinary Surgeons Bill was promoted to open once more the Supplementary Veterinary Register. This time, the legislation had rather crept upon the profession unawares. In June 1962 the Association had noted that the Royal College intended to suggest to MAFF that Section 7 of the Act (that governing the Supplementary Veterinary Register) should be rescinded. The idea was to tidy up the situation whereby some 500 existing unregistered practitioners (many of whom had been in practice overseas) were still working as vets. They would be admitted to the SVR and subjected to the appropriate discipline. The BVA had supported the move. Little comment was aroused at the time; but it was not realised that MAF would draw up an entirely new Veterinary Surgeons Act.

There were indignant complaints from the membership at the reopening of the SVR, in the form of letters to the journal, alleging that the membership had, in effect, been sold down the river. There had been no publicity about, or any mention of, the publication of this new Bill until it was printed on 2 December 1965.[57]

It was Harry Steele-Bodger's son, Alasdair, who now led the Association into the fray. He first took the blame for the lack of notice, saying it had arisen because of a misunderstanding of the advice that he had given the editor. He called a special meeting of council, at which the RCVS was represented, to discuss the matter and clear the air. Before that, however, the BVA was able to have discussions with MAFF at which it raised matters in the new Bill with which it disagreed. First among those concerned the reopening of the SVR which, said the Association, had been considered closed in consequence of the 1948 Act: Why should it be reopened to admit more names? MAFF had explained that no new licences for existing practitioners had been issued since 1952 although technically that could have

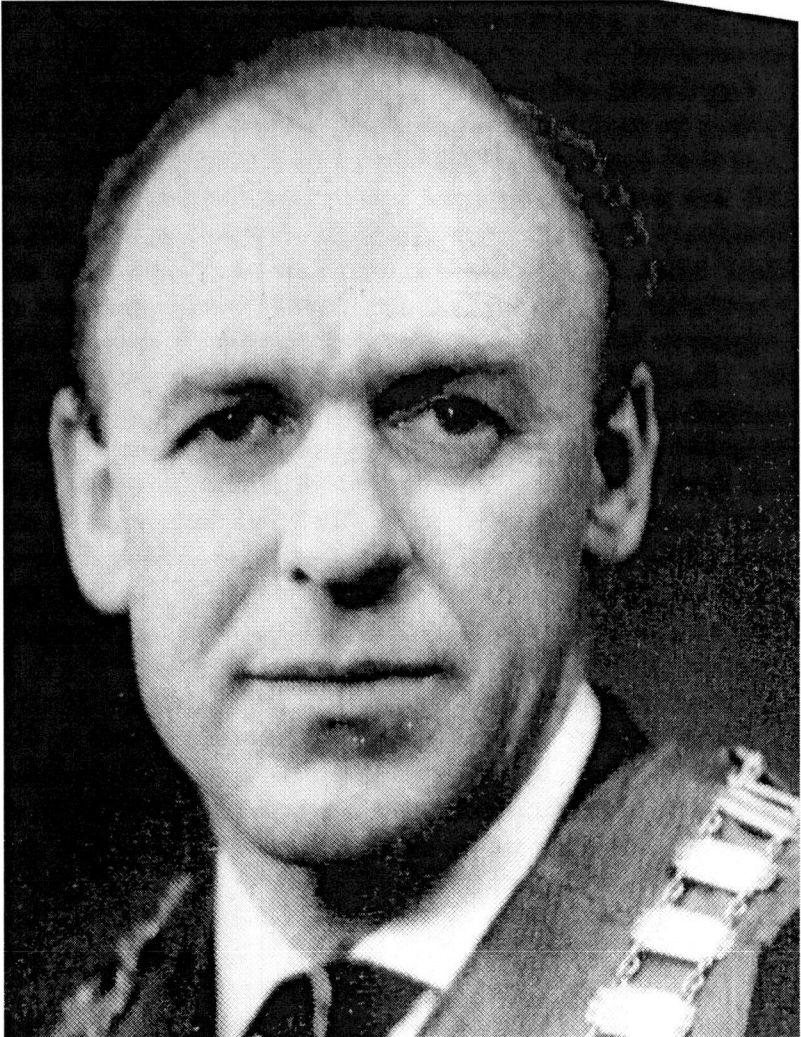

Figure 13. Alasdair Steele-Bodger, son of Harry and cast in a similar mould, followed in the president's chair in 1966.

been done. If the relatively few current licensees became registered in the SVR they would immediately come under the discipline of the Royal College, which was not the case at the time.

The *Record* [58] carried a verbatim report of the council discussion of the Bill. In spite of the vociferous opposition, council, having looked into all the circumstances in the light of full discussion and some clarification given by the government, recommended its acceptance. It was bowing to the inevitable. And the fact remained that 'by and large, the right to practise veterinary surgery is already more protected than is the right to practise human medicine'.[59]

In a final word on the events which had caused such ructions within the Association during the year, the secretary, John Anderson, said that, as the Bill was a government one, its contents could not be known in advance of publication either by the Royal College or by the BVA. He said that a combined exercise by the officers and others in the Association had had 'such remarkable success' that the authorities had been persuaded to accept the majority of the BVA's recommendations in the face of what must have been considerable opposition. He invited the 'vociferous minority' to contrast the original Bill with the Act as passed.[60]

And as time went on, the decline in numbers of those unqualified veterinary practitioners placed on the Supplementary Veterinary Register working in the various charities' clinics dwindled, to be replaced by veterinary surgeons. The last few additions to the SVR were made under the Veterinary Surgeons Act 1966; by 2009 the supplementary register contained only nine names. The principle of professional veterinary treatment solely by veterinary surgeons had been finally established.

CHAPTER EIGHT

A HOME OF THEIR OWN

When it was founded, the organisation that grew into the British Veterinary Association was tiny and without resources. Its first accommodation was in shared premises with the Royal College of Veterinary Surgeons in Red Lion Square, London WC1. It was to be forty years before premises of its own were acquired: two rooms in Buckingham Palace Road. Then in 1925 slightly larger accommodation was rented, at 10 Grays Inn Square, followed by a move to Verulam Buildings, also in Gray's Inn Square, in 1931.

The growth in membership and consequent administrative and editorial work and of course, staff, soon made it essential that suitable premises should be found in which council meetings could be accommodated as well as staff. The search for suitable accommodation for the Association was delayed by considerations of the possibility of finding shared accommodation with the Royal College. The apparent advantages of one central building for the whole profession with shared facilities and costs seem obvious and that possibility has regularly been reconsidered. However, supposed savings in costs were largely illusory and both parties concluded the advantages were far outweighed by disadvantages.

So it was that in 1937 the Association acquired premises of its own at 36 Gordon Square WC1. The property was an attractive Georgian house in a convenient location; in fact, only a few yards from the headquarters of the British Medical Association in Tavistock Square. The twenty-year lease cost £2,500 and the rent was £275 a year. The NVMA had six full-time members of staff, including a caretaker who was paid 10 shillings a week in addition to his accommodation. The president of the day, Robert Simpson, said that the premises they acquired 'stood in a commanding situation . . . [and] the building as a whole was in keeping with the influence and prestige of the Association'. The house offered ample accommodation, with the Association occupying the basement, ground and first floors, leaving the two upper floors available for rental until such time as the Association expanded to occupy them.[1]

The Association had hardly settled into the new accommodation when it was forced to evacuate the building because of enemy action in 1940. The house had a narrow escape. Two incendiary bombs pierced the roof and fell into an office on the top floor. One failed to ignite but the other burned through the floor boards and was extinguished as it lay beside a live gas pipe.[2] Although the building was not badly damaged it was surrounded by devastation and unexploded bombs; it was some time before the area was made safe and the roof patched up to allow the house to be used again. In the interim, the editorial office moved to Welwyn Garden City, after finding temporary accommodation in the British Medical Association building across the road, and the administrative office moved to Lichfield to be housed at the premises of the president, Harry Steele-Bodger, until the house could be patched up.

After the war, the ground landlords (the University of London) gave notice that the lease would not be renewed when it expired in 1956 and in 1953 a search began for a new headquarters in central London. Suitable premises in the 'consultants' district' centred on Harley Street proved to be available. Located in Mansfield Street, No 7 was an Adam house which had been the residence of a doctor, now retired. A 999 year lease from the Howard de Walden estate would cost £15,000 and the ground rent £350; some repairs and renovation would be necessary – the house had suffered bomb damage – bringing the total expenditure to some £20,000. As by 1953 the Association had accumulated reserves of some £66,000, a subscription income from some 3,750 members, at £4 4s. each, plus the substantial financial input of the *Veterinary Record*, the undertaking does not seem excessive. Nevertheless, BVA legend has it that the treasurer, H. E. Bywater, did not sleep for three nights before the signing the lease, worrying about committing the Association to such a large expenditure. In the event, inscribing his signature on the lease document represented the most important act in Bywater's distinguished seventeen-year stint as treasurer. First elected in 1937, he did not relinquish the office until 1955. Few investments can have proved so valuable over the half-century since Mansfield Street was acquired as that 999-year lease. The two fine Perry chandeliers in the main first floor rooms are themselves now worth more than the original purchase price. In 1954 the Duke of Norfolk officially opened the house that is still home to the Association.[3]

Number 7 is reckoned to be the most typical Adam house in Mansfield Street; it is featured in a 1922 monograph by A. T. Bolton, curator of the Sir John Soane museum. Its first tenant was one Robert Burdett who took it in 1774 at a rent of £300 a year, a very considerable sum at that time. General Sir James Walker, a Peninsular War veteran, lived there in the 1830s and from the 1880s to 1932 a family called Waters (Mr Waters being 'a translator and wood carver') occupied the house. When Dr Geoffrey Evans bought it in 1934, No 7 had been empty for a couple of years and was somewhat dilapidated. Evans made extensive alterations and improvements, including replacing four lost original Adam fireplaces through the good offices of Lord Howard de Walden, who gave four similar Adam fireplaces from houses being demolished in nearby Portland Place. It is a nice coincidence that the original fireplaces had been removed by the first tenant, General Walker, who happened to be the great-great-uncle of Dr Evans.

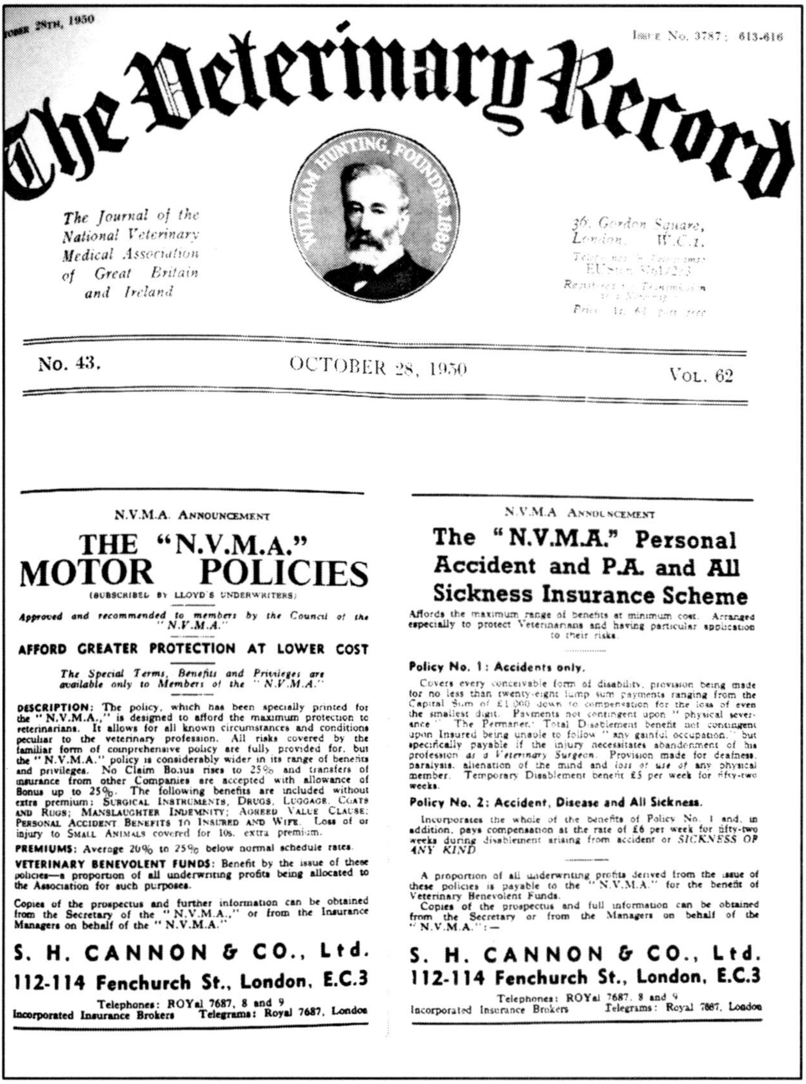

OBER 28TH, 1950

ISSUE No. 3787 : 613-616

The Veterinary Record

The Journal of the National Veterinary Medical Association of Great Britain and Ireland

36, Gordon Square, London, W.C.1.

No. 43. OCTOBER 28, 1950 VOL. 62

N.V.M.A. ANNOUNCEMENT

THE "N.V.M.A." MOTOR POLICIES

(SUBSCRIBED BY LLOYD'S UNDERWRITERS)

Approved and recommended to members by the Council of the "N.V.M.A."

AFFORD GREATER PROTECTION AT LOWER COST

The Special Terms, Benefits and Privileges are available only to Members of the "N.V.M.A."

DESCRIPTION: The policy, which has been specially printed for the "N.V.M.A.," is designed to afford the maximum protection to veterinarians. It allows for all known circumstances and conditions peculiar to the veterinary profession. All risks covered by the familiar form of comprehensive policy are fully provided for, but the "N.V.M.A." policy is considerably wider in its range of benefits and privileges. No Claim Bonus rises to 25% and transfers of insurance from other Companies are accepted with allowance of Bonus up to 25%. The following benefits are included without extra premium: SURGICAL INSTRUMENTS, DRUGS, LUGGAGE, COATS AND RUGS; MANSLAUGHTER INDEMNITY; AGREED VALUE CLAUSE; PERSONAL ACCIDENT BENEFITS TO INSURED AND WIFE. Loss of or injury to SMALL ANIMALS covered for 10s. extra premium.

PREMIUMS: Average 20% to 25% below normal schedule rates.

VETERINARY BENEVOLENT FUNDS: Benefit by the issue of these policies—a proportion of all underwriting profits being allocated to the Association for such purposes.

Copies of the prospectus and further information can be obtained from the Secretary of the "N.V.M.A.," or from the Insurance Managers on behalf of the "N.V.M.A."

S. H. CANNON & CO., Ltd.
112-114 Fenchurch St., London, E.C.3

Telephones: ROYal 7687, 8 and 9
Incorporated Insurance Brokers Telegrams: Royal 7687, London

N.V.M.A. ANNOUNCEMENT

The "N.V.M.A." Personal Accident and P.A. and All Sickness Insurance Scheme

Affords the maximum range of benefits at minimum cost. Arranged especially to protect Veterinarians and having particular application to their risks.

Policy No. 1: Accidents only.

Covers every conceivable form of disability, provision being made for no less than twenty-eight lump sum payments ranging from the Capital Sum of £1,000 down to compensation for the loss of even the smallest digit. Payments not contingent upon "physical severance." The Permanent Total Disablement benefit not contingent upon Insured being unable to follow "any gainful occupation," but specifically payable if the injury necessitates abandonment of his profession *as a Veterinary Surgeon*. Provision made for deafness, paralysis, alienation of the mind and *loss of use of* any physical member. Temporary Disablement benefit £5 per week for fifty-two weeks.

Policy No. 2: Accident, Disease and All Sickness.

Incorporates the whole of the benefits of Policy No. 1 and, in addition, pays compensation at the rate of £6 per week for fifty-two weeks during disablement arising from accident or *SICKNESS OF ANY KIND*.

A proportion of all underwriting profits derived from the issue of these policies is payable to the "N.V.M.A." for the benefit of Veterinary Benevolent Funds.

Copies of the prospectus and full information can be obtained from the Secretary or from the Managers on behalf of the "N.V.M.A.":—

S. H. CANNON & CO., Ltd.
112-114 Fenchurch St., London, E.C.3

Telephones: ROYal 7687, 8 and 9
Incorporated Insurance Brokers Telegrams: Royal 7687, London

Figure 14. A *Veterinary Record* cover from the 1950s, which carried the image of its founder, William Hunting, from the 1920s to the 1960s. The advertisements represent the Association's attempt to promote services for members.

Eventually, the BVA outgrew the existing accommodation and acquired further space in No 9 for the editorial and press relations offices and main boardroom. It was able to relinquish this additional space in 2009 when the *Veterinary Record* staff moved to BMA House and BMJ Publishing assumed the role of publisher (the BVA retains ownership of the journal).

Following that move, No 7 Mansfield Street was extensively restored and refurbished, making the accommodation more suitable for both the general and administrative functions of the headquarters of a major professional association. As well as elegant meeting rooms, offices with up-to-date equipment, and a small flat for the use of the president are provided.

BVA INITIATES NEW ANAESTHETICS ACT

A clinical matter that had caused some concern to the BVA was the existing restriction on the use of anaesthetic procedures to those listed in the 1919 Anaesthetics Act; this outdated measure excluded, for example, cats and dogs, the animals most frequently operated on, and pigs. The matter had first been broached some twenty years previously, when the rigid conditions laid down in that Act became outmoded by developments in anaesthetic and surgical techniques. The veterinary surgeon had been put in the position of not legally being able to do what he or she knew to be in the best interests of the patient. After years of fruitless attempts to get the government to amend the Act, the BVA took matters into its own hands and decided to promote its own Bill. Parliamentary counsel was engaged and a draft Bill prepared. Lord Stamp introduced the Bill in the House of Lords where discussion in that House indicated why the government had previously resisted changes to the 1919 Act. This led to some modification being made before the Association's Bill was put before the Commons.

Viscountess Davidson, who had won a ballot for private members' time, agreed to introduce and sponsor the Bill.

She did so 'with a skill and lucidity which secured its passage', commented the *Record*. Viscountess Davidson explained that the 1919 Act had made the use of anaesthetics compulsory for certain operations on animals, Since its introduction, however, many important advances in anaesthetics and new surgical techniques had taken place. Some operations for which general anaesthesia was compulsory under the 1919 Act could now be more humanely performed with nerve block or spinal anaesthesia. And while anaesthesia was compulsory for the removal of tumours in horses it was not in the case of dogs, the species in which it was most often performed.

In other words, the 1919 Act was too specific in its provisions; it gave a limited list of animal procedures in which anaesthesia should be used. The new Act took the opposite approach, making anaesthesia compulsory except when specifically excluded.

G. R. H. Nugent, parliamentary secretary, MAF, welcoming the Bill, paid tribute to the veterinary profession: 'It has developed during the last few decades into a profession of very high standing not only from the humanitarian but from the economic point of view. Their particular concern to extend the protection which this Bill gives to animals is only what we would expect.'

MP Fred Willey pointed out that it 'would make legal what was the general present practice of the veterinary profession. It was a real tribute [to the profession] that their own professional bodies had assisted in promoting the Bill.'[4] In fact, the BVA had done more than 'assist' the Bill; it had initiated, drafted and ensured its introduction to the Parliamentary process. When it passed back to the Lords, Lord Stamp's championship secured its safe passage by an almost unanimous vote.[5]

That Bill, which became the Protection of Animals (Anaesthetics) Act 1954, was a small but important measure. It was indicative of the Association's interest in the welfare of the veterinarian's patients. That would be a growing concern of the Association.

PRACTICE COMMUNICATIONS

During the 1950s, while farm practices tended to be busy, communication between the vet out on his rounds and the practice base was still haphazard. The conventional way for the practice to communicate with clients was to leave a list of the day's calls at the practice base. Any urgent messages would be telephoned to the farms on the list to be relayed to the vet when he visited. This did not always work; it was not unusual for a vet to return to base only to find there was an urgent call from a farm close to one he had just left. The introduction of the in-car radio telephone system (long before the mobile phone), which enabled the practice to contact the vet directly on his rounds, and vice versa, brought immense benefits in time saving.

In 1957, the BVA, through the *Veterinary Record*, asked a member who had experience in the system to advise others on its use. The member whose advice was sought was E. C. (Eddie) Straiton, a Staffordshire vet with an extensive practice. In an article in the *Record* Straiton extolled the radio telephone's virtues.[6] He wrote: 'During the last twelve months since it was installed in the five practice cars, I estimated that the radio telephone installation has saved this practice some 75,000 road miles.' The reaction was one of disbelief.

In the following week's issue, Edward Wilkinson commented that Straiton's estimate of saving 75,000 road miles in a five car practice in twelve months meant a saving of 15,000 miles per car per year.[7] For many practices, he said, the usual annual mileage is about 22,000 and rarely more than 25,000. Straiton responded[8] that the mileage per car in his practice ranged between 46,000 and almost 55,000 miles per year for the farm practice vets. Straiton also noted that in one year his own personal mileage had reached just over 96,000. He said he had worked 'really hard' that year.

Another correspondent, P. R. Greenough,[9] wondered how Straiton had totted up such a large mileage. 'At an average speed of 32.5 miles an hour one would cover 260 miles' – the daily total to make 96,000 – 'in some eight hours. Presumably during such a day one would make about thirty visits and giving a reasonable service would no doubt spend about fifteen minutes with each client. Thus would be spent fifteen and a half hours of Mr Straiton's day to which we should add a further one and a half hours for natural processes such as eating, washing and shaving.' It would be most interesting, wrote Greenough, to learn how the remaining seven hours of Mr Straiton's day would be spent.

In the same issue P. J. Dingle commented on the 260 miles a day which would be needed to travel 96,000 miles in a year at a slightly lower speed, thirty miles an hour: 'That gave him ten hours in driving alone.' Dingle also noted that 'in the old days' Straiton had said that he'd many times spent six to ten hours on embryotomy cases.[10] Other correspondents in that issue made similar points.

Responding to his critics, Straiton said:[11] 'During the tough years such luxuries as sleeping, eating and other "natural processes" had to take a very back seat. I had a ten minute breakfast at 5:45 am and a twenty minute meal any time between 11 pm and 4 am next morning. To stop for food during the day was unthinkable.' He repeated his claim to have covered 96,000 miles in one year and was dismissive of remarks about travelling at speeds as low as thirty miles an hour: 'Good heavens! Has he [Dingle] never been busy?' he wrote.

The correspondence exchange ended with a letter from J. Deans Rankin, a contemporary of Straiton's at Glasgow veterinary school, who said he had succeeded Straiton as assistant in a practice in 1942. He wrote: 'One day the boss said to me: "You're a Glasgow man. Do you know a chap called Straiton?" Guardedly, I admitted to knowing him. "Queer fellow," he said, "you couldn't kill him with work." '[12] Straiton established a lifelong reputation as a controversialist. A letter stating that 'the veterinary world offers little or no opportunity to women and yet we continue to accept female students'[13] brought dozens of letters, both men and women vets pointing out that women made a valuable contribution to the veterinary profession. Straiton alleged that the female 'struggled through her years at university, in many cases losing her femininity in the process' only to 'come up against a blank wall of prejudice and disillusionment'. He said that in most parts of the country farmers would not accept a female veterinary surgeon and that in all parts of the country female pet owners preferred a man. He went on to maintain that 'precious places in the veterinary schools should be reserved for men only'.

Throughout this period there was numerous correspondence criticising the broadcasts by the 'television vet' who was, of course, also Eddie Straiton. He continued to arouse, and amuse, his fellows over a long career. His media broadcasts ended after he fell foul of the RCVS by relating over the air the story of how he and a colleague had a 'race' to see who could spay a cat more quickly. Straiton's punch line was that he had mistakenly operated on a male animal. The resulting (public) Royal College disciplinary committee hearing was something of a show trial, as he called in his defence stars from the television series based on the James Herriot tales of a country vet, on which Straiton had been a veterinary adviser. He was let off with a reprimand.

CHAPTER NINE

NEW IDEAS, NEW ENTHUSIASMS

The period of relative prosperity experienced by agriculture and therefore the veterinary profession during the 1950s, together with rapid advances in therapeutic and surgical treatment, had been matched by new ideas and new enthusiasms among veterinary surgeons who wished to develop special interests. From the start of the 1960s there was a rapid development in species specialisation and with it the formation of thriving new specialist divisions of the Association, some of which would come to threaten the status of the BVA itself. Relationships between the practising vet, as local veterinary inspector, and the state, waxed and waned. The fluctuating fortunes of the State Veterinary Service continued to cause concern and the Association continued its efforts to bring veterinary public health and meat hygiene services up to accepted Continental standards. The growth of intensive livestock farming techniques brought increasing awareness of the need for veterinary preventive medicine schemes but conflicting views on how they should be organised. Potent new animal medicines and more stringent regulation of their use brought benefits but also problems of illegal sales. While recognising the new trends, the BVA's leaders were chasing the dream of government financial support for preventive veterinary medicine schemes involving LVIs in an on-farm advisory service.

The president at the 1961 congress was a man who had divided his career almost equally between practice and teaching. A popular member of the BVA, Sidney Jennings was well qualified to review in his message to the congress the present situation of the profession and to suggest how it might develop in the future. He predicted a situation in which the veterinary general practitioner would increasingly call upon the services of the specialist; he argued that veterinary hospitals for large animals, as well as small animals, would make the work of the practitioner more effective; laboratory services would increasingly be utilised to help make diagnoses more accurate. Preventive medicine schemes, which included advice on animal husbandry, were the way forward for farm practice, he maintained. In the running of the veterinary practice there should be proper charging for services, which took into consideration the veterinary surgeon's time spent in travelling as well as in consultations.

He spoke of the difficulties faced by practising veterinary surgeons from extraneous sources: MAFF veterinary officers were taking over tuberculin testing of cattle; free advice was offered to farmers by veterinarians employed by pharmaceutical companies, and animal charities provided free services to almost anyone. To overcome the 'slow strangulation by many inroads into veterinary practice' he suggested the ultimate inevitability of some form of national veterinary service – that recurrent theme of presidential addresses.

This could, he said, take the form of an extension of the group practice. 'Let it be imagined that a large group of practices amalgamated in a defined area', he continued, 'and negotiated with the NFU a *per capita* fee on all farm animals in the area. The group would jointly own a central hospital and its equipment and employ clinicians. If MAFF was represented in the group, it would be reasonable to ask it to provide veterinary investigation officer services and a laboratory.' He went on to suggest that the groups could be coordinated by a central board. That would form the basis of a national veterinary service for farm practice without the fear that one day a nationalised veterinary service could be thrust upon the profession.[1]

His views may well have been influenced by the successful culmination of the MAFF-led scheme to eradicate bovine tuberculosis. After years of veterinary tuberculin testing of cattle, culling of reactors and establishment of attested (i.e. TB-free) herds, Britain was declared free from the disease. In a 1960 meeting held to celebrate the fact, the Minister of Agriculture, Christopher Soames, described the eradication of bovine TB as 'a great agricultural achievement brought about by the cooperation of veterinary surgeons in the government service and in private practice, farmers and the ministry'. BVA past president George Gould reminded the meeting that the preliminary steps had been taken by vets in private practice and that their work had made the official scheme possible. He added that the chief veterinary officer, John (later Sir John) Ritchie 'could justly be described as the chief architect of the eradication scheme'. Gould also commented on 'the harmony and unity which existed between private practitioners and veterinary surgeons in the ministry service'.[2] Fifty years later, Britain was struggling to maintain that TB-free status as tuberculosis spread in Wales and the west country.

Jennings's Utopian vision of a wholly coordinated veterinary service reflected not dissimilar ideas put forward by predecessors including W. R. Wooldridge.[3] Like most Utopian schemes, those proposed for the veterinary profession were not to be realised. Jennings's predictions of increased use of specialists and of laboratory services were, however, fulfilled when the wide establishment of referral practices and veterinary laboratories, privately owned as well as government operated, became a fact. And group practices, some of them very large, are now the norm – if not in the way Jennings suggested they might come about. Nor did he foresee that small animal work would become economically predominant in the typical veterinary practice.

While vets were doing relatively well at the time, changes in the country's economic climate and in agricultural practices brought fears for the future. The creation of some system of practice organisation that could cope with changes, and help shield the veterinary professional from growing competitive commercial pressures, had long been a recurring theme among BVA members. Meetings such as that organised by SPVS and the Southern Counties Veterinary Society had as their theme 'The next thirty years'. Growing specialisation, the growth of multi-vet practices and the decline of single-handed ones were among the forecasts made. After the meeting, D. Fenwick Jones commented that for the past fifteen years the profession, most of whom were contracted as local veterinary inspectors (LVIs), had enjoyed 'pleasantly substantial ministry cheques [for LVI fees]'. In 1946 LVI fees amounted to £300,000; by 1964 the ministry paid out fees of approximately £1,700,000 (at 1946 rates).[4] At the same time, continued Fenwick Jones, there had been 'an ever increasing demand for veterinary services that has until now comfortably exceeded supply of veterinary surgeons', but would the next ten years see supply outstripping demand? Aggregation of farms into larger units would certainly cause a decrease in work. 'Everybody in agricultural practice knows which they would prefer to have on their books – ten 50 acre smallholdings or one 500 acre farm.'[5]

Another factor causing concern was the policy introduced by some animal medicine companies of selling direct to farmers many products previously restricted to supply through vets. Such sales were often accompanied by veterinary advice provided by the companies' own qualified staff: how was the profession to combat this? 'Is it not time we forgot restrictive practices and sought better payment for our surgical skills and advice, particularly in the fields of preventive medicine and meat inspection?' argued a correspondent. Sales should be left to others such as chemists and pet shops, he maintained.[6] In the same issue, another correspondent felt that such problems could be solved by 'a scheme of state veterinary service which would be acceptable to the great majority'. He explained: 'This service could be paid for by a levy on the agricultural community. The ministry would take over all existing practices and put them under the control of the Animal Health Division. The ministry would be responsible for fees and travelling allowances. The farmer could still be responsible for the purchase of drugs and would have a choice of veterinary surgeons.'[7]

One solution offered was that practices within an area should combine to form a centralised body for administration without interfering with the day-to-day running of the 'truly veterinary' side of the practices. 'The business side of such a group practice could be managed by personnel trained in business methods and be situated at a central office at which accounting, drug supplies, special equipment and, perhaps, laboratory and hospital services provided.'[8]

J. B. White addressed the question during his presidential address at the annual general meeting in 1963. He said that provided the vet was thoroughly conversant with farming practices in his area, nobody else in the whole agricultural field was better equipped on the control of diseases such as mastitis, parasitism and metabolic disease. White was speaking at a time when the farmer had access to free advice from MAFF's National Agricultural Advisory Service (NAAS, later Agricultural Development Advisory Service), from veterinary pharmaceutical companies, the Milk Marketing Board and from some large animal feed manufacturers. So, he asked, would farmers pay for such veterinary advice? 'In many cases the answer is no,' acknowledged White. But he felt some would; 'This is a new approach to the control of disease and I do not feel we can expect it to be generally accepted overnight.' While the idea of a nationalised scheme was repugnant to many, he continued, they should 'give thought' to the possibility of such a service in case the government should decide to introduce one.[9]

In response to such pressures, the BVA set up a committee to look into ways and means of increasing the role of the profession in the field of preventive medicine. It was faced with the problem of how best to provide the farmer with a service of preventive medicine, which would be basically advisory, that could be operated by the practitioner and yet be within the normal fee-paying structure of veterinary practice. The Royal College set up a similar committee 'to look into the question of the future of animal health services in the United Kingdom, particularly on all aspects which concern the Royal College, with the intention of cooperating with the BVA in producing any report'.[10] The BVA president, J. B. White, said: 'The thoughts of both committees are still very fluid.' They were not under any pressure, nor were they in any negotiations about a possible national veterinary service.[11]

In fact, the concept of State subsidised preventive medicine had already been trialled by the so-called 'survey scheme' during the 1939–45 war, when it had been supported by MAF. And for reasons of its own, MAF was also looking at the question of paying for veterinary advice on preventive medicine. For one, it would help make agriculture more efficient. For another, the proposed entry of Britain into the EEC, being considered in 1961, would mean the end of the system of guaranteed prices for farmers: the provision of free veterinary advice, it was thought, would be a form of compensation for that. As it was thought that such a service could only be delivered by a nationalised veterinary service, an internal working party was set up to consider the structure and cost of such a measure. When it reported in 1963, the impetus was gone: not only were the cost of such an operation and the supply of the appropriate veterinary manpower major limitations, but Britain's joining of the EEC had been blocked by General de Gaulle. That proposal was shelved but consideration was continued of more modest possible support.[12]

Throughout the year debate continued on means of combating competition on medicines sales and promoting preventive medicine. Direct sales of medicines to farmers continued to generate correspondence. One member felt that 'the changes which are rapidly occurring in agriculture will have profound effects upon the nature of future practice. Together with an increasing number of colleagues I believe that there is now a golden opportunity to formulate long-term plans through the medium of a State veterinary service which would be of inestimable value to the farming community and increase the livestock farmer's profitability. At the same time, a happy and contented veterinary profession would be ensured; one fully employed in its true vocation, including preventive medicine and its wide ramifications, together with opportunities for specialisation, refresher courses and further research to the advantages of all concerned.'[13]

Putting another view, Hugh Kay argued that vets should sort out their difficulties for themselves. As LVI fees had been reduced, attendance fees should be increased. The sale of drugs by 'travellers' should be met by charging the 'face price' for all drugs. Kay noted that 'a very fair margin of profit is received by us'; the farmers would have no further cause for complaint about prices changed by vets.[14] Speaking from the small animal practitioner's viewpoint, V. A. Harrison referred to competition from so-called 'free clinics'. He maintained that private practitioners should agree on a scale of fees for standard procedures as, he believed, many members of the public were 'put off visiting the private sector because of concern about the fees they might be charged'. He proposed that veterinary hospitals should be financed by a private company whose shares would be owned by the principals of cooperating practices. The staff of the hospital would be paid by the company and agreed fees charged to each participating vet for hospitalisation and other services provided.

Within such proposals lay the germ of developments, such as stakeholder involvement and company-run group practices, that lay in the future. Trying to counter direct sales by refusing to buy from companies that used such techniques was a popular option for some members. Such a course was clearly ineffective: unless universally adopted, it was merely 'spitting into the wind'.

In 1964, the National Farmers Union asked the government to set up a study group 'to consider ways of encouraging the application of veterinary research on the farm'. MAFF provided the modest funds required and the BVA joined with the NFU and the National Agricultural Advisory Service (NAAS) in setting up regional groups to organise talks, demonstrations and publicity material, hoping to raise farmers' awareness of local animal health problems and how to control and prevent them. The Association's leaders saw these initiatives as vital in building goodwill and educating farmers in the need for veterinary advice. They, and the farmers, also hoped that the study groups would evolve into a system of regular state funded veterinary visits to farms.[15]

At the same time, the BVA's Mid-West Division, with Bristol veterinary school and the local NFU branch, set up a pilot scheme on fifteen farms to demonstrate the benefits (assuming there were some) of the application of preventive medicine over a three-year period. The twelve vets participating made four visits to each farm every year, each visit being of at least two hours duration. In their visits they would tackle any health and husbandry issues arising. There were hopes that the initiative might foreshadow a national development in preventive medicine. All the farms in the scheme improved their performance, even though, paradoxically, only half the farmers thought the scheme had been of value. Valuable lessons had been learned, including that of a formal relationship with NAAS advisors – and the need for the farmer's own willingness and capability to be involved.

The pilot study led in 1969 to the BVA persuading the Animal Health Department and NAAS to participate in a joint exercise ('jointex') in which practising vets and NAAS advisers would together visit two hundred farms, three or four times a year, with MAFF paying the vets' fees. Again, the BVA hoped that this would be a forerunner of a national advisory scheme[16] with the vet 'as the hub of the wheel whose spokes comprise all the scientific, clinical and technical aspects of livestock production'.[17] It was also hoped that joint meetings between the BVA and BMA divisions, already held occasionally, would become meetings at national level to discuss matters of common interest, such as public health.

The next development followed the setting up by MAFF in 1971 of yet another committee (the second Swann committee) to consider the future role and education of the veterinary profession. This was done, at the request of the RCVS, in the light of the massive changes in livestock management and knowledge of disease since the two Loveday committee reports of 1938 and 1943. The Swann committee launched the most detailed study of the veterinary profession ever carried out. It took the opinion of every interested party and individual who cared to offer one and visited the USA to see how vets there were organised.

When its report was eventually published in 1975, it concluded (as had the earlier Northumberland report) that preventive veterinary medicine would be important, and that 'past experience has shown that preventive medicine will not develop to the best advantage if left to make its own way'. It supported the BVA's request for a system of state subsidy for vets' advisory visits to farms. It recommended that the 'jointex' programme should be continued and practising vets employed part-time within NAAS (now Agricultural Development and Advisory Service [ADAS]) at an estimated cost to MAFF of £6 million to £8 million a year, to enable the formation of advisory teams. Thus it seemed that the BVA's long sought system of State supported advisory visits to farms was about to be realised.[18]

However, times had changed; there was less enthusiasm among vets and farmers for the study group meetings. The massive epidemic of foot-and-mouth disease in 1967–68 had interrupted the continuity of the exercise. Cost cutting and changes to ministry advisory services (NAAS having been subsumed into ADAS) meant there was no longer funding available. The Swann recommendation for the employment of practising vets within ADAS was not taken up.

Nevertheless, the 'jointex' exercise continued for four years, after which it was said to have provided firm evidence in favour of joint action on the farm by the practising veterinary surgeon and ADAS officers.[19]

There was also the fact that the situation for farm animal vets' veterinary services such that their enthusiasm for extension of a state-funded preventive medicine service had waned. There was still full employment for the practising veterinary surgeon with things as they were. 'Fire brigade' emergency services, medicine sales and, importantly, LVI fees (which contributed 46.5 per cent of practice profit), provided a reasonable basis on which to run a veterinary business.

The by now faint flickering of enthusiasm for some form of nationalised service was finally extinguished by the Swann report on the profession. Swann considered nationalising the profession but rejected it (a similar conclusion had been reached in 1963 by an internal government inquiry)[20]: 'We could see few advantages and a great many difficulties.' Not least, 'even a government that might see a point in nationalising farm practice would hardly be anxious to spend public money on nationalising small animal practice'. And a measure that would 'cause a split down the middle of practically every practice in the land was scarcely a realistic thing to recommend'.[21] But if nationalisation was a dead duck, the pressures to retain, and if possible increase, government support in the form of the LVI scheme would continue.

WELFARE IMPLICATIONS OF INTENSIFICATION

The growth in intensification of livestock production caused increasing concern among members of the public about the welfare implications of the systems being introduced for the animals involved. In response, the government set up the Brambell committee of enquiry into intensive livestock husbandry. The BVA, which had always regarded itself as a main promoter of animal welfare, submitted extensive oral and written evidence to the inquiry. Detailed opinion and advice was given on all aspects of the handling of farm animals kept under intensive management. The Association's evidence concentrated primarily on those systems which had been the subject of public criticism: such criticisms had all been based on indoor housing of stock but the Association noted that the term 'intensive' could be applied to some outdoor husbandry techniques developed to increase the productivity from grassland such as paddock grazing. It also noted that many of the systems under review had been introduced too recently to permit the long-term observation needed to provide the factual information on which to base a judgement.

In its conclusions the Association felt that most of the commonly accepted practices of intensive husbandry could be carried out without cruelty and without detriment to the welfare of the animals concerned, provided that – an important proviso – they were operated with care and concern for the stock. Cruelty, where it entered into the picture at all, was mainly attributable to inexperience and ignorance of the potential risks involved, or to accidents such as power cuts, air conditioning failures or ventilation breakdowns.

It pointed out that the larger livestock units, against which a good deal of uninformed public criticism had been levelled, were not necessarily the worst offenders; those managing such units could afford both better housing and equipment and regular professional advice. The extent and value of such advice was not always recognised by the smaller establishments.

Not surprisingly, the BVA felt that designers of intensive system animal houses should ensure that they had up-to-date information on disease control and prevention; and that more use could be made of professional advice on the relationship between disease control, stock management and building before the unit was in production, and preferably before new buildings were erected or old ones adapted.

Specific recommendations were that salmonellosis in cattle should be made a notifiable disease; that, in veal production, total darkness and close confinement in boxes were both undesirable and unnecessary; that declaration of the addition of non-nutritional additives in feedingstuffs should be made compulsory. Close confinement in two- or three-bird battery cages was deplored; and birds should be effectively stunned before slaughter.

In an appendix on the addition of non-nutritional products to feedingstuffs the Association strongly condemned the indiscriminate inclusion of drugs, hormones and other non-nutritional additives, because misapplied use of such substances might delay proper veterinary attention to ailing animals and render diagnosis and treatment more difficult. Further, there was the possibility of danger to the health of the animals concerned, to other stock and to the animal attendants or the consumer.[22] It was as a result of the Brambell recommendations that the Farm Animal Welfare Advisory Committee (superseded in 1979 by the Farm Animal Welfare Council) was set up and the 'Five Freedoms' of animals established. These were: freedom from hunger and thirst; from discomfort; from pain, injury and disease; freedom to express normal behaviour; and freedom from fear and distress. It was to formalise the Association's concern to make a positive contribution to those aims that it established a charity, the BVA Animal Welfare Foundation, in May 1983.

GROWTH OF SMALL ANIMAL PRACTICE

For years, an increasing number of vets had been exploring the potential of small animal practice. There had long been a number of the profession, mainly town-based, whose activities since the demise of horse-drawn transport as a major veterinary concern had concentrated on dogs and cats. The BVA's concern for such members, however, had been in those aspects of small animal work which were of interest to the animal welfare charities and the competition such bodies created by the offer of free or heavily subsidised treatment; of particular concern, as has been seen, were the activities of the PDSA. Such matters had traditionally been dealt with by the Association's organising committee, which in 1956 had changed its name to the small animals committee as more and more of its agenda was taken up by small animal business.

But political and financial concerns continued to dominate farm practice. Influential parliamentarians such as Fred Peart, long-serving member of RCVS council and a one-time Minister of Agriculture, had the ear of the profession. Some senior members of the BVA were thought to be patronising in their attitude towards those treating pets. J. C. MacKellar, BVA president 1973, was typical of the 'hard men' whose main concern remained with agricultural animals.[23] Nevertheless, there was a solid and growing core of involvement in small animal work. The number of vets deriving a substantial part of their practice income from the care of pet animals, and seeking ever improving standards of treatment for them, was increasing rapidly – and they felt their interests were being neglected. Already by 1935 every case referred to the Veterinary Defence Society, which provides liability insurance, involved a dog.[24]

There was also international interest in small animal medicine, mainly from the USA. The UK initiative was sparked by W. Brian Singleton, who worked at the Animal Health Trust's Canine Health Centre. He wrote: 'It has been suggested that an international Association of Small Animal Specialists should be formed. . . . It is proposed to hold an exploratory meeting, preferably in London, in early autumn.' Interested colleagues were invited to write to him.[25] There was an immediate response. Pressure was thus increasing for the BVA to deal more fully than it did with the issues of companion animal practice.

A group of veterinarians, mainly members of the London-based Central Veterinary Society, had already realised that an organisation to deal with the small animal veterinary matters was needed. They took action; in 1957, the *Record* published a letter announcing the formation of the British

Small Animals Veterinary Association (BSAVA).[26] The founding members of the new association included C. E. Woodrow, Bruce V. Jones, John Hodgman (head of the AHT Canine Health trust), Joan Joshua and G. N. Henderson; all belonged to the Central Veterinary Society and had, according to Brian Singleton, expressed 'a certain degree of disenchantment' with the [limited] activities of the BVA small animals committee. The following year, the fledgling BSAVA held its first conference, at which were presented scientific and clinical papers, with a trade exhibition. The event was declared a 'huge success': 'The BSAVA was well and truly launched,' with 335 members signed up.[27] That first launch was the beginning of a revolution in veterinary practice.

An important factor in the early progress of small animal practice was the growing use of prophylactic vaccination of pet animals. Spurred by the introduction in the mid-1950s of an effective vaccine against canine distemper, the most common disease of young dogs, Burroughs Wellcome's Epivax, the routine administration of vaccines became accepted. Distemper vaccines were followed by a vaccine for a new virus disease, parvovirus, in 1978, which created an additional demand. Feline vaccines against such diseases as panleukopenia and viral rhinotracheitis followed. The regular use of booster doses meant that vets had a source of income higher and more stable than before and were thus able to plan the development of their practice business, economically and technically. New clinical facilities and equipment became affordable. It was also a pragmatic example of a privately operated and financed preventive medicine exercise.

The BSAVA realised there was an unsatisfied appetite for clinical information. The new association's congress fed a demand for specialist courses which soon grew into more formal training in continuing practice development (CPD). Such 'life long learning' schemes have become a permanent feature of the BSAVA's, and other BVA divisions', activities.

The BSAVA's annual congress became a major international event. Attendance (2010) grew to over 7,000, of whom 3,000 (some eight times the figure for the BVA's own congress) were vets, making it by far the largest meeting of its type. The conference venue in Birmingham became host to a programme encompassing scientific, social, trade and professional interests, with satellite meetings to cater for specialist activities. Accompanied by the burgeoning growth in small animal practice, the finances of the small animal association became a serious business. By 2010, it had its own headquarters, named after one of its founders ('Woodrow House') and assets of over £8 million: its annual revenue totalled £5.4 million (£0.5 million net) and the congress income was £2.5 (£0.3 million).[28] Clearly, the fledgling quickly became fully grown.

Parallel with the BSAVA's educational activities was a long-standing part of the BVA's small animal activities: the operation of a number of canine health schemes run in association with the Kennel Club. The first of the schemes was that for veterinary examination of abnormal development of the hip – canine hip dysplasia. Since the scheme was established in its present form in 1984 more than 100,000 animals have been assessed. Each is scored on a point scheme which indicates the degree of dysplasia present. Another scheme examines canine elbows which are similarly graded for signs of abnormality. A third scheme, run in collaboration with the International Sheep Dog Society as well as the BVA and the Kennel Club, examines eyes for abnormal conditions such as cataracts, glaucoma and Collie eye anomaly.

The formation of the BSAVA was followed by more specialist divisions and 'clinical clubs' catering for virtually every branch of veterinary endeavour. The British Equine Veterinary Association, led by Col. John Hickman, was formed in 1961; the British Cattle Veterinary Association and the British Sheep Veterinary Association established thriving divisions; eventually there were nine species specialist veterinary societies. The extent of this increase in special interest organisations caused some concern among the leaders of the Association. In 1960 the president, Sam Hignett, feared that the rising number of veterinary groups could bring the risk of duplication of effort, so that the profession could not 'face the public on a united front'. The increase in the 'vocational' (i.e. specialist) divisions 'all of which', he said, 'have a big membership and are increasingly active', had been accompanied by poor attendances at many meetings of the territorial divisions.

Unlike the BSAVA, which had acquired divisional status almost as soon as it was formed in 1957, many of these new groups were not at first affiliated to the Association. Hignett argued that it would be in the interest of the profession as a whole if the specialist divisions became 'part and parcel of the Association'. He added that that would call for a complete overhaul of the present system of representation on council; but that was something the more progressive members had long realised was overdue.[29]

All the new specialist groups did, in fact, become divisions of the BVA with an important input to council meetings and the policies of the Association. Commenting on the proliferation of the new divisions a few years later, the *Veterinary Record* remarked that the emergence of specialist divisions was an inevitable result of the rapid evolution of the veterinary profession. 'As knowledge increases, veterinary medicine will almost certainly follow the path of human medicine with the specialist standing behind the elbow of the general practitioner; the creation of BVA divisions having interest centred either on a single species or pertaining to some esoteric discipline, will provide an atmosphere that is peculiarly favourable to the increase in the spread of knowledge.'

The specialist divisions had an important part to play in the advancement of the BVA as a national professional organisation, continued the article. To an increasing extent the Association's advice and opinion was sought by government or other official bodies on a great variety of problems covering the whole spectrum of domesticated animals. The value of being able to refer such enquiries to bodies of experts provided by the specialist divisions needed no emphasis, it pointed out. And members who wished to widen their knowledge of specific areas of practice were naturally attracted to bodies offering them facilities to do so; many vets became members of two or more specialist divisions in addition to the BVA.

The *Record* did sound one warning note. The veterinary profession was small in numbers and would suffer grievously from fragmentation, it pointed out. 'If the new, and essential, specialist divisions are to contribute their full potential it must be as divisions of the BVA. Any tendency to separatism would be as inimical to their best interests as it would be injurious to the parent body.'[30]

In time, as some specialist divisions became influential in their own right there were occasions upon which some of their members have felt such divisions should plough their own furrow rather than apply their influence through the parent body. Such divisions have, at times, included the BSAVA, because of its size and commercial influence; the British Cattle Veterinary Association, because of its agricultural and public health connections; and the British Equine Veterinary Association, because the horse held its place as the origin of the veterinary profession and its members represented the most affluent clients owning the most valuable animals. In fact, some years later the BSAVA, riding the crest of a wave of popularity and under pressure from some influential members, came close to seceding from the parent body; the threat dissipated, however. At the BSAVA conference in April 1976 the president, Roger Green, said that 'unity in such a small profession as ours is of paramount importance'. He affirmed that 'in spite of the view of a small number, BSAVA wished to remain a division of the British Veterinary Association'.[31] One small matter that helped to emphasise the overall cohesion of the specialist divisions was that of liability for insurance claims. The Association itself takes third party insurance cover on behalf of all the divisions.

Naturally, 'single interest' groups feel they can best respond to questions relating to their own particular area. But the value of directing their specialist expertise through a national body, where matters of public interest are concerned, is unarguably more effective than that of a numerically small veterinary profession having a multiplicity of voices.

It would, however, take some time before the historically sensitive relationship between the parent organisation and its lusty offspring would really settle down. From time to time, complaints surfaced in BVA council that the views of divisions were not recognised by the executive to the extent some of them believed they should be.[32] In time, aided by improved electronic communications and enhanced cooperation by both sides, things improved greatly. Input to national BVA policy by a particular division was always acknowledged. The current situation is now more akin to that of a federation, with each division sharing its views with those of the head office and jointly formulating policy.

SOME PRESIDENTS OF THE 1960S AND 1970S

Nineteen sixty-seven saw the election of the Association's first woman president, Mary Brancker. Her year of office was a tough one for the veterinary world in the UK. A massive outbreak of foot-and-mouth disease swept the country and Brancker was centrally involved in the task of marshalling the practising arm of the profession in combating that scourge; she rose to the challenge. All veterinary services were desperately overstretched. Virtually all the ministry veterinary staff, the Royal Army Veterinary Corps and a great many private practitioners were drafted into service, diagnosing infected animals and supervising the slaughter and disposal of carcases.

The disruption to ordinary life and business was immense, with cattle markets closed and the countryside virtually shut down. The need for help from the private sector was so great that the president personally appealed to practices to release members who were licensed veterinary inspectors (LVIs) for duty with the Animal Health Division to help combat the outbreaks.[33] MAFF placed an advertisement detailing how vets could offer their professional help during the disease emergency. One of

Mary Brancker's less arduous presidential duties was to represent the BVA at the Norwegian veterinary association's congress. Her Norwegian hosts had not realised that the Association's president was a woman. In fact, among veterinary delegates from the whole of Europe, she was the only woman. Her acceptance was, however, assured when during a tour of Oslo the visiting vets were shown a memorial to British servicemen who had been killed during World War II. Among the names listed was that of Mary Brancker's brother; she became, by association, the heroine of the hour.[34] Miss Brancker continued her work for the BVA and the profession long after her formal retirement. She instituted the profession's involvement with fish medicine, being influential in obtaining a Nuffield Trust grant to set up the Institute of Aquaculture at Stirling University. She was keenly interested in zoo medicine. She worked for the (former) Animal Nursing Auxiliary scheme. She was the recipient of the BVA's two highest honours: the Dalrymple-Champneys cup and medal, in 1972, and the Chiron Award in 2005.

The Dalrymple-Champneys Award

At the 1934 AGM Sir Weldon Dalrymple-Champneys presented a cup and medal to be awarded annually to a member of the NVMA in recognition of 'scientific or clinical work of outstanding merit'. He made the award 'as a mark of the esteem in which he held the veterinary profession'. An ancestor, an exiled French aristocrat, had practised as a veterinary surgeon to the governor-general in India.[35] Sir Weldon was a Ministry of Health medical officer (later deputy chief medical officer) with a particular interest in zoonoses, especially brucellosis. He was a governor of the Royal Veterinary College and a member of the Animal Health Trust. He, with his wife, Anne, were for many years regular visitors to the Association's congresses. Sir Weldon died in 1981; his award is still made annually.

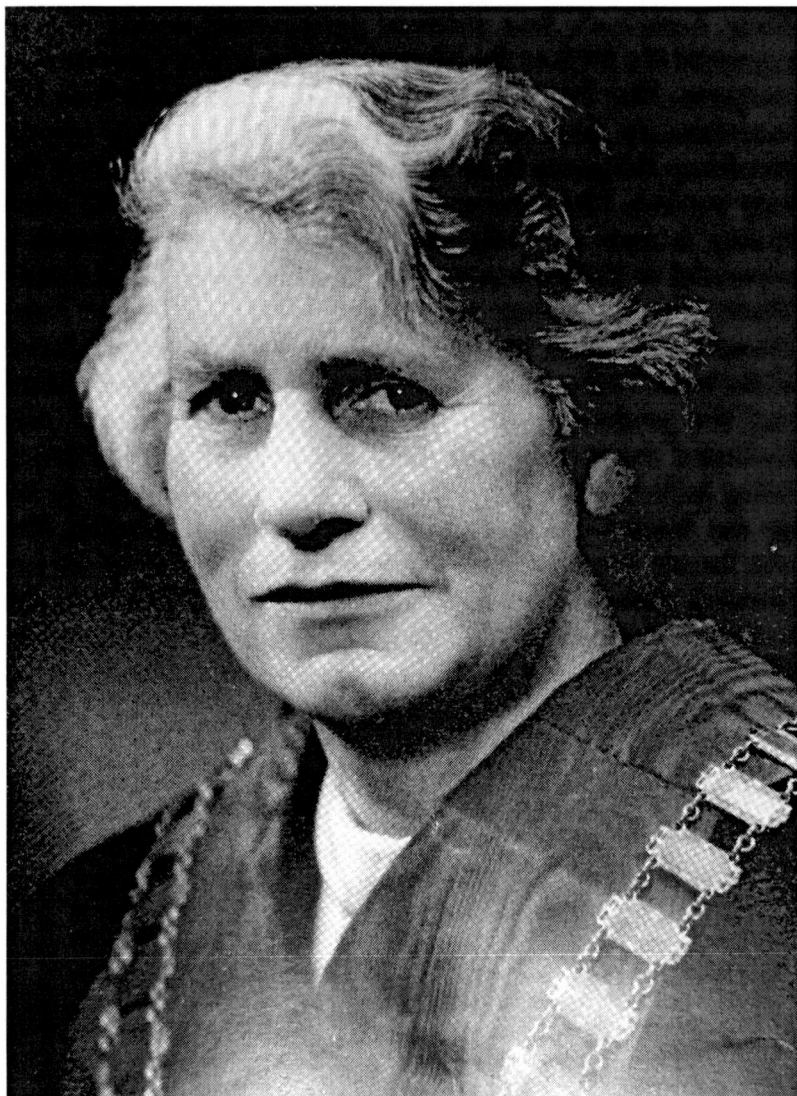

Figure 15. Mary Brancker became the first female president of the BVA in 1968, and was the only woman to hold the presidency until 2006.

Awarded the OBE in 1969, she proceeded to CBE in the year 2000. Well into her nineties, in 2010 Mary Brancker was still an active part of the Association's scene.

Chapter 9

Dr Peter Storie-Pugh, who, in 1968–69, succeeded Mary Brancker as president, was exceptional in almost every way. His father and grandfather were both eminent veterinary surgeons; his grandfather David Pugh, FRCVS, founded a notable practice in Sevenoaks and his father, Professor L. P. Pugh, CBE, FRCVS, was the first professor of veterinary clinical studies at Cambridge. Storie-Pugh first studied (human) medicine at Cambridge, where he was a foundation scholar of Queen's College, but immediately on the outbreak of the 1939–45 war joined the army. By the end of the war he had risen to the rank of colonel, had won decorations including the MC, MBE (military) and TD, to which three clasps had been added. He had been wounded and captured at Dunkirk, escaped from his first prison camp, was recaptured and sent to Colditz, the Saxony castle from which escape was reckoned impossible, from which he also attempted to break out.

Returning to civilian life in 1945, he qualified MRCVS from the Royal Veterinary College in 1948, then spent four years as a research scientist, gaining his PhD for a thesis on ovine pregnancy toxaemia, before taking up a university lectureship at Cambridge veterinary school, which he held for thirty years. Along the way, he became DL, CChem and FRSC, and was elected FRCVS in 1982. Storie-Pugh continued his military career in the Territorial Army, including commanding the 1st Battalion, Cambridgeshire Regiment.

This dynamic man became a member of the BVA council in 1954 (and of the Royal College council two years later). He was twice president of the BVA and leader of the College in 1977. A leading member of several specialist national and international veterinary bodies, which would later include MAFF's Farm Animal Committee and the home secretary's Advisory Committee on the Cruelty to Animals Act 1876, he was one of the first UK vets to become involved with the EEC. A delegate to the Veterinary Liaison Committee since 1962, and later president of the Federation of Veterinarians of the EEC (FVE), over twenty years he helped to establish

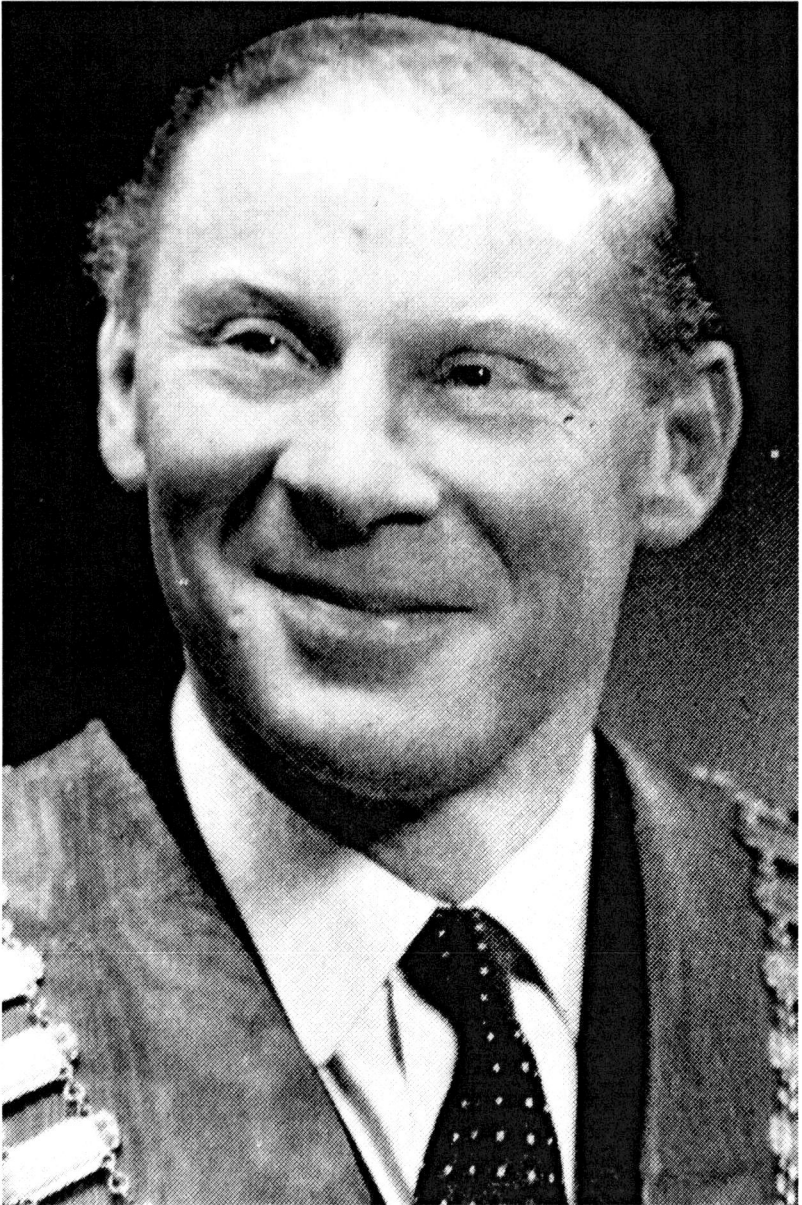

Figure 16. Dr Peter Storie-Pugh, Colditz escapee, veterinary polymath and twice president of the BVA (1969 and 1971) and of the RCVS in 1977.

a tradition of British leadership in European veterinary and animal health matters.

Chapter 9

In the early 1970s he was joint editor of a book, *Eurovet: A veterinary anatomy of Europe*, which presented the first description of what the EEC would come to mean for the profession and those who served it, and the first cataloguing of the organisations and government departments involved. His keen interest in Europe must have been inspired by his wartime experiences; his links with Germany, initiated by his involuntary residence as a prisoner of war, strengthened in peacetime. Involvement with his veterinary colleagues in that country was recognised in 1972 by his award of the Robert von Oerstetag medal by the German Veterinary Association. Storie-Pugh was also behind the introduction of 'The European Scene', which became for some years a regular feature in the *Veterinary Record*. The piece gave short news items about veterinary matters in continental Europe 'having regard to the possible entry of this country into the EEC'.[36]

As a personality, Storie-Pugh had great charisma. Not tall, his dapper figure, crowned with strikingly ginger hair, could always be spotted in a crowd. He would be talking at the centre of a group of colleagues, making his points with lucidity and wit, adding emphasis with a jab of the pipe he always carried.

Storie-Pugh's successor as president for 1972–73 was Angus Taylor, a man who had spent virtually his whole career in the State Veterinary Service. He was elected at a time when, after a period of relative stability, there was serious concern over the salaries of veterinary surgeons employed by the government. Things had reached such a pitch that the Association issued a notice advising any member intending to apply for a ministry post to check with the Association of State Veterinary Officers, via the BVA, before doing so – a similar action to that it had taken during the pay dispute twenty-five years previously.[37]

The situation for state veterinary officers was very different from that described by the minister of agriculture, James Prior, only two years before Taylor's congress speech. Speaking at the time of the formation of the Agricultural Development and Advisory Service (ADAS), into which the

SVS had been incorporated, Prior said the status of the veterinary staff had never been higher and they could look to the future with confidence. Their career prospects would be improved: the new service would 'open up opportunities for individual officers to widen their knowledge and experience and there would be increased opportunities both for those who wished to specialise and in the management field both within ADAS and the wider regional organisation'. He added his thanks to the practising arm of the profession for their help in implementing the brucellosis eradication scheme then in progress. 'Ministry veterinary surgeons alone could not handle the blood sampling of 35,000 or more herds and that is why well over 80 per cent of the blood sampling has been undertaken by LVIs,' said the minister.[38]

The period was one of great unrest in the UK. Inflation was rampant, government support had failed to maintain the stability of sterling and there were strikes, including by civil servants, against prime minister Edward Heath's introduction of a pay freeze which restricted any wage increases to the amount by which the cost of living had risen, 7 per cent. To add to the government's difficulties, the IRA had stepped up its terrorist activities in response to the 'Bloody Sunday' shootings in Londonderry, 30 January 1972. It was not, therefore, an auspicious time to be seeking an improved pay scale.

Nevertheless, when Taylor gave his September 1973 presidential address to the congress, he argued the case for his State Veterinary Service colleagues very strongly. He began by recalling that when he had joined the service, in 1943, it was a powerful service. It had recovered from the trauma of amalgamation with local authority veterinary services in the late 1930s and was invigorated by the young recruits who had joined since 1938. In those days there had been fifty applicants for some twelve posts.

'What do we find today?' he asked. 'An ageing service with most of its members over forty-five.' Morale and enthusiasm were practically non-existent. There was no longer any pride in belonging to the SVS. There was a threat that some activities would face withdrawal. Young, and not so young, officers were looking for opportunities to leave. The problem was not new, Taylor pointed out. As long before as 1951 the unsatisfactory state of recruitment had been acknowledged by the ministry but to fill the gaps temporary veterinary inspectors had been recruited at a daily salary equivalent to the basic grade salary of a veterinary officer. That failure to recruit permanent staff had resulted in 'the sorry state we have reached today'.

The BVA, he said, had to bring all the pressure it could muster to make the powers that be aware of the changes that had taken place in veterinary education, in the opportunities available to the veterinary surgeon and the growth in prosperity of the profession. There had to be a good career structure in MAFF for vets, with salaries comparable with those of the medical and dental officers in the civil service.[39] That plea, of course, had been made by presidents of the Association since almost the beginning of the century. Taylor put the blame for the 'sorry state' largely on the civil service management which had ignored representations of its veterinary staff and the recommendations of the Northumberland and other committees on recruitment. Management had, too, 'failed . . . to take heed of the narrow escapes the livestock industry had experienced' during the FMD outbreaks of the 1960s.

That criticism of his employers (of which the above is just a sample) was strong stuff, coming from a regional veterinary officer some way from retirement. Taylor drily commented that 'the great shortage of veterinarians in the SVS makes my instant dismissal unlikely'. He was not dismissed; but the unheard of criticism by a civil servant of his masters did not please his superiors. The chief veterinary officer sent Taylor a formal letter of complaint about his speech.[40]

Efforts towards ameliorating the situation of the SVS officers continued. An eagerly awaited report of a MAFF working party on veterinary career development was not published, being 'for internal use only'. That direction is usually applied to medicines intended to have a curative effect; there was no cure effected in this instance. The

Association's own memorandum on the subject was widely circulated; it noted a shortage of a hundred field veterinary officers out of a basic grade complement of 330. Half the staff were due to retire in the next ten years, and the ministry's own estimate showed that an additional ten would be needed when the UK joined the EEC. Pay and conditions of employment were unsatisfactory and promotion prospects were poor. There was a risk of being unable to cope with disease outbreaks. Among the remedies suggested was that 'it may be more realistic to establish a service less in numbers but higher in calibre and to delegate more work to LVIs and more routine work to technical assistants'.[41]

Meetings were held with politicians, the minister of agriculture, his permanent secretary, and senior civil servants. Questions were asked in the House of Commons and two Parliamentary debates held. LVIs were asked to support 'certain action' by SVS veterinary officers. The BVA kept in close contact with the body responsible for formal negotiations on SVS pay and conditions of service, the Institute of Professional Civil Servants. But all to little avail. A modest pay award to civil service scientists was 'not likely to solve the serious problems of the state service.'[42]

By 1975, however, in spite of a continuing poor economy, the situation for veterinary officers was better. Revised salary scales for the State Veterinary Service, it was felt, 'should remove most of the justifiable grievances which had existed'. The SVS salary and career structure 'was now comparable with most other areas of the profession'. And remuneration for private vets on LVI contracts was improved: the Association announced that it had agreed with MAFF that fees should be raised to £9 per hour.[43]

INFLATIONARY PROBLEMS

The BVA's own finances, in common with the rest of the country, were in need of improvement; inflation was running at a frightening 24 per cent[44] and costs were racing ahead of income from both membership subscriptions and the *Record*. In the short space of three years, while subscription income had doubled, from £65,000 to £135,000, so had related overheads and staff costs. For the *Record* the situation was even worse; postal, paper and printing charges had jumped from £98,000 to £206,000, in spite of all practical economies, and staff costs and overheads had also almost doubled. Even though advertising income and sales had increased over the same period from £126,000 to £215,000, from being a net contributor to the budget, the *Record* now cost each member £10 a year.

Giving those figures at the 1976 annual meeting, the treasurer, J. B. Walsby, set them in the context of the value to members of the services, including the *Record*, which the Association provided for its members. He reminded them that the BVA was regarded by the government as the authoritative voice of the profession, and 'many must be aware of the bargaining power of the Association in continuous negotiations with outside bodies, particularly the Ministry of Agriculture'. Walsby was so convincing that instead of an increase in the annual subscription from £15 to £27, which he had asked for, the meeting voted to double the existing fee, to £30.[45] Doubling the fee did not discourage membership; it only reduced the numbers members by twelve, to 6,776, the following year.

John Parry, elected in 1976, was ideally suited to the presidential role; Cambridge educated, dignified of mien, a natural chairman. Son of a vet with farming interests, he practised in Wales, and occupied a prominent position in the affairs of the principality. He was a member of the boards of various Welsh and UK agricultural bodies, including the Agricultural Advisory Council and the AFRC, chairman of the Hill Farming Research Organisation and became BBC national governor for Wales.

His successor could hardly have been more different. D. L. Haxby – 'Don' to everyone – was a man of remarkable attainments and prodigious energy. He qualified from the Royal Veterinary College after completing his two years' National Service, during which he rose from eighteen-year-old recruit to Warrant Officer First Class, a rank usually reserved for long serving non-commissioned officers. His veterinary interests were wide; they ranged from a large practice in the East Midlands to lecturing at veterinary schools and consultancies with a major poultry producer and pharmaceutical companies.

Handing over to Haxby, Parry said of the incoming president that 'his diligence is such that meetings occasionally started at six o'clock in the evening and finished at seven-thirty in the morning';[46] such meetings were not, of course, all about business. But Haxby was an effective representative of the profession; he became something of a legend both for his facility in cutting red tape and his ability to break through the barriers of vested interests in the different bodies with which the BVA had to negotiate. Those who worked or socialised with him, it is said, never forgot the experience. His colleagues compiled a commemorative memoir, The Great Haxby.[47]

In Haxby's address to the 1979 congress he told his audience, and the minister of agriculture, John Silkin, who was present, that animal welfare, disease control and preventive medicine were areas in which the veterinary profession had to lead. He reminded the minister that more than 3,500 practising veterinary surgeons, as licensed veterinary inspectors, 'were actively supporting his policies and were an integral part of his ministry's activities'.

The following year's congress, at York, saw the president, Dixon Gunn, preside over a new format. Instead of what had become a traditional Monday to Friday event, the proceedings were condensed into a long weekend. The idea was that members who found it difficult to give up work days would be able to find the time to attend at least some of the programme on Saturday and Sunday. That aim was not realised: attendance was down to about 700 and the congress, for the first time ever, made a loss. The president and his wife confessed to having been 'rushed off their feet' to keep pace with all the functions they had to attend. However, a similar format at Exeter in 1981 saw numbers revive, and in fact peak, to close on 2,000 including day visitors, although the programme was still felt to be hectic.

THE PROFESSION UNDER SCRUTINY

The Association had been prompted in 1961 to consider its views as to how the veterinary profession was likely to develop, when it was asked to submit evidence to the Duke of Northumberland's committee of inquiry into recruitment into the veterinary profession and the development of postgraduate studies. The resulting memorandum, in fact a report running to some 5,000 words, gives a picture both of the current veterinary state of play and the shape the BVA thought it might take in the future.

The Association identified the need for the more positive maintenance of health in farm animals that would follow the increasing intensification of production in livestock farming. This, it was felt, would require the greatly extended application of veterinary preventive medicine, although the vet's role in providing emergency and curative treatment must continue. The Association acknowledged that the wider adoption of preventive medicine was hindered by the existing method of payment on a 'fee per case' basis.

It was cautious in its comments on future manpower requirements, noting that there did not, at the time, appear to be any acute shortage of veterinary surgeons for country practice. Veterinary work was still related to the emergencies of farm life and there were accordingly peaks of activity at autumn calvings and spring lambings. It warned, however, that 'a deficiency could very quickly arise if by some change in the pattern of veterinary practice work on the farms was markedly increased'.

While the Association's memo noted that small animal practice was 'non-essential from the point of view of the nation's economy' (a comment that must have raised quite a few eyebrows), its future prospects looked 'extremely good'. The statement that small animal practice was 'non-essential', so out of kilter with the facts, reflected the contemporary Association view; in spite of the galloping progress of the BSAVA, the BVA was still reluctant to accept that small animal practice had become a major force in the profession.

But it was accepted that a higher level of investment in the facilities offered to the pet-owning public would encourage greater public awareness and use of those facilities. The report also predicted that many mixed practices would in future almost certainly employ a 'full-time small animal man' (*sic*). However, it did not think the expansion in small animal practice would necessarily mean more graduates were needed: the necessary vets would be available from shrinkage in large animal practice, if patterns from the United States were any guide.

There was also likely to be a need for suitably trained veterinary surgeons to be concerned with the increasing number of animals used in research. The report notes that the number of veterinary surgeons engaged in meat inspection was small but 'should England and Wales adopt the Scottish and European' system of meat inspection, there would be a case for increasing their numbers. That eventually happened, as we have seen, in 1995.

The interests of the considerable number of veterinary surgeons in membership of the Association who served in the Colonial veterinary service of former Empire (present Commonwealth) countries had always been an important concern of the BVA. The overseas division, and later the overseas committee, represented them on council. The granting of independence to most of those areas had affected the demand for British vets drastically. While there was urgent need in those emergent independent countries, especially in Africa, for skilled veterinary advice it was unlikely to be met at the required level until conditions of service offered greater security and better salaries. Until those countries achieved a reasonable degree of stability there could be no justification for an increase in the number of veterinary graduates from Britain to meet their particular needs, it was believed.

Nevertheless, the UK veterinary schools should continue their practice of accepting academically suitable students from the developing countries and serious consideration should be given to the need for greater encouragement of postgraduate training in veterinary tropical medicine at suitable centres in Britain.

On postgraduate training to meet the needs of the future, the BVA argued that the increasing complexity of veterinary science, and the need for specialist advice in applying preventive medicine, underlined the need for more specialists for teaching, research, investigation and advisory posts. Those were all seriously hampered in their proper development by a shortage of personnel. But the creation of more specialists could be achieved only by postgraduate training in the veterinary schools, which could not happen until their staff numbers were increased and their facilities for teaching and research further improved. The report called for an immediate and substantial improvement in the value of postgraduate awards to veterinary graduates.

Summing up, the Association said the overall position at present suggested that supply and demand for veterinary surgeons were likely to achieve equilibrium in the near future. 'Unless there is some radical and unforeseen demand for more graduates we do not anticipate the need for an increased output within the next decade. Indeed, in view of the variable factors to which attention has been drawn in this document it is conceivable that a surplus will rise the next few years. We feel therefore that there is at present no need to consider the foundation of another veterinary school; but this matter should be reviewed again in ten years time.'[48]

Northumberland took account of many of the BVA's comments. It recommended no change in the level of admissions to veterinary schools but said the position should be kept under review. Grants should be made available so that the facilities for postgraduate training and research could be 'brought up to an acceptable level. It was more positive on the question of overseas veterinary involvement, recommending that a scheme should be introduced to allow UK graduates to serve 'in the field, in research and in the universities overseas, and for senior British vets to be able to act as consultants to institutions in developing countries'.[49]

What neither the BVA nor Northumberland took into consideration was the possible effect on the work patterns of the profession of an increasing number, and ultimately a preponderance, of women graduates; nor could it have foreseen the greatly increased number of applications for places in veterinary schools following a sudden rise in the attractiveness to young people of a career working with animals: what might be called the James Herriot syndrome. That author's books, films and, particularly, television series with its sentimentalised nostalgic view of a country vet's life was in no small way responsible for a sudden swamping of the veterinary schools with applicants.

'James Herriot' honoured

A popular event at the 1976 congress was the election to honorary BVA membership of J. A. (Alf) Wight, otherwise the author James Herriot. The books on his fictionalised experiences as a Yorkshire country vet in the 1930s, and the film and TV versions of them, had brought immense interest in the profession, to the extent that the veterinary schools became overwhelmed with applications. One result was that academic grades needed for acceptance became the highest of any profession. The BVA's long held aim of producing a promotional documentary film became redundant. When the presentation was made, one of Wight's former colleagues, John Crooks, quoted a remark made by a farmer client who had said to Wight 'Alf, tha's a useful vetin'ry - and tha can write a bit, an' all'. Alf Wight himself retained an innate modesty; he said that he would never have been able to become a vet nowadays – he would not have been able to pass the exams.

Professor D. L. Hughes in his presidential address to the 1964 congress said the Northumberland report 'will certainly become a landmark in our professional history'. He added 'but its ultimate effect will depend on the extent to which the government is prepared to heed its advice and act upon its recommendations'.[50]

The Association itself had conducted a survey of members' opinions on their professional future. A questionnaire sent to 7,500 vets in 1963 generated a response of 3,376 – a very high level. After three years' analysis, no very clear conclusions were forthcoming. There was 'a general feeling that a change was desirable', preferably in a way that would allow the veterinary surgeon to be able to undertake a greater role in preventive medicine. Most practitioners felt this could not be achieved under the existing practice structure. The three schemes 'likely to provide practitioners with these stated objectives' were:

1. Private group practice, in which several practices combined to provide a central hospital, laboratory and administrative services;

2. A corporation scheme, in which a controlling organisation composed of representatives of such bodies as the BVA, the RCVS, MAFF and the NFU with central, regional and local committees to supervise local veterinary arrangements, financed by a levy on farmers;

or (perhaps surprisingly in view of 'a general feeling that change was desirable')

3. No change.

What the survey did provide was an indication of how practice finances had changed between 1958 and 1963. While turnover had increased from a base of 100 in 1958 to 150 in 1963, profitability (not defined) had fallen from 39 per cent to 37 per cent.[51]

CHAPTER TEN

ANOTHER SWANN REPORT

Yet another committee of inquiry into the veterinary profession had been deliberating for four years when its report was finally published in 1975 by its chairman, Sir Michael Swann. The Swann report was undoubtedly the most important event of the 1975 conference, at York. Opening the event, Dr Gavin Strang (Parliamentary Secretary, MAFF) commented: 'If we were Chinese, we would declare it the Year of the Swan.' He hoped the BVA would be ready for discussions on the report 'by the end of the year', but warned that 'any measures involving additional government expenditure would be difficult to introduce'.[1]

The report[2] had been published only a few weeks previously, on 29 July 1975, some four years after the inquiry had been set up. The *Record* said 'no more important study of the profession is likely this generation' and the report had been well worth waiting for. It was indeed a substantial document, running to two volumes. In the main, it followed the lines the BVA had long maintained. These included greater veterinary involvement in public health and meat hygiene, the development of state-subsidised preventive medicine on farms, and better research facilities in veterinary schools. Better funding and facilities were *sine qua non* for those recommendations.

The fact that the ten-man committee contained four BVA vets (John Parsons, John Reid, Professor Sir Alexander Robertson and Brian Singleton) ensured the profession's views were well represented.

Sir Michael Swann, in an exposition of his report, said that in his committee's inquiries 'they had listened to every conceivable interest within Britain and compared the profession with those in a lot of other countries'. He would like to think, he said, that 'what we say will stand for quite a long time – at least until 1995'.[3]

In the sessions that followed, four eminent veterinary surgeons, representing practice, education, research and the State Veterinary Service gave their initial reactions.

Nigel Snodgrass, a past president of the Association and a very senior practitioner, noted that the report publicly recognised, for the first time, that a greater amount of practice time was devoted to small than to large (i.e. farm) animals. It was clear, he pointed out, that 'if small animal practice becomes unhealthy, then so does the profession'. While Swann had recognised that no government department or research institute had primary responsibility for veterinary research in small and recreational animals, Snodgrass was more concerned that, in spite of the fact that there was a government department with primary responsibility for veterinary matters, it was 'not competent' to exercise that responsibility with regard to the profession's small animal involvement. In matters affecting the health of farm livestock, a vet could consult the Ministry of Agriculture with expectation of receiving some support. But if the matter involved small animals, there was nowhere to turn, other than in the restricted fields of rabies and exports. He saw that as a serious weakness. That statement by Snodgrass was the first unequivocal acknowledgement of the importance to the profession as a whole of the companion animal.

Turning to farm animal practice, Swann had recognised the problems faced by the practitioner in the small farm area. While the main demand for preventive medicine schemes came from the larger units, many vets would continue to be concerned mostly with small farms. It recognised that in such a situation the practitioner might be fully occupied in reacting to calls and have little time for the initiation of health service schemes. The report recognised 'what the BVA had been preaching and pleading for years'. Swann recommended the interaction of husbandry and management advice from the ministry with [veterinary] advice from practitioners as an extension of licensed veterinary inspector (LVI) – i.e. state funded – activity.

Snodgrass argued that what the practitioner required to extend the LVI function were laboratory support, consultative support and adequate remuneration. And that remuneration, he emphasised, must be in a form that did not 'leave the practitioner as the only fee-charging member of the team'. On postgraduate training, while the report had referred to the subject, he felt it had not given sufficient thought to refresher courses (he was speaking in the context of preventive medicine). The veterinary schools should be involved in organising such courses for practitioners so that the practitioners' direct experience could feed back through the tutors to the undergraduates.

He accepted the argument that some tasks could be carried out by trained lay personnel. Snodgrass felt, however, that while they had a place in a 'very large' practice, in a smaller or single-handed practice, routine tasks 'such as calf foot trimming or dehorning' could be done in conjunction with professional work while a lay technician would be making a separate (charged-for) visit. And lurking behind any proposal to include lay personnel in veterinary legislation was the suspicion that it might lead 'by another back door' to admission of technicians to the register.

The Swann committee's recommendations on meat hygiene led Snodgrass to comment: 'Yet again an outside body has examined the evidence and come out with a powerful argument for veterinary supervision and central control.' But he suspected that, once again, nothing would be done.[4]

Chapter 10

The report's recommendations on education were considered by Professor W. I. McIntyre, dean of Glasgow University veterinary school. McIntyre felt that Swann had been 'less than fair' to the achievements of the veterinary schools since 1945. 'Despite the fact that not one of them ... had adequate buildings or staff to carry out the tasks expected of them in teaching and research, they had transformed the whole prewar scene.' The report had given them too little credit for that. It had discussed changes such as integration in the preclinical courses and developments such as recovery surgery, but made no mention of developments which had been carried out. These included new ways of presenting subjects, involving cooperation between anatomists and surgeons, physicians and pathologists; and the creation of a whole new standard of scientific information.

Nor had the report recognised some of the outstanding research programmes in veterinary schools that had helped put veterinary research on the map of world science. He instanced Plowright's rinderpest vaccine, and the lungworm (*Dictyocaulus viviparus*) and feline leukemia vaccines being developed at Glasgow. They had to give credit to the Agricultural Research Council (criticised by Swann) for its support, particularly in development of the lungworm vaccine.

McIntyre welcomed the recommendation that consultant groups should be developed. 'For too long', he said, 'the veterinary profession had been the only one of any significance without consultants.' But the concept that one was a consultant once one had gained a higher degree or FRCVS had to be quashed: 'These were but initial training schemes on which to build professional experience.' The 'biggest disappointment' in the report was the section on university salaries. He welcomed the report's 'concern and strong language' about ministry vets' salaries. But 'what of the people who are supposed to train practitioners and to arrange refresher courses and invent new programmes of preventive medicine?' Academic salaries were now far below state service salaries. While McIntyre welcomed many of the

199

ideas in the Swann report, they would remain a dream, he felt, unless the whole question of salaries for vets in universities was tackled immediately.[5]

Taking up the report's comments that it wished to see more research in veterinary schools and that the Agricultural Research Council should be 'put in a position' to substantially increase its support for such research, Dr (later Sir) William Henderson, Secretary of the ARC, queried whether that was 'a threat or a promise'. He said he would be happy to receive additional funds earmarked for the support of veterinary research in the universities; but he 'felt obliged' to point out that there had been a time when some universities had 'declined to retain the research opportunities they had in their grasp'. He also noted that that the ARC was the Agricultural, not the Veterinary, Research Council. The initiative, he continued, rested with the schools; the approval rate for research grants from veterinary schools was 66 per cent. He approved Swann's 'sensible' suggestion that there should be a joint policy of attempting to secure a steady expansion of research in the veterinary schools by the universities, research councils, government departments, and the University Grants Committee.[6]

The deputy chief veterinary officer of MAFF, (A. J. Stevens), broadly welcomed the report's conclusions on the salaries, staffing and functions of the State Veterinary Service. This, he said, had 'just come through a dismal period of acute staff shortage' but the more that seventy new staff – 'young, energetic and handpicked' – had given the service a wonderful new opportunity. He also approved Swann's comments on disease surveillance and the SVS involvement in that, and its coordinating role with the private practising veterinary surgeon.

Where he differed from Swann, said Stevens, was in three points essential to good preventive medicine. He felt the best person to act as a mediator between the farmer and the technical adviser was the practising vet, who knew the local conditions (Swann had recommended that MAFF advisers should combine husbandry advice with that of the vet).

200

While more use should be made of lay assistants, they should be used as part of a 'team approach', rather than deciding 'which jobs can be given over in their entirety to lay assistants'. Stevens said he hoped that the SVS could extend its use of lay assistants in providing assistance in the field and setting an example for the rest of the profession. He was sorry that the Swann Committee had not 'grasped the nettle' of the use of lay assistants for 'at least part' of the tuberculin test for bovine tuberculosis.[7]

What the report also tried to do was to predict future manpower requirements for veterinary surgeons, the extent to which a male dominated profession would become one in which women were increasingly represented and how that would affect recruitment. In its evidence to the committee, the Society of Practising Veterinary Surgeons claimed that 'a difficult and imponderable position will arise, especially in farm practice, if a high proportion of graduates are female'. The Society recommended that, to cope with the increasing demand for veterinary surgeons, an additional one hundred undergraduate places should be provided 'as soon as possible and that for at least five years these should be filled by male students'. If there was no male bias, considered SPVS, 'we may need as many as two hundred more undergraduate places'.[8] SPVS was assuming a shorter working life for women. In fact, an RCVS survey in 1973 showed that almost 65 per cent of all women who had graduated were working in practice. The committee based its recommendations for future numbers on the assumptions that the proportion of women graduates would rise from one third to one half. It estimated that raising the annual student intake from the current 290 to 360, the number of graduates would reach 9,600 by 1985, with 'an ultimate plateau of 11,400'.[9] The actual figure was in fact over 23,000, with two-thirds of new graduates being women – a proportion that would rise to three-quarters.[10]

Not everyone agreed that preventive medicine should be a state-financed operation. R. G. Eddy, an influential farm animal practitioner and BVA member, had a different view. He acknowledged that the implementation of preventive medicine required 'initiative and organisation . . . from the profession, farmers and agricultural departments' but felt that 'Government organisation . . . will inevitably lead to mediocrity'. In his view, that could not be good for the profession 'when considering the selling of sound advice based on the analysis of accurate information'. Eddy advocated the extension of the then current BVA/ADAS ('jointex') scheme and bringing in another 200 farms 'on a free basis'. Computerised recording and analysis, recommended by the report, could then create a cost-benefit database quantifying the advantages of preventive medicine. He argued that it was the lack of such information that prevented many practitioners and farmers from embarking on such schemes. A state financed scheme, said Eddy, would apply too many constraints to allow the practitioner to tailor a scheme to suit individual vets and farmers.[11]

Twelve months later, the Association published its interim observations on the report. There were few major points of difference from its conclusions and recommendations. It disagreed that 'routine' tasks in farm practice (dehorning, foot trimming, etc.) might prevent the vet following up opportunities for 'more advanced' veterinary work. On the contrary, such tasks often provided 'the opportunity to make a general appraisal of herd health and to promote the preventive medicine strategy' advocated in the report. Although accepting that 'it is conceivable that in the future trained lay assistants could be used for . . . technical work at present reserved to the veterinary surgeon', he thought a stronger case should be made for any expansion in their use. But if such a case was made, the Association said it would accept that there should be a statutory register of lay assistants. However, as a very large number of the profession was of the opinion that there was 'no value in the extension of the use of lay assistants'. The recommendation that 'vigorous steps should be taken' to extend the employment of lay assistants in farm practice was not accepted.

It was felt that the extent of preventive medicine in small animal practice was underestimated. The BVA argued that 'the position of the small animal veterinarian is similar within a pet-owning family to that of a family doctor. Over the years', said the Association, 'a personal relationship is set up and a wealth of advice and information is given, besides the straight medical care, on the pets of the family.'

On public health and meat hygiene, the Association strongly endorsed the report's recommendations; they were very similar to its own long held policies.[12]

It would be another twelve months before the government gave its own statement on the report. The statement, presented by the agriculture minister John Silkin to the House of Commons on 5 May, 1977, might be summarised, flippantly, as 'Thanks' to Sir Michael Swann and his committee 'for services rendered' and to the BVA and the RCVS for their 'thorough and constructive examinations' of the report; but 'No thanks' to those of its recommendations that would involve additional government funding. The concept of preventive medicine, it said, was recognised by such important activities as the pig health scheme and the mastitis awareness campaign. While agreeing that the Government should 'stimulate the progress' of preventive medicine on farms, it did not agree that public funds should be provided for that purpose – a point with which R. G. Eddy (above) would agree.[13]

The tone of resignation in the BVA's response to the Minister's statement was palpable. President, John Parry, said: 'The Association was, of course, disappointed that the [Government's] views came at a time of financial stringency which inevitably curtailed any action arising from the recommendations.'[14]

A very modest official contribution to the preventive medicine process advocated by Swann was, however, made in 1978, when government funding was provided for a series of paired booklets on animal health topics issued under the joint auspices of the BVA, which prepared the texts, and ADAS. The first pair was 'Respiratory diseases in housed calves' and 'Pneumonia in housed calves', and the second pair, 'Diseases of the lamb and the post-parturient ewe' and 'Diseases before and after lambing'. The first title in each pair was distributed to farm animal practices and the second to farmers.[15] However, the response was disappointing and the project dropped.[16]

The Swann Report, taking five years from conception to closure, was the most important of the several studies of the profession since the Loveday report in the 1930s. It comprehensively surveyed the situation at a particular point in time. Its prognostications, as all such exercises must be, were based on the situation at that time. It remains an important historical document. But not least because of the financial constraints consequent on the economic conditions in the 1970s, the report's recommendations would have little effect. And Swann's expressed hope that its findings would stand 'at least until 1995' were not to be realised.

FURORE OVER THREAT TO VETERINARY SCHOOLS

By the mid 1980s, questions of the supply, and education, of qualified veterinary surgeons had been debated by a succession of official bodies. As has been described in earlier chapters, the aim of their investigations had been to ascertain whether too many or too few vets were being produced to cater for the likely demand for veterinary services.

In 1985, yet another manpower review of the veterinary profession was produced by a working party chaired by Lord Stodart. His report[17] recommended that the student intake for the ensuing five years should be reduced from 335 to about 306. The slimming down process was taken a stage further when the University Grants Committee (UGC), concerned about the rising cost of veterinary education, and believing that veterinary undergraduate numbers would fall, imposed a funding cut of 2 per cent per year from October 1985 for five years, with a further cut of 10 per cent to follow. Towards the end of 1987 the UGC decided to investigate the whole question of veterinary education. It set up a committee – the Riley Committee – 'to consider the provision of veterinary education in the six veterinary schools in Great Britain and the scope for its rationalisation and to make recommendations'.

The BVA, working closely with its divisions (especially the Association of Veterinary Teachers and Research Workers and SPVS), after what it called 'almost certainly the most thorough examination of the requirement for veterinary manpower ... that has ever been undertaken', prepared its evidence for the committee. In spite of this thorough examination, however, it had to own that its conclusion that the six UK veterinary schools should be maintained, derived from inadequate data. There were no precise figures of the number of vets not in veterinary work, the extent of part-time work or the age distribution in the various sectors of employment. Predictions of the future numbers of vets that would be needed had therefore to be based largely on assumptions. The Institute of Management Studies was commissioned by the Association to analyse the figures and to make predictions from them. The results showed that the predicted numbers of students required varied widely when only small percentage changes were made in those assumptions. For example, taking the median level of the assumed requirements, a decrease of 1 per cent in the working hours of all vets would increase student numbers from 291 to 383.[18]

The figures used for the study, prepared from RCVS records and the BVA's own data, are given in the table overleaf.[19]

When the Riley committee issued its report in January 1989 it was met with dismay by the BVA and the profession in general. Riley recommended that there should be a single veterinary school in Scotland, with Glasgow amalgamating with Edinburgh, and that Cambridge veterinary school should close its clinical departments – effectively ending veterinary education there – and leaving only four veterinary schools remaining, together with major changes in Scotland and substantial adjustments in England. The restructuring proposed would cost about £20 million

Distribution of Veterinary Employment in the UK	
TOTAL NAMES ON REGISTER	13,626
Less:	
Retired	1,406
Overseas and Food and Agriculture Association	2,379
Republic of Ireland	1,639
Supplementary retired	33
Temporary list	9
Sub-total not in whole-time employment	5,406
TOTAL IN WHOLE-TIME EMPLOYMENT	8,160
Employed in:	
Government and municipal service	628
Universities	313
Research	144
Industry	285
Cattle breeding	19
Animal welfare	175
General practice	6,596

The veterinary argument against such a drastic move was that, if the Riley recommendations were to cost 'at least' £20 million, that sum injected into the existing veterinary schools would go 'a very long way indeed to correcting the imbalances that Riley had found'. Riley did however urge that the University Grants Committee should make it clear that 'a restricted [veterinary] educational establishment will be restructured in the future at a level that will fully maintain the national capacity that will have been created'.[20]

Walter Beswick, the BVA president, enlarging on those comments, regretted that the Association's case – that there should be six fully funded veterinary schools, taking in at least 335 students a year – had not been accepted. And the report failed to examine what £20 million could do for the status quo; that was wrong. The proposals, he said, would appear to limit the profession's ability to respond to market forces. Circumstances had changed radically since the enquiry had been commissioned. 'Veterinary science today and the completion of the European market tomorrow needs more, not fewer, vets,' he argued.

The Royal College expressed its dismay at the recommendations that Glasgow and the clinical departments of Cambridge should be closed. It pointed out that that would represent a loss of 25 per cent of the country's capacity to produce veterinary surgeons in the numbers and of the quality required, adding that it was only forty years since it had been decided (following the Loveday committee's report) that the way forward in veterinary education was to increase the number of veterinary schools from four to six.[21] It was as a result of that recommendation that the Bristol and Cambridge schools had been established in the 1970s.

A large and highly critical correspondence was published in the *Record* following publication of Riley's recommendations. More than twenty letters were published; more were received for which there was no space. Only one was not highly critical of the proposals to close two veterinary schools. The dissenting correspondent, M. J. Chapman, said he had travelled widely around veterinary schools in northern Europe. He had previously noted what he called 'the poor state of veterinary education in the UK' and one factor in that lack of quality, he argued, was the number of small isolated academic communities. The British Isles had the smallest schools in Europe; the UK average was 287 students per school; the EC country with the next lowest number of student was France which had an average of 577 students per school. Spain had 1,551 students, the Federal Republic of Germany 1,450, and the Netherlands 1,260.[22] That was a valid point which should have merited discussion but was swamped by the wave of opposing views.

Predictably, there was a particularly strong reaction to the Riley proposals from those connected with the Glasgow school. Graduates, staff and students joined in mounting a vigorous campaign against the closure. Posters, stickers and other publicity material were produced and a national petition organised. Similar processes were mounted on behalf of Cambridge veterinary school. In the House of

Lords, peers from all three main parties attacked the proposals to close the two schools although it was accepted that the report did contain some useful recommendations, including the strengthening of clinical teaching. Lord Molloy (Labour) said that the closure plans would be opposed by 'many millions' of farmers and ordinary people who valued the curative and preventive work of the profession

The RCVS, holding (jointly with the BVA) its first press conference in ten years on 9 March 1989 said that Britain was facing an acute shortage of veterinary surgeons and the situation would be exacerbated if the Riley recommendations were accepted. It argued that the UK was already reliant on European Community and Commonwealth vets to make up the shortfall in the existing supply. Alistair Porter, the College registrar, criticised the Riley report's assumption that the intake of the remaining veterinary schools could be increased from the optimum level of between sixty and eighty, which had been recommended by the Swann committee on veterinary education in the 1970s, to 110 without ill effects. The larger classes needed could not, according to Porter, receive the same quality of education.

Beswick pointed out that some 150 situations vacant for vets seeking staff were advertised every week in the *Veterinary Record* and some practices were placing advertisements for veterinary staff directly in foreign publications. He explained that Lord Stodart, in his earlier manpower review of the veterinary profession, had greatly underestimated the growth in number of vets in practice. Beswick acknowledged that the BVA had to accept some responsibility for recommending a cut in intake to that review, but pointed out that it was not possible for the Association to have foreseen the increase in small animal work or the simultaneous relative buoyancy of farm animal practice. Further, by 1992 – in three years – Britain's abattoirs would have to meet European standards (a development expected to involve the employment of many more veterinary surgeons).

A joint submission from the presidents of the BVA and the RCVS to the chairman of the University Grants Committee, Sir Peter Swinnerton-Dyer, accepted that Sir Ralph Riley's working party had not actually been asked to consider the manpower needs of the profession, other than being asked to address the needs for an annual entry of 302 students, but to allow for the possibility that overall entry could be expanded to 335. The earlier figure was that recommended by the Stodart manpower review; the higher figure that recommended by the 1970s Swann report. The BVA and RCVS went on to argue that it would be inappropriate to rely upon the projections made by Stodart's review body when those projections were clearly proving to be erroneous. Stodart's report, published in 1985, was based on evidence submitted and obtained in 1984 with a view to assessing the manpower situation five to ten years ahead of that. It was only now (five years later) that the accuracy of the forecast could be assessed and disproved. Figures for registration with the College in 1988 showed that an annual admission rate to the UK veterinary schools of 302, with Stodart's estimated 7 per cent wastage rate, would produce about 280 graduates a year 'and that number will manifestly not meet the current manpower requirements of the country'. Even an intake of 335, producing 312 graduates, would be 'quite insufficient'.

The barrage of protests must have had some effect: the next development was an announcement in April 1989 by the Universities Funding Council (UFC, formerly the University Grants Committee) that it had shelved any decision on the future of the Cambridge and Glasgow veterinary schools until the results of the next review of manpower requirements were available.23 This review was in the hands of yet another working party on veterinary manpower needs and the demand for veterinary education. This new group was chaired by Dr Ewan Page; its terms of reference were to assess 'the need for veterinary manpower and in UK, both for the public service and the private sector; and the demand for veterinary education from home and overseas students'.

The working party was also asked to make recommendations on 'how any increased manpower requirement might be met having regard to constraints on public funding and to the potential funding from the UFC and other sources'; and 'what future arrangements should be developed to assess the demand for veterinary manpower and determine the number of student places'.

The BVA argued that those terms 'sounded reasonable but might not be easy to satisfy'. Two of the terms of reference were actually outside the profession's control. First, the demand for places in veterinary schools was 'self generating': the number of potential students eligible for places far outstripped the availability of such places. Second, was the matter of 'more stringent' funding. In principle, it was argued, educating veterinary surgeons should be no different from educating other professionals and funded on the same basis. 'Why, then, question sources and availability of funds for one small profession? Why pick on the vets?'[24]

There was a further step forward later in April when the University Funding Council agreed that the 10 per cent cut in admissions to veterinary school which had been scheduled to be imposed for 1989 had been abandoned. Sir Peter Swinnerton-Dyer in a letter to the president of the BVA noted that the UFC had agreed that admissions should be based on a notional intake of 335 'in the light of the acknowledged shortage of vets'. He added that it was 'of course' without prejudice to the eventual outcome of the manpower review. The sting in the tail was the warning: there would be no more cash to fund the higher intake.[25]

That constraint became irrelevant with the advent of the student loan scheme to fund tuition fees in 1998.[26] The number of veterinary students grew apace. It was further spurred by the opening of a new veterinary school in Nottingham in 2006. The annual intake grew to 846, with a total of 4,345 students.[27] This growth was achieved in spite of undergraduate courses lasting five years, student fees continuing to rise, and a worsening economic outlook.

CHAPTER ELEVEN

THE ASSOCIATION'S CENTENARY

When the BVA celebrated its centenary in 1982, it was able to do so in some style. By now a solidly successful body, with over 8000 members, an income of around £1 million a year and an elegant headquarters building in a favoured part of London, the Association felt it only appropriate to invite the Association's patron, H. M. the Queen, with Prince Philip, to visit Mansfield Street, an invitation that Her Majesty was 'graciously pleased' to accept.

The visit took place on 9 February. After being welcomed by the president, Dr Tom Gibson, the royal visitors were shown round the building, being introduced to all the staff, before being entertained to tea in the boardroom. The visit, planned to last one hour, ran well over that time as the president and his colleagues answered many questions from the Queen and Prince Philip on veterinary matters (particularly those of an equine nature) and explained the work of the Association. At the termination of her visit, Her Majesty unveiled the commemorative plaque that is displayed in the lobby at Mansfield Street.

A more public event was the splendid centenary banquet, held in the City of London's Guildhall a month later, on 10 March. Some seven hundred members and guests attended; the guests included the Home Secretary, Sir William Whitelaw, with the minister of state, Timothy Raison and his permanent secretary; the Earl Ferrers, minister of state,

Ministry of Agriculture; Lord Peart (former Minister of Agriculture, and an honorary member of the BVA) and Lords Winstanley and Balerno. The last named was an academic at the University of Edinburgh with a long history of working with veterinary research workers and students. The presidents of the British Medical Association and the British Dental Association attended; also present, of course, were the president of the RCVS, P. G. Hignett, and the registrar, Alastair Porter.

At the start of the proceedings the president of the West of Scotland division presented the Association's president, Dr Gibson, with a scroll to mark the occasion. The scroll read: 'The West of Scotland Veterinary Society, which was founded in 1848, Lancashire Veterinary Society, founded in 1862, and the Yorkshire Veterinary Society, founded in 1863, send their loyal greetings to the British Veterinary Association on the occasion of its centenary.' It concluded: 'The child is the father of the man.'

The toast, 'The British Veterinary Association', was proposed by Sir David Napley, chairman of the UK Interprofessional Group and past president of the Law Society. He spoke of his 'enormous admiration' for veterinary surgeons; they gave dedicated service of great importance to anyone who cared for animals. He praised the skill and dedication with which the veterinary profession was run by the BVA and the RCVS; it was a model for any profession, he maintained. Sir David, who was speaking at a time when the Monopolies Commission was seeking to liberalise the professions' attitudes towards advertising, was of the opinion that if the professions were brought into the realms of commercialisation 'of the type which some people wished' it would destroy them.

Responding, the president said that the BVA was celebrating one hundred years of veterinary political activity which had contributed not only to the welfare of the profession itself but, significantly, also to the welfare of society. Dr Gibson went on to review the history of the profession from its earliest beginnings to the foundation of the Association and then spoke of the way veterinary

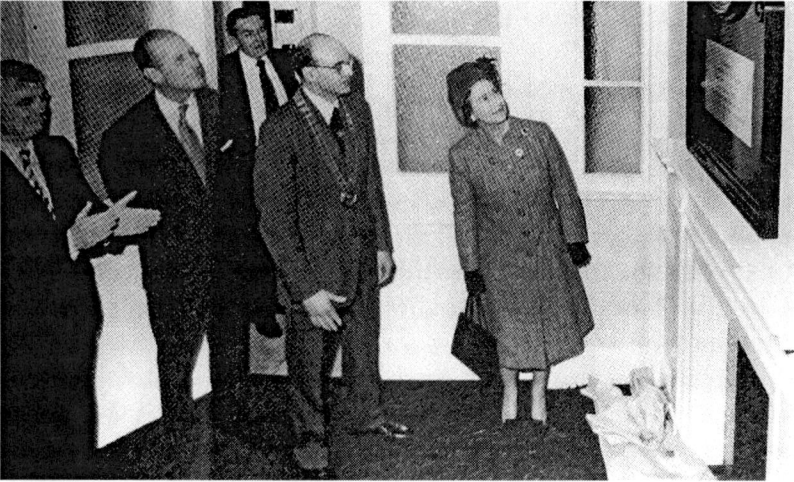

Figure 17. HM Queen Elizabeth and HRH Prince Philip visited Mansfield Street in 1982 on the occasion of the Association's centenary. Her Majesty unveiled a commemorative plaque to mark the occasion. The photograph shows the Queen with the president, Dr Tom Gibson, Prince Philip and senior vice-president John Tandy (left).

practice, and the Association itself, had changed and developed. 'If we keep before us our ethical principles, if we never let the word "vet" mean anything other than to examine carefully, then I predict that in 2082 the then president of the British Veterinary Association will be standing on this spot in the Guildhall, and he will be looking back on a very successful second century of the BVA's existence and looking forward to the third,' was Dr Gibson's optimistic conclusion.

Earl Ferrers also praised the veterinary profession. He said that whether one was a big or a small farmer, or 'just one of the cat and dog brigade', all had cause to be grateful for the profession's great knowledge, expertise and wisdom – as well as its friendliness. Commenting on the changing face of agriculture, Earl Ferrers said the more intensive it became, the bigger the risk; as agriculture sought to fulfil its duty to the world, farmers relied on the veterinary profession to care for and protect their animals, to prevent, detect and cure disease. Although the town dweller did not realise it, he depended on the veterinary profession as much as the countryman, for he relied on wholesome products to eat.

'Yours is a respected and responsible profession,' he concluded.[1]

Centenary banquets were also held in Scotland and Wales.

During the centenary year, the *Veterinary Record* published a series of articles on the history of the Association, by Nigel Snodgrass,[2] and on one hundred years of companion animal practice by Trevor Turner and Dick Lane, who outlined the changes in status and techniques of that branch of the profession and described some of the influential personalities involved.[3] Colin Vogel covered similar ground for equine practice[4] and David M. Jones dealt with the history of veterinary involvement with exotic animals.[5] Other features covered the changes in farm animal practice and the relations between the animal health industry and the veterinary profession.[6]

BEHIND THE SCENES

With the appointment as general secretary of Fred Knight, in 1925, the Association had accepted that its team of volunteer officers needed the underpinning of a competent administration with a full-time head, under whatever title, to provide continuity of experience for the growing amount of work generated within the NVMA and through its contacts with government and other outside bodies.

Fred Knight came to the Association from the Royal College, where he had been assistant to Fred Bullock, the registrar. He held the post of general secretary for thirty-five years, throughout the Second World War, until his retirement in 1960; he died a year later. Knight was the unsung catalyst who helped to put flesh on the bones of the ideas and schemes promoted by officers and the various committees. The increasingly numerous requests for the NVMA's views on proposed legislation, or for documents promoting or defending the Association's interests on behalf of its members called for a wide knowledge of the veterinary world and the political and professional environment in which it operated. Knight established the tradition of dedicated competence from its staff on which the Association came to depend.

He was succeeded by John Anderson, a widely experienced Scottish vet. He had wartime service in the Royal Air Force, followed by administrative roles in the veterinary pharmaceutical industry and had latterly run his own practice. Anderson brought a wider view of the secretary's role; in effect, he acted more as a chief executive than a general secretary and was well-known personally throughout the profession and those organisations with which the BVA had dealings. His early and unexpected death, from a heart attack, in 1968 deprived the Association, in the words of the serving president, Peter Storie-Pugh, of 'an experienced, efficient and devoted servant'. He had, said an obituarist, laboured literally day and night to promote the interests of the veterinary profession. 'Hours meant nothing to him. . . . and long continued overwork took a heavy toll on his health.'[7]

This excessive workload had led to the appointment of a deputy secretary, P. B. Turner, just less than a year previously. Pat Turner was not a vet; he was an Oxford graduate in his thirties whose previous career had been in business administration. He had been appointed to supervise reorganisation of the administrative facilities at Mansfield Street, a task he had completed to general satisfaction, and on Anderson's sudden death had taken over the day-to-day management of the BVA. In the ensuing eleven months, Turner had carried out his unexpected new responsibilities with 'assured competence'.[8] He was now appointed to succeed Anderson.

As general secretary Turner had to implement the recommendations of a working party on the Association's council and general administration. These, like similar efforts in the past, mainly effected some streamlining of the committee structure but made little change to council's unwieldy format. The main committees were powerful in their own right; some members felt they were almost autonomous bodies, with too much power vested in the chairmen.[9] This remained the case. What Turner did do was to bring within his own personal oversight all the reports and papers, internal and external, issued by the BVA. His capacity for work was prodigious but as time went on and the Association's activities and involvements expanded, the amount of material to be processed began to be overwhelming for the administrative structure then in place. Providing responses to governmental proposals affecting veterinary matters demanded more research and awareness of how MAFF operated and what its priorities were. There was, too, a growing need for firmer control of a larger staff and its diverse functions, with the responsibility of managing an annual budget increasing to exceed £1 million by the early 1980s.

The amount of input required by the president of the day – who was the executive, as well as the titular, head of the BVA – was such that it became more and more difficult for a working practitioner to devote the time needed for the post. One past president (let's call him Smith) told the author that when he took up the office his practice partnership was known as Smith & Jones. After a year as president, he said, it had become Jones & Smith. Another effect of the system was that successive presidents might have very different priorities towards promoting particular policies pursued by the Association. This might mean, for example, that if negotiations on a particular issue with MAFF had stalled when one president was in office, the ministry would wait to see if his successor was more amenable. Turner saw his role in relation to the incoming president as to 'prepare the stage for the principal actor'.[10]

Neal King, president 1982–1983, was a young and busy practitioner; he was concerned that the situation might limit the Association both in its selection of presidents and in its effectiveness as a membership organisation. As a first step towards change, he arranged, with council's approval, the appointment as a consultant of Charles Shillito, a recently retired permanent under-secretary, MAFF. Shillito was widely respected as an administrator and had great experience of the veterinary profession. The following year, council took matters further by appointing a working party with the task of reviewing the Association's management structure and the formulation and execution of policy. The review was prompted by the inquiry into the misappropriation by the Association's then accountant of £25,000 of BVA funds.[11] The loss was made good but that it had occurred was an indication that more rigorous controls were needed in the way its financial matters were managed.

The management review group was chaired by past president Nigel Snodgrass, with another past president, Dixon Gunn, the president-elect, Brian Hoskin, the treasurer, John Richardson and Shillito as members. The report they produced was far more comprehensive than anything that had gone before.

Its first recommendation, perhaps surprisingly, was that the basis of the existing system of council representation, with its historical links with divisions – and 'with its recognised imperfections' – should remain. These 'imperfections' included the complications introduced by members belonging to several divisions, each of which had representation on council. The complications had been noted often in the past; in 1919 the honorary secretary, Colonel J. W. Brittlebank, had said: 'The machinery of this Association is the most cumbrous machinery it is possible to devise.'[12]

But it was necessary, the working party felt, to reduce the size of council. As others had claimed previously, the representative body was unduly large and too cumbersome to be effective. The system of appointing members by divisions – one representative for up to 100 members, two for 100–200, three for 200–300 and four for more than 400, together with officers, committee chairmen and all past presidents having the right to sit on council in perpetuity, resulted in a body with, at that time, 137 members. No similar professional body had so large a council. The BMA, with 60,000 members, had a council of sixty; the Pharmaceutical Society, with 29,000 members, had only twenty-four on its council. The working party could see no compelling reason why the Association, with a membership of around 8,000, should not be able to conduct its business 'to the entire satisfaction of the membership' by appointing only one representative per division.

The working party recommended that that level of representation should be introduced, except for those divisions with more than 1,000 members, who should be allowed two representatives. And only the four immediate past presidents should have the right to attend council, unless specially invited. The Scottish Branch and the Welsh Branch, which comprised the regional divisions, should not send representatives to council. As organisations which existed to coordinate the views of the divisions in their countries to deal with any separate legislative or other issues specific to their own countries, they should, if necessary, contact the executive committee direct or arrange for their divisional representatives to raise the matter in council.

That reorganisation would reduce the size of council to sixty-seven members (at that time) and make for a more manageable and effective decision making body. The report added the comment that 'except on the most vital issues' it hoped council members would not be mandated to support a particular view rather than being allowed to consider the points made by others.

The 'inordinate amount' of paperwork produced for council meetings came in for criticism. What were needed were summaries of committee meetings, a report from the executive committee and separate papers on significant matters requiring a council decision. The committees themselves were in need of reorganisation, with their remits more clearly defined. The general purposes committee came in for particular attention: its role had become uncertain and its membership was too large. That committee should be replaced by a committee of chairmen of the standing committees. These should be reduced to a membership of six, plus an officer, with individuals called in to advise on specific items when necessary.

The working party felt strongly that the executive committee (the five officers and senior members of staff) was the part of the management structure most in need of attention. A greatly increased workload had fallen on its members, and particularly on the president. Changes at officer and senior staff level were needed to relieve the president of some of the day-to-day burden, to enable him or her to concentrate on the most important issues and to provide continuity and greater administrative expertise. That could only be achieved, in the working party's view, by a new appointment: a chief executive officer. This individual would be responsible to the president for the 'effective discharge of the Association's business and for control of the staff'. The existing post of BVA secretary would continue, servicing council and committees and acting as company secretary.

When the BVA management structure report was put to council there was a long and detailed debate. At the end of it, all the working party's recommendations were accepted. There were, however, those who considered the proposals on modernising council were not sufficiently radical. Roger Green thought that the possibility of a totally elected council might have been considered.[13]

During the debate, past president John Tandy was one of the few members speaking against the recommendation that a chief executive should be appointed. He said that the job description for this 'powerful' post must be absolutely clear, otherwise 'there might be a good deal of trouble and many headaches'.[14]

The appointment of a chief executive followed quickly. The first individual to hold the post, J. Buckley, a former civil servant, was appointed in 1985. He made some changes to the staffing arrangements but after only two years left to take up another post. His successor was James H. Baird, an experienced administrator with a background in agricultural science, who joined the Association in October 1987. He was familiar with the BVA, having been brought up in a veterinary household; his father was a respected practising vet in Cumbria.

Baird came with a set of priorities: to develop a coherent national policy for the BVA; to establish sound finances; to generate effective publicity for the profession; and to renovate 7 Mansfield Street, which had become rather shabby after years of hard use. One of the first, and most visible, areas to be refurbished was the downstairs front room. This, which had been used as a general office and stationery store, was transformed into an elegant sitting room for the use of members. The main boardroom, on the first floor, was redecorated, as was the first floor drawing room in the accommodation leased at 9 Mansfield Street, which became the council chamber. Staff accommodation was rearranged and the whole building freshened. The result was a headquarters that members could be proud of. Financially, a major boost to the Association's assets was given by an updated valuation of the lease of 7 Mansfield Street, which was reassessed at about £1.5 million at that time.

The new chief executive, supported by the Association's officers, was eager to introduce changes. Moves to make the administrative structure and organisation of the Association more efficient were proposed. In September 1988, introducing what would be a long discussion on the executive committee's draft proposals and the reasoning behind them, Baird told council that the current system was unnecessarily wasteful of time and resources. It was not well equipped to produce the rapid responses to important documents that were demanded by government. Increasing involvement in Europe, via the Federation of Veterinarians of the EEC (FVE), added another dimension to the BVA remit.

Changes were necessary, Baird felt, so that the Association could better tackle the issues facing the profession and to improve the relationship between the divisions and headquarters. He put forward a number of options for consideration, ranging from maintaining the status quo to the radical idea of doing away altogether with the committee system and replacing it by members with specialist knowledge. It would take some time for his proposals to be refined and put into a new structure acceptable by council: the first step was for council to set up a working party to review the issues.[15] This reported initially in May 1989[16] and finally in September of that year.

Eventually, in December 1989, it was agreed to cut down the number of committees and refine their remits. Instead of the old system, where most committees were species-based, the new committees would be created to service three main functions: company services (broadly, business related matters); veterinary policy (broadly, political matters) and veterinary services (professional, practice and scientific matters).[17] Several recently retired senior MAFF personnel were retained as consultants on matters where their specialist knowledge would be useful. The new structure meant that there was a source of expertise available to provide data across the whole field in which the BVA was engaged and that council was presented with cogent papers on topics for discussion. Corporate plans were produced annually, reviewing the Association's performance and setting out its aims.

Subsequently, BVA internal affairs ran relatively uneventfully for some years; then there began to be rumblings in council. By 1996, there appeared to be some confusion about the way policy papers were developed and reached council, and about communication between committee members, council and the divisions. The vice-president, Paul DeVile, acknowledged that situation at the July council meeting but said the executive committee did not propose changing the present system; they were, however, 'open to suggestions for making improvements'.

However, the time had come for another look at the Association's internal workings. A review of the committee structure in 1997 noted that, while performance had 'markedly improved' since the 1989 changes, 'criticisms had been received' of 'deficiencies in democracy including lack of consultation and clarity in decision making and a gulf between BVA headquarters and its membership'.

Some council members held the view that policy was centred in too few hands; Dr Tony Andrews argued that too much power resided with the executive committee. Stephen Ware said that the existing system had been in place for six years and the time was ripe for a review of how it was performing. He said: 'You must take the profession with you and allow for divergences of opinion.' Dick Sibley, for the British Cattle Veterinary Association (BCVA), put it forcefully: 'We want access to the decision-making process.' Peter Jinman pointed out that policy decisions often had to be made quickly: specialist divisions should get onto the BVA straightaway if a problem arose.

The chief executive, James Baird, said it was not always feasible to contact members for their opinion when, for example, the president or a vice-president was required for a television interview at an hour's notice. But he accepted that after six years of the new committee system it was appropriate for it to be reviewed.[18]

The ensuing review said the BVA had an effective system of governance and administration; any improvement lay not in more sectional interests but mainly in communication and consultation. The modifications, agreed at the next meeting, on 25 March 1998, were that two committees, veterinary services and company services, should be replaced by a 'members' services group', drawn from the 'employment-based' divisions and geographical regions. The chairmen of the new bodies would be elected by the group. But there was to be further scrutiny of the administration. An 'internal audit group' was to be set up with these terms of reference: 'At the request of council/executive to investigate any case where in the interests of the Association a structural, scientific, legal, financial, policy or procedural audit should be carried out, and make specific recommendation for the benefit of the Association.'[19]

At the behest of Professor John Bleby, the long standing representative of the Central Veterinary Society and a keen scrutineer of the executive committee's doings – he had previously alleged a lack of financial control and disregard of the Articles of Association by the officers[20] – the internal audit group was appointed. It consisted of 'four members of council of whom only one shall be a past president or officer. The members shall be re-elected annually and shall normally serve for a period of up to three years. The group shall appoint its own chairman who will not be a past president or officer. The chairman shall have a casting vote.'[21]

Professor Bleby proposed that the new group should investigate his allegations. However, his suggestion that a 'wide ranging review of the role of the executive committee and its relationship with the standing committees' should be carried out was not taken up. Instead, it was agreed that the executive committee and the veterinary policy group should have a meeting, independently chaired, and report back to council.[22]

A report of the meeting was duly presented to council by Howard Hellig, the past president who had chaired the meeting. A number of recommendations (unspecified), aimed at improving communications between the executive and the veterinary policy group, were made. Professor Bleby then reintroduced his proposal, withdrawn at the earlier meeting, that the internal audit group should carry out regular monitoring of the activities of the BVA and the executive and other committees. The proposal was defeated; instead, a paper on the subject of internal audit would be prepared.[23]

That paper became a review of the corporate governance of the BVA, prepared for council by the executive committee. The document reviewed the state of the Association's progress in relation to best management practice, discussed the scope and implications of internal audit, identified areas that still had to be addressed and suggested ways in which this could be done. When the paper was discussed by council, policy committee chairman, David Catlow, pointed out that the committee chairmen's responsibility included consideration of feedback from members and monitoring their own committee's actions – as well as those of the Association. He could not see the value of the internal audit group in the present situation.[24]

However, a report was duly produced by the audit group – but not presented to council. According to an unofficial account in a press article generally critical of the BVA, it disclosed staff problems and 'loss of trust' in the executive team.[25] The BVA itself aired the staff situation in a full page article under the title 'BVA officers are not above the law' in the members' supplement to the *Record* in October 2002.[26] It indicated that 'any such matters' [i.e. staff problems] had been resolved. It explained that the audit group's full report could not be presented to council 'because of the way it had been sought and also because natural justice requires that a member of staff against whom a complaint has been made knows details of the complaint and ... the name of the complainant'. It also set out the way staff complaints would be handled, much being made of the need for the 'preservation of natural justice' and the need to follow (no doubt expensive) legal advice.

The document must have seemed quite extraordinary to the majority of BVA members, who would have had little interest in the internal affairs of the Association. The staff – the civil servants of the organisation – were, as civil servants are, mostly uncomplainingly efficient, unseen and unheard. In fact, there was seething discontent among some of them, mainly relating to aspects of personnel management.[27] If the intention was to clear the air, it did nothing to deter those BVA members who felt that radical action was called for and who had already indicated their intention to propose a vote of no confidence in the Association's executive committee.

While these procedural matters were rumbling on in the background, the BVA, its executive committee, its head office staff and many of its rank and file members were having to deal with the biggest nationwide outbreak of foot-and-mouth disease the country had ever experienced; many of them were active in the field assisting the State Veterinary Service; not to mention the matter of dealing with the Competition Commission investigation into the supply of veterinary medicines and other ongoing business. It is not surprising that the chief executive felt that this vital work detracted from the efforts to deal with the dissatisfaction some members of council felt in regard to the executive committee's handling of its affairs.[28]

'NO CONFIDENCE' MOTION

So it was that in August 2002 a letter was published in the *Record* giving notice that the authors (seven prominent vets) intended to propose a motion of no confidence in the executive committee. In the same issue was another letter, signed by sixteen past presidents, who expressed 'concern at the adverse publicity being attracted on the matter of staff relations and administration at BVA headquarters'. The letter pointed to a lack of open discussion in council and failure on the part of the executive to communicate with the membership. The signatories urged that the matter be resolved before the coming annual general meeting in October; to this end, a special meeting of council would be held the following month on September 25. Finally, BVA president Andrew Scott appended a letter refuting the allegations of lack of consultation. The executive, he wrote, had followed expert legal advice at every stage; the matters had been discussed, in camera, at every council meeting in the past year and on each occasion the executive had been supported by an overwhelming majority.[29]

Other letters, supporting the executive and otherwise, appeared in subsequent issues.[30] Then, shortly after the extra council meeting, a letter from the original proposers confirmed that the motion of no confidence would be presented at the annual general meeting on 6 October.[31]

There matters rested until the meeting took place. Then everything suddenly changed. At the start of the proceedings, the junior vice-president (and president-elect), Peter Jinman, announced that Baird, the chief executive, had retired the previous day. Jinman went on to describe the changes the Association needed to make in order for it to function successfully. While its aims and objectives had not altered, society had radically changed, as had the knowledge that had been the key to the development of the specialist divisions. There was, he said, a need to review the Association's structure and function so that it could cope with all the demands made on it for consultation, comment, lobbying and representing the profession. Overall, there was a need for 'one clear voice to present the profession of this country'.

To achieve this, he said there should be an expanded management board, a 'political action committee', and an improved internet communications network for officers and staff. The pay and conditions of officers should be reviewed to reflect changes in their workload and prevent any barriers to obtaining 'candidates of choice' to serve the Association. Finally, Jinman said the system of electing officers should be reviewed 'to reflect the needs and transparency of a democratic election process'.

Dr Barry Johnson, speaking following the vice-president, said the motion of no confidence which he and his colleagues had notified was to effect changes that would provide a platform for the 'development of a strong and vibrant BVA', and outlined what those could be. His seconder, Professor Neil Gorman, said the intention was to make a BVA structure that was 'appropriate to 2002 to 2010'.

There was a long debate, during which there was much support for those ideas; many members felt that the action felt necessary was already in hand; the proposals made by Peter Jinman were little different from those put forward by Dr Johnson and Professor Gorman. The motion of no confidence was withdrawn.[32]

At the meeting of council which followed the debate, it was decided to set up a project team to evaluate the way forward for the restructuring.[33] Peter Jinman, by now president, took interim charge of executive matters with a senior member of the existing staff, Henrietta Alderman, acting as head of administration. The desired changes were implemented, a board of management selected and a more structured system of organisation introduced. The position of chief executive was discontinued and a new head of staff appointment, that of BVA secretary-general, made. Henrietta Alderman was confirmed in that post in 2007. The resulting administrative structure has endured to the present; the final, and important, organisational tweak in

2011 was the long sought for reorganisation of council to reduce its size (to forty-one) and include a nucleus of twelve directly elected members.

Not everyone, however, was happy with the manner in which events had developed. Past president, and long-serving officer, R. C. Young, thought council had behaved 'disgracefully' in the way the matter had been dealt with.[34] Young wrote to the *Record*. He said that the chief executive, Jim Baird, had left the BVA after fifteen years of dedicated service to the Association. 'Those past presidents who had the privilege to work with him are those best qualified to pass judgment on his commitment to the affairs of the BVA during that time,' he maintained. He praised Baird's 'obsessive' dedication to the BVA and his constant endeavour to 'uphold the dignity of the president and with it the credibility of the veterinary profession'. He continued: 'Over many years council has been complimentary about the quality of the papers that have been presented to it and it should be remembered that Jim Baird was the author of nearly every one. Jim did much to promote the influence of the BVA beyond our shores and was instrumental in improving the credibility of FVE. He was the catalyst to setting up regular meetings between the executives of American and Commonwealth Veterinary Associations. The healthy state of our finances and the refurbishment of 7 Mansfield Street are a memorial to his dedicated service. At the recent AGM it emerged that last year every budgetary target approved by council has been exactly met or improved despite difficult trading conditions.'

The letter was not published.

Several of the past presidents who held office during the tenure of the chief executive held an annual reunion, together with Baird, for many years. But as far as the BVA was concerned officially, the contribution of its long-serving chief executive officer remained unacknowledged.

The subsequent years saw the administrative machinery of the Association brought into line with modern business practices, and the application of effective internet resources. These greatly facilitated rapid communication between the

BVA head office and the specialist divisions, enabling the Association to produce a prompt, informed, response to parliamentary, government and media queries. An example was given by past president Nicky Paull. Leaving a meeting in Liverpool she was telephoned with an urgent request to give a BVA comment on a topic on which she had no specialised knowledge. Using information supplied by colleagues in the appropriate division via email, by the time she reached Mansfield Street two hours later she was fully briefed on the matter in question.[35]

CHAPTER TWELVE

TENDERING FOR VETERINARY CONTRACTS

Negotiations with government over local veterinary inspector (LVI) fees had always been difficult. The BVA sought what it considered a reasonable fee for a professional service; the government had a responsibility to the taxpayer to negotiate the lowest price it could. The process had been particularly complicated in times of economic depression and spiralling inflation.

In 1987, the ministry had been criticised for its dilatoriness in coming to terms on new rates for local veterinary inspector work; the *Record,* seeking a reason, asked 'Is there something we should be told?'[1] MAFF then sprang a surprise – 'dropped a bombshell' might be more appropriate – by proposing to discard negotiations and invite tenders for testing for bovine tuberculosis and brucellosis. Tendering was the Government's common procedure for selecting contractors for most outsourced services, so why not use that well established system for some routine veterinary services? That, presumably, was the Treasury's thinking behind the proposal.

The first hint was given when, in informal conversation at that year's Royal Show, the chief veterinary officer, Keith Meldrum, said to the editor of the *Record* (the present author) and the Association's press officer, Chrissie Nicholls¸ 'What do you think the BVA reaction would be if we put out TB testing to tender?'

When the proposal was made public shortly thereafter, the BVA reaction, predictably, was one of appalled disbelief. There was to be a pilot scheme in eight counties from April 1988 when bids would be invited, initially for bovine TB and brucellosis testing. 'This extraordinary move' struck at the heart of professional ethics and practice, thundered the *Record*. Tendering went against the provisions of the RCVS guide to professional conduct. But, no doubt bearing in mind that the profession had been forced to concede to the government over the lifting of restrictions on advertising, the government proposed, in effect, to offer LVI work up for auction.

The BVA council opposed tendering; farmers opposed it. There were fears of 'testing only' services springing up to the detriment of established practices. The profession's opposition to tendering was not based on special pleading to protect self-interest, it was argued, it sprang from the conviction that it would not work to the benefit of anyone – animals, farmers, vets or the ministry itself, ruled council.[2]

A letter from the president of the RCVS protesting against the proposals, and emphasising that tendering was unethical, described the measures the College had taken to object to them. The FVE supported the College's stance. Divisions and individual members voiced their displeasure.[3]

Then, after keeping the profession on tenterhooks for the best part of a year, the tendering proposal was dropped. A letter received just before the Association's 9 March 1988 council meeting offered an 8 per cent increase in LVI fees from April 1. The offer was subject to an independent assessment of LVI rates based on fifty 'representative practices'. Not without some misgivings by the BVA, the offer was accepted.[4]

That was not to be the end of the affair. The award of contracts by tender became the norm for provision of official veterinarian (OVS) duties in the Meat Hygiene Service from 1995 (see below). In 2000, MAFF announced it was to explore competitive tendering for LVI work, which was described as a major service to the farming community, 'as a way to improve the quality of its on-farm veterinary service'.

The total annual cost of LVIs fees in Great Britain at the time amounted to £12 million, still a considerable sum in the practices' budget.

A pilot study was to be set up by the Preston office of the SVS. It would cover Cheshire, Lancashire, Greater Manchester and Merseyside. From 1 July 2000, TB testing, the collection of blood samples for brucellosis testing and abortion inquiries in that area would be subject to competitive tender.[5] As had happened on the previous occasion when tendering for LVI work had been mooted, rural practitioners protested at the perceived threat to the established system. The loss of opportunities to visit farms routinely, missed opportunities for disease surveillance, not to mention a risk of losing a valuable contribution to practice income, were among the reasons.[6]

In March, advertisements for the scheme appeared inviting interested parties to apply for a tender document. Potential contractors were invited to submit bids for twenty-six 'lots' (areas) within the pilot area. The BVA, on behalf of its members, was among those bidding for work and through a company set up for this purpose submitted a comprehensive tender for all the lots. If its bid was successful, the Association intended to contract with local practitioners in the area to carry out LVI duties in particular lots.

MAFF questioned the BVA's bid on the grounds that it might be uncompetitive. That was vigorously disputed by the Association. It said it had at no stage discouraged any local practices from submitting their own tender; nor had the Association's proposed tender price been disclosed to any local practitioners. The scheme was originally planned to start on 1 July but MAFF wrote to the BVA on 26 June 2000 that it had been delayed in evaluating tenders and did not expect to be able to make a decision until the middle of July. The start date for the scheme would therefore be postponed until October.[7]

The BVA had serious reservations about the proposed scheme; not least, it said, because of the importance of local knowledge in disease monitoring and of maintaining a healthy veterinary surgeon/client relationship if monitoring was to be successful. That was why it had submitted its own tender. David Catlow, representing the Lancashire Veterinary Association which covered the area of the proposed tender, was concerned that neighbouring practices might win tenders and thus gain access to another practice's farms with the risk that they might take work away. Or 'corporate bodies might come in and take over the whole area'.[8]

The chief veterinary officer, Jim Scudamore, said that the tendering exercise was a way of 'seeing that the LVI service MAFF paid for with taxpayers' money' was giving the best value. There were, he said, many issues to be considered in evaluating the scheme: the cost of setting it up and the impact on rural practices were two of those. But 'just because something had run well for years, as the LVI system had, did not mean there was no need to investigate it to see if there might be a better way'.[9]

Eventually, as had happened in 1988, MAFF decided not to proceed with the pilot project on tendering for LVI services. In a letter sent to LVIs on 17 August 2001, MAFF said that 'after careful examination of the bids received, the Department has concluded that none of them would deliver clear improvements over the existing arrangements in terms of quality of service and value for money'. MAFF had therefore decided not to award a contract under the tender but to retain the existing system for the provision of local veterinary services. Four bids had been received, two proposing partial coverage and two full coverage of the pilot area. What had happened was that all the practices in the pilot area had been consulted by the BVA division and agreed to present a united front in their approach to the tender bid.[10]

BVA president, Eifion Evans, naturally welcomed the decision, commenting 'the LVI system as it stood represented the best kind of interaction between the public and private sectors and provided an efficient, cost-effective service. It also provided an important resource on which the state veterinary service can draw in the event of disease emergencies.'

Then once again, in 2009, the government tried to introduce the process for certain LVI functions. Negotiations had stalled by 2010 when the BVA, not without criticism from some members, had in effect walked away from the table leaving the tendering situation in limbo. In the intervening years, veterinary practices had changed; there were many group and corporate practices; inter-practice competition had increased; it was unlikely that a united front could have been presented.[11]

But the move to tendering had not been abandoned, only postponed. Animal Health Veterinary Services (the most recent manifestation of the government's veterinary arm) confirmed its intention to 'move towards the procurement of professional veterinary services through fair and open competitive tendering'. As well as testing for bovine TB, DEFRA, and the Welsh and Scottish devolved governments would seek to establish a cadre of 'veterinary reserve personnel' who could be called upon to supplement government vets in an emergency such as a major outbreak of exotic disease. Holders of this new title for what had once been called licensed veterinary officers would also be appointed by tender.[12] That, however, lay in the future.

Somewhat paradoxically, the award of contracts by tender had, without too much fuss, become accepted as the norm for provision of official veterinary duties in the Meat Hygiene Service from 1995. The Royal College had offered no objection. Its excuse was that tendering for the meat hygiene service did not conflict with College guidelines as the treatment of live animals was not involved.[13]

CONFLICTING VIEWS ON MANAGING MEAT HYGIENE

The campaign by the BVA for the establishment of a national meat hygiene service in England and Wales, with full veterinary supervision, was an ongoing saga. It had been one of the first aims of the Association. The meat hygiene service in Scotland had long been under professional supervision and was regarded as a model to be emulated. With the expansion of the production of meat and meat products that followed the ending of meat rationing in July 1954, fourteen years after it was introduced in the 1939–1945 war, and the boost to livestock production given by the Agriculture Act 1947, the Association renewed its efforts in that direction. It was prompted by anxiety about the facilities and conditions in the newly opened and newly licensed slaughterhouses established to meet the increased demands for meat products following the government relaxation of controls on the production and distribution of food.

Throughout 1953 a working group was devoted to drawing up a comprehensive scheme for the organisation and control of meat and meat products which set out proposals for the more efficient utilisation of all aspects of the meat industry. These included, as would be expected, arguments for a centralised meat inspection service overseen by officers of the Animal Health Division.[14]

To help research data for the project, the BVA sponsored a delegation consisting of Dr W. R. Wooldridge and H. Thornton, from the Association, and two MPs, one Conservative and one Labour, to explore the systems of meat inspection in western Europe. The delegation reported: 'In all the countries visited the standards of inspection and of hygiene and the consequent protection of public health are so much superior to most of the standards here at home.' The delegates were unanimous in the opinion that 'the meat inspection services in England and Wales should definitely be brought under veterinary control'.[15]

Before finalisation, the draft memo was discussed by the BMA/BVA liaison committee. The BMA was apparently lukewarm, as ever, towards any veterinary involvement in public health matters. The report back to BVA council on the discussions notes merely that joint discussions had given the Association 'a clearer idea of where the memo conflicted with BMA policy'.[16]

The memo itself was concise, but comprehensive. It began by asserting the validity of the veterinary profession to proclaim its views on meat hygiene and production. Although the Ministry of Food closed many of the original small abattoirs, which were both inefficient and uneconomic, and initiated a 'skeleton' centralised veterinary advisory service, this had merely emphasised 'the utter inadequacy' of the majority of abattoirs. While (veterinary) technical advisers had been appointed, there were few of them and they lacked legal powers. Either the power of the local authorities, whose veterinary officers had been absorbed into the state service, should be restored, or a national meat inspection service established, argued the BVA.

It went on to deal with the economic utilisation of abattoir by-products and how cooperation between the different branches of the veterinary profession could utilise the information obtained from abattoirs in the control of animal disease. The memo proposed specific measures for coordinating the efforts of all sectors of the meat industry. This, the BVA claimed, would lead to more effective control of animal diseases, initiation of new lines of research and treatment of disease, and would stimulate better production methods. Finally, effective cooperation would provide information useful in connection with eradication schemes for tuberculosis and other diseases.[17]

In a speech on the proposals to the veterinary hygiene section of the Royal Sanitary Institute congress that year, the BVA president, A. Thomson, emphasised that in suggesting the value of veterinary services at the abattoir 'my profession has no thought in mind that non veterinary inspectors should be displaced. They have done and are doing very valuable work. It is only that such work, we feel, could be of still greater value had they more veterinary colleagues.'[18]

Two years later, another BVA president, Edward Wilkinson, would complain that there had been no progress in the field of meat inspection in England and Wales. 'It is evident', he said, 'that most medical officers of health still appear to think that they have no need of the assistance of public health veterinarians. Yet the public health veterinarian is considered essential in almost all other countries the world over where a serious attempt is made to safeguard public health in the matter of foods of animal origin.'[19]

The Association's case for a national hygiene service was not supported by the meat producers or the government. Lay meat inspectors and environmental health officers (EHOs) were fiercely opposed to any system of meat hygiene which increased participation by the profession. They felt that would diminish their responsibilities and therefore career opportunities; they also knew that, although a few vets had always held prominent positions in the organisation and management of municipal meat hygiene facilities (where they existed), there were not many practitioners who had experience of the meat trade and working in abattoirs.

Swann in his 1975 report had recommended that 500 to 700 vets would be necessary for a system that matched Continental standards of handling the procedures involved in ensuring that animals for slaughter were healthy and the resulting meat and meat products uncontaminated. The Environmental Health Officers Association (EHOA) found his recommendations unacceptable; they felt that the United Kingdom 'should not be forced to follow blindly systems which operated on the Continent'.

While the protection of public health was the overridingly important factor in the securing of effective meat hygiene services, there was an element of territorial warfare in the conflicting attitudes of the EHOA and the BVA on how best to achieve that goal. The one was concerned to defend its existing position, the other to expand theirs. The EHOA's president said the 'necessary spirit of cooperation which must exist' could not be developed so long as the veterinary profession insisted that it should control meat inspection. But the BVA was determined to secure a position it had long sought to establish. It argued that, in most European countries, vets had the senior role in the health and hygiene aspects of the processing of meat and meat products and the UK would have to match that.

Britain's entry into the Common Market, however, forced the authorities to begin to comply with EEC hygiene requirements for meat products. At first, changes were introduced only for products exported to Europe. While the new rules, which specified veterinary supervision of abattoirs producing certain types of meat and meat products for export to the EEC, were felt to be an improvement on existing arrangements, the BVA was not happy about the way it was intended to administer them. Administration and enforcement of the regulations would be done by individual local authorities rather than one central body. The BVA pointed out that: 'There would almost certainly be differences in interpretation of the regulations by different authorities.'[20]

Some progress was made when it was ruled that, from January 1976, a 'public authority' – typically a county borough or municipality – would have to 'employ and instruct' veterinary inspectors to carry out the supervision and certification of meat for export. In effect this meant little change to existing procedures where a local veterinary inspector was already employed by a local authority; the only result was some grumbling about fees. Meat producers complained that the BVA recommended fees were too high, while some LVIs pointed out that in fact they actually represented a reduction in the previous BVA recommended rate.[21]

The Association's policy on meat hygiene was enunciated as follows:

The hygienic production of foods of animal origin should be supervised by veterinary surgeons.

A central, Government controlled meat hygiene service under veterinary control should be established. The service should employ veterinary and lay meat inspectors and should be responsible for the licensing of slaughterhouses, training of personnel, animal welfare, meat inspection and the hygienic production of foods of animal origin.

There should be a national slaughterhouse policy; adequate technical laboratory and other facilities enabling the achievement of veterinary specialist supervision should be provided.

The appropriate EEC directives on health problems concerning intra-Community trade in fresh meat and poultry meat should be applied also to the home market.

The supervision of the hygiene of meat-based products should be a veterinary responsibility with appropriate lay assistance.[22]

The government did not agree that vets should be appointed to supervise EHOs. It sought to allow EHOs themselves to carry out supervision and certification under the directive on meat-based products. In view of that official policy it was paradoxical that the Minister of Agriculture at the time, Fred Peart, endorsed the BVA view on meat inspection. Speaking at the Royal Agricultural Show in 1976, he said: 'I cannot see why some people are against veterinary control of meat inspection:' both veterinarians and EHOs had their parts to play. He said that he saw no reason for rivalry between the parties.

The EHOs maintained their opposition to BVA policy. At their annual meeting on 3 July 1976 in London they voted to 'accept a need for noncooperation' with MAFF if the government did not 'satisfactorily amend' a proposed Bill intended to satisfy regulations which would give effect to the EEC directives on poultry slaughter. The Bill would introduce measures that put vets in control of poultry meat inspection and hygiene. The EHOs did not accept either the validity of the directives or their interpretation by MAFF.[23]

For the BVA there was, however, progress, albeit slow, in the case of poultry meat inspections. Following the implementation of the Poultry Meat (Hygiene) Regulations 1976 in August 1979, 340 vets had completed the courses qualifying them to hold official veterinary surgeon (OVS) appointments in poultry processing plants (the fact that such courses were necessary might have been taken by EHOs as support for their anti-vet stance). Although there were some problems in establishing uniform standards of inspection in different local authorities, this was addressed by consultation between the BVA, the EHOs and the British Poultry Federation.[24]

While some sort of concord on poultry meat hygiene had been achieved, the disagreement on responsibilities for red meat inspection rumbled on. In 1978, a new minister of agriculture, John Silkin, speaking at the BVA congress at Lancaster, said that when he became minister he had immediately been confronted with differing opinions as to who should do what in meat hygiene. He felt the three disciplines involved (vets, EHOs and meat inspectors) could do more to improve meat hygiene if they pulled together. Accordingly, he had set up a meat hygiene working group with the aim of improving the relationship between the three disciplines and their contacts with government departments.

Silkin emphasised that the government had no intention of changing existing food hygiene arrangements for British meat plants whose output was entirely for the domestic British market. But for export-approved slaughterhouses the government took a pragmatic view that it must 'satisfy the requirements of the customer'. Other member states and most countries outside the European Community required that slaughterhouses exporting to them should be under continuing veterinary supervision. 'We cannot afford to put at risk our considerable export trade in meat by failing to satisfy that requirement,' he said

The requirements of the EEC rather than the wishes of the BVA continued to direct the government's slow acceptance of the need to bring UK meat hygiene services into line with those of the rest of the Community. Two years later, another Minister of Agriculture, this time the Conservative Peter Walker, made a statement in the House of Commons, following discussions with representatives of the EHOA and the BVA, about their respective roles in meat hygiene. The minister said he wished to secure recognition in Brussels that EHOs as well as vets were qualified to carry out supervision and provide public health certification of meat products under the directives on intra-community trade. He also aimed to gain similar recognition in relation to supervision and certification in poultry cutting premises and cold stores. The meat would 'in all cases have been produced in accordance with the relevant directive in a slaughterhouse under veterinary supervision and the EHOs would be designated by the minister, who would have to be satisfied as to their qualifications'. The criteria for being satisfied were not specified.

From the BVA's point of view, there was better news in the case of red meat export slaughterhouses. Work was continuing on the preparation of regulations which would require EC standards for intra-community trade; these included a requirement for veterinary supervision to be maintained at all times. Local authorities would be responsible for the maintenance of such standards and for the appointment of official veterinary surgeons but MAFF would be responsible for the approval of export abattoirs and the maintenance of the national standard.

But there was no such requirement for those red meat slaughterhouses which operated solely for the home market. Although the BVA had reasserted its view that in the longer term there should be a centralised MAFF-administered meat hygiene service, the minister confirmed that the government had no intention of altering the existing arrangements, by which the enforcement and the execution of legislation on slaughterhouse hygiene and meat inspection would remain a local authority function, which was what the EHOs wanted. Their entrenched view was that there should be a minimum of legislation, and associated added cost, in the process of meat hygiene.

It remained the government's policy to oppose any EC proposal to extend veterinary involvement in those duties which were the responsibility of EHOs beyond the poultry meat or red meat export slaughterhouses. It remained convinced, apparently, that a policy of minimum interference with the legislation was in the majority interest; it was certainly to the meat industry's financial advantage. The only crumb thrown to the Association was the statement that further discussions would be held with the BVA and EVHOA on those matters.[25]

A hard-bargaining meeting between the two associations and the minister brought agreement by the BVA to accept that 'suitably qualified' EHOs should be able to carry out the inspection and certification of meat products for intra-Community trade, subject to 'certain provisions'. In return, the EHOA would support the red meat export regulations that required the full-time veterinary supervision of export slaughterhouses. At a further meeting between MAFF, the BVA, the EHOA and the Association of Meat Inspectors, it was suggested by the ministry that the three latter bodies should jointly draw up codes of practice; the BVA welcomed the proposal.

Although the abattoir owners, through their representative body, the Association of British Abattoir Owners, could see advantages in full-time veterinary supervision, they were concerned about the financial consequences if they had to pay for supervision by both vets and other local authority officials. It was noted that the UK was the only country in the EEC where the processor was expected to pay for the meat inspection service.[26]

TOWARDS A CENTRALISED SERVICE

It was not until 1984 that the government decided it would pay for veterinary inspection in abattoirs producing meat for export. The meat trade had always resented this addition to their costs which was felt to give their Continental competitors, where such charges were met by governments, an unfair advantage; the Minister of Agriculture said the new scheme would apply to the costs of employing vets for supervisory duties in export approved red meat slaughterhouses and cutting (i.e. butchering) plants, cold stores and in export approved poultry slaughterhouses and cutting plants. The scheme would apply both where it was carried out by official veterinary surgeons appointed by local authorities and by local veterinary inspectors appointed by MAFF. The cost was estimated at about £2.5 million a year. This was an exceptional measure, the minister emphasised, and in no way prejudiced the general principle that costs of meat inspection would be charged to the industry.[27]

The slow progress towards introducing full veterinary supervision of meat inspection for the domestic market received some advancement on 5 February 1988, when regulations bringing procedures for post-mortem inspection for red meat were brought into line with those for export to EEC countries. However, the real breakthrough, so far as the BVA was concerned, came with the announcement by the agriculture minister, by then John Gummer, on 9 March 1992 that he had agreed that a central service was the best option for implementing EU meat hygiene legislation. The service would be an agency of MAFF, accountable to ministers. He said that MAFF would be working closely with local authority associations and organisations representing the veterinary profession, environmental health officers and meat inspectors to ensure a smooth transition to the new arrangements.[28]

Commenting on the decision the *Record* recalled that as long ago as 1903 the then National Veterinary Association passed a resolution that: 'The members of the NVA, recognising that the sanitary supervision of the meat and milk supplies is of vital importance to the health of the general public are of the opinion that the time has now arrived when such supervision should be conducted on uniform and scientific lines, under the direction of a national board having at its head a responsible minister of public health and on its permanent staff expert medical and veterinary surgeons.'

At last, it continued, it looked as if one of the main aspects of that resolution – that the government should set up some form of centralised meat hygiene service – was about to be realised. The setting up of an independent agency to form the service was the preferred option of the

BVA; for one thing, it would do away with the piecemeal nature of individual local authorities. The fact that the government had also planned for an agency structure was cause for some satisfaction within the Association.[29] That decision was not, however, the first choice of every group consulted on the issue; unsurprisingly, the Institute of Environmental Health Officers was among the bodies opposing a centralised service.

Already at that time a number of veterinary practices were negotiating for contracts to carry out veterinary duties in connection with meat inspection; some of those contracts were, it was said, being tendered for at rates as low as £6.50 an hour.[30] However, a BVA survey indicated that the average hourly rate for such work was £25.70 which was close to the government agreed LVI rate for meat hygiene, roughly £26 per hour.[31]

The chief veterinary officer, Keith Meldrum, said that the veterinary input into the new meat hygiene service would be substantial. Until the centralised service was established it was anticipated that practising vets would largely fulfil the demand. Meldrum hoped that when the centralised service was fully operational more vets could be employed full-time but that there would still be a need for a substantial input from practitioners.[32]

Progress towards the promised goal of a fully centralised service was not to be without snags. In June 1993 MAFF, concerned about the costs of the improved meat inspection service, imposed a cap on charges. A limit of £40 was set for the first four livestock units – animals, in common parlance – presented for inspection on the same location and £6.30 for each additional unit presented with the first four. That maximum had to cover the cost of all the duties chargeable to the abattoir operators carried out by local authorities and slaughterhouses. Those included ante mortem inspection, taking of samples, health marking and local authority costs.[33]

MAFF acknowledged that the new pricing arrangement might cause difficulties in low throughput slaughterhouses. The ministry suggested that costs might be contained by controlling slaughter times in order to restrict attendance times, renegotiating official veterinary surgeon and meat inspector contracts and employing local large animal practitioners and 'retired vets' to carry out ante-mortem inspections or 'in exceptional cases' – the ministry's words – relying on meat inspectors to perform the initial ante-mortem inspection. It added that local authorities would have to take account of the veterinary surgeon's professional opinion in determining the appropriate level of attendance.

Given the financial pressures, it was questionable how much notice local authorities would take of that opinion, commented the *Record*. From the point of view of public health it was essential that veterinary attendance was at a sufficiently high level. If savings had to be made in the meat hygiene service it was administrative costs that should be curtailed, it maintained.[34]

There was vociferous opposition to the veterinary position on meat hygiene (and, indeed to a national meat hygiene service) from meat producers, because of perceived additional costs, and from EHOs concerned for their status. The Association's position was set out in a letter from the president, Francis Anthony, to the Minister of Agriculture. There was now a new incumbent in post, Gillian Shepherd, and Anthony was concerned to set out the situation, as he saw it, to the new minister. He pointed out that a long standing decline in the number of abattoirs was an occurrence caused by market trends rather than meat hygiene regulations. Ninety per cent of the national kill was processed by 20 per cent of abattoirs. There was potential for rationalisation of procedures and improvements in efficiency and economy.

The opponents of the current proposals had had 'such an impact' because neither MAFF nor, presumably, the BVA itself, had been successful in putting over the case for veterinary involvement in meat hygiene. Anthony found it necessary to explain to the new minister that the official veterinary surgeon (OVS) was not a meat inspector but the supervisor responsible for maintaining quality, with an input into the management of the plant. They were leaders of the team, organising and supervising, training and maintaining the competence of the meat inspectorate; it was they who had to take responsibility if anything went wrong. And much of what was planned in England and Wales was already in place in Scotland and Northern Ireland.

It is not known whether the minister took much account of Anthony's lesson but the introduction of the national Meat Hygiene Service (MHS) went ahead on 1 April 1995. Vets would be central to the new arrangements either as employees or as official veterinary surgeons employed on a contractual basis. As well as advertising for permanent staff, MAFF had written to all veterinary practices asking them to indicate whether they would be interested in tendering for contractual work. The BVA was concerned about that move, continuing its objections to tendering. It queried whether appointing OVSs on the basis of competitive tendering was the best way to proceed. Tendering might be appropriate for large projects, it commented, but many of the OVS contracts amounted to only a few hours a week. It argued that it would be better to set a realistic fee for the work rather than have the appointments based on tendering.[35]

In spite of its reservations about the process the BVA had drawn up guidelines for vets who wished to tender for the provision of meat hygiene services. It noted that it was government policy to require tendering when contracting services out and the BVA sought to provide the best advice possible in the circumstances.[36] The tendering process itself was not clear cut. The BVA president, now Paul DeVile, said it was regrettable that the invitations to tender provided inadequate information of the plants for which the tenders were invited. He advised members proposing to submit tenders to visit the plant concerned, to make their own assessment of the standard to which it was operating and the likely OVS input required. They should, advised DeVile, generally evaluate for themselves how the plant was run before compiling a tender.[37]

By the time the initial contracts expired in 1996, two events had occurred that threw into greater prominence the vital need for an efficient meat hygiene service. One was the bovine spongiform encephalopathy (BSE) crisis, which had greatly increased the pressures on the system even before the revelation in 1996 that human cases of Creutzfeld-Jakob disease had their origin in BSE-infected meat. The other was an outbreak of food poisoning in Lanarkshire caused by meat products infected by *Eschericia coli*: some 400 people were made ill and twenty died.

Public concern about the incidents led to government action to raise standards of meat inspection and staffing levels of the MHS. Douglas Hogg, the Minister of Agriculture, told Parliament that new contracts for official veterinary surgeons would ensure sufficient time was spent at each plant. Four hundred and fifty additional staff (not all vets) had been appointed to the hygiene service. Former health minister, Dr Gavin Strang, criticising the government's past record in relation to meat hygiene and veterinary supervision, said that the number of vets employed by the State Veterinary Service had fallen in the previous three years from just under 600 to 289.[38]

When the BVA council discussed the tendering operation for the new contracts on 9 April the veterinary head of operations for the MHS, Peter Soul, addressed the meeting. He emphasised that it was government policy that the contracts had to be allocated by tender. When some members of council expressed concern that tenders were being awarded on the basis of cost to the neglect of other factors they were assured that it was not the case that the cheapest bid was always a successful one. Another criticism was about the number of foreign graduates being employed by the MHS. This was, perhaps, less a criticism of the quality of overseas vets than the UK profession guarding its territory. Past president Howard Hellig (himself South African trained) pointed out that, for example, Spanish veterinarians could spend three years out of their five-year course specialising in meat hygiene. Council member John Williams said that while the Yorkshire division had been critical of it in the past their criticisms had been taken very seriously by the BVA and they were now broadly satisfied with the tendering process.[39]

It is interesting that the decision to put out contract work for meat hygiene services to tendering, although not welcomed, did not cause the adverse reaction which the proposals to introduce that procedure for LVI work had brought in the 1980s, nor the difficulties caused when DEFRA proposed in 2010 that some other official veterinary work should be allocated on the basis of tendering. The RCVS had taken the view that when tendering for the MHS was originally introduced, the treatment of live animals was not involved so there was no conflict with its professional guidance.

Finally, in 2010, the Meat Hygiene Service was absorbed into the Food Standards Agency. At that time the service employed, full-time, twenty-one official veterinary surgeons and had under contract, as OVSs or LVIs, 292 vets. So the BVA's aim for a national, veterinary-supervised meat hygiene service had, eventually, been achieved – but not, perhaps, in quite the manner it had anticipated. Rather than an integral part of many practices, meat hygiene veterinary services were in the hands of relatively few firms specialising in the work. And the OVS personnel employed were to a large extent those trained in EC countries. Most English vets had little interest in meat hygiene and public health work, in spite of the importance of those aspects of food production in an age when zoonoses and new strains of microorganisms pose a major risk to health.[40]

CHAPTER THIRTEEN

DISEASE CONTROL

From its very foundation, the BVA and its members have been closely involved with official schemes to control diseases, particularly those affecting farm livestock. While this volume is a history of the BVA and not an account of animal diseases in the UK, the one cannot be told without some reference to the other. Diseases such as foot-and-mouth disease and BSE which created massive social and economic perturbations are dealt with in the context in which they occur. Bovine tuberculosis, an ongoing and intractable problem, is described here. Other diseases which proved more amenable to eradication on a less devastating scale, are dealt with below.

TUBERCULOSIS, BOVINE AND HUMAN

The continuing prevalence of bovine tuberculosis with its threat to human as well as animal health was a matter of great concern to the entire profession. The programme of the 1925 annual meeting at Cambridge included a paper on the reintroduction of the 1914 Tuberculosis Order (which had been suspended on the outbreak of war) and recent legislation on food inspection. The Order said that where human infection was suspected as a consequence of animal infection the 'consultant in public health medicine' – unspecified, but usually a medical practitioner – had to be informed. The reintroduction of the Tuberculosis Order came in response to rising concerns about quality of milk and its potential for the spread of TB to the human population. During the inter-war period various groups such as the National Association for the Prevention of Tuberculosis lobbied the government to take action against the disease and ensure a pure supply of milk.[1]

J. W. Brittlebank, who was chief veterinary officer for Manchester, said that to keep the Tuberculosis Order, with its 'restrictive provisions' for controlling the disease by testing and isolating infected cattle, was 'however limited, better than doing nothing'.[2] At the 1925 congress, Arthur Gofton, Brittlebank's opposite number in Edinburgh, welcomed the introduction of the Milk and Dairies Acts which would, at long last, 'accord the veterinary officer a definite place in the public health machine in which he is peculiarly fitted to render service to the community' by his role in milk and dairy inspection. These measures specified that to qualify as producers of Grade A (TT) milk, cows had to undergo the tuberculin test, performed by a veterinary surgeon, twice yearly and reactors removed from the herd. Compensation was paid for cattle slaughtered because of tuberculous udders, those which were emaciated and those suffering from 'TB cough'.[3]

The commercial production of tuberculin, an extract of *Mycobacterium tuberculosis*, was pioneered in the UK by Sir John McFadyean, principal of the Royal Veterinary College 1894–1927. Although a valuable diagnostic tool, its unregulated production had led to accusations by the NVMA of a 'far reaching system of fraud in its use'.[4] During 1928 representations were made by the Association to the Ministry of Agriculture and the Ministry of Health urging that the distribution and use of tuberculin should be controlled and its distribution should be limited to the veterinary and medical professions. However, 'no replies have yet been received'.[5]

The general concern about the risk to the bovine population of human tuberculosis is perhaps indicated by the fact that during the 1927 NVMA conference a lecture for the general public on the prevention of tuberculosis in animals was given by McFadyean.[6] Control of the disease remained problematic throughout the inter war years. Efforts by the Ministries of Agriculture and Health to protect the interests of their respective constituencies (the producer and the public) led to much wrangling over milk pasteurisation, while the depressed state of the economy prevented any concerted efforts to tackle the disease in cows.[7]It was not until 1935, with the introduction of the Therapeutic Substances Act, that a degree of standardisation was introduced. At the same time, a voluntary herd testing scheme was launched, testing was made compulsory in 1950 and the production of tuberculin purified protein derivative (PPD) established. The tuberculin test, also known as the Mantoux test, is still used both in human and bovine patients.

Nevertheless, the growth of attested herds, and the gradual improvement in the health status of cattle through the herd testing scheme meant that the United Kingdom, since the 1950s, had enjoyed the status of being officially free from bovine tuberculosis. However, localised pockets of the disease continued to occur, particularly in parts of the West Country and Wales, and in the 1970s, the incidence of outbreaks was increasing. By 1980 there was growing concern over the possible involvement of badgers in the spread of tuberculosis infection among cattle. This led the government to commission a report on the problem from Lord Zuckerman, a former chief scientific adviser. His report recommended the selective culling of badgers in areas of high incidence of bovine TB, a proposal that aroused strong opposition. The subject of badger culling was controversial at the time, and remains so.

The BVA supported the badger cull in the following terms:

'The British Veterinary Association endorses the findings and recommendations of the Zuckermann Report on Badgers and TB. We regret the continued unconstructive criticism of those who will not accept the findings of the report and its endorsement by MAFF. We believe the tubercular badger population is a major reservoir of bovine TB in those localities

which satisfy the stringent conditions imposed by MAFF before
badger gassing is instigated. We challenge those who dispute
the findings of the report to provide acceptable alternative
scientific evidence for their case and to suggest alternative
strategies for the control of TB in cattle and badgers in the
interests of the health and welfare of cattle, badgers and man.'

The Association was quick to support the decision to
stop the killing of badgers by gassing with hydrogen
cyanide, a method then used, on welfare grounds.[8]

The Zuckerman report was but the first of a series of
investigations, trials and recommendations which continued
to seek solutions to the problem – so far without success.
The next investigation was by the scientific review group on
bovine tuberculosis in cattle and badgers chaired by
Professor John Krebs, in 1997. The Krebs report
recommended that culling of badgers to control tuberculosis
in cattle should end in most parts of the country and be
replaced by husbandry methods aimed at reducing the risk
of infection. In areas where bovine TB was endemic,
however, it was recommended that experiments should be
set up to assess the impact of different badger culling
strategies; these should include the culling of lactating
female badgers.[9]

The BVA was disappointed that Krebs's recommendations did not suggest an immediate solution to the problem
of bovine TB. With the disease firmly established in the
south-west and apparently spreading to the north and east
the situation was urgent. The Association believed that the
balance needed to be redressed by the next investigation, by
an expert group set up to oversee the experiments suggested
by Krebs. It was critical that this group, to be chaired by
Professor John Bourne, did not include a vet with practical
experience of the disease.

Krebs had acknowledged that infected badgers were a
cause of infection in herds and the Association feared that,
given that badger removal operations would be confined to
only twenty 10 km x 10 km areas during the course of the
experiment, the disease would continue to spread. The BVA
was concerned also that the report placed relatively little

emphasis on the growing problem the disease was creating for cattle farmers. It pointed out that the goodwill and cooperation of farmers would be essential to the effectiveness of the trials. If there was any non-compliance by farmers in those areas included in the trials the validity of the experiment would collapse. It concluded: 'The expert group will face a daunting task in attempting to obtain meaningful data while trying to ensure that the disease is contained.'[10]

The House of Commons agriculture committee on badgers and TB noted the difficulties of dealing with a problem where so many different interests were involved. It was critical of delays in implementing some of the recommendations in the Krebs report. While the committee emphasised the urgency of the need to find a solution to the problem of bovine TB it was disappointed that, having drawn attention to the fact that the culling trial might take five or perhaps seven years to complete, Krebs had not provided much in the way of practical suggestions as to what might be done to ameliorate the problem in the meantime.[11]

Investigations by Bourne's independent review group into this ongoing disease dragged on for over nine years from its establishment in 1998, during which period it produced five reports. One of its first recommendations was that randomised badger culling trials should be introduced. These began in six areas where there was a high incidence of tuberculosis in cattle; the trials were intended to answer questions about the contribution of badgers to bovine TB infection and whether proactive or reactive culling strategies would result in a significant reduction in the incidence of such infection; whether other badger control strategies (such as maintaining badger populations below a certain threshold) could be used effectively; and whether such strategies would be cost-effective. Other areas of investigation would seek to determine whether modifications could be made to farm management practices that would reduce the transmission of tuberculosis to cattle.[12]

The BVA responded to the setting up of the Bourne investigations in a letter from the president, Ted Chandler. While the Association was pleased that an epidemiological study was, at last, to be set up, the Association still had serious concerns about the disease and its control. The proposed study, Chandler pointed out, would take between six and seven years to complete; analysis of the results and implementation of the control policy would occupy a further period. Meanwhile, the spread of the disease was likely to continue to have devastating effects on the value and health status of the UK cattle population. Farmers would suffer further losses to their livelihood. The Association argued that action should be taken in new and existing disease areas not included in the trial. It asked the government to carry out testing and movement control of cattle herds together with a total cull of badgers in those areas. The principle of culling for disease control in specified areas had been established for many years and had been effective in controlling and eliminating disease and maintaining a high health status of British livestock, it pointed out. Chandler concluded: 'We must not allow the tuberculosis problem to escalate into another disaster.'[13]

In due course, an audit panel chaired by Professor Charles Godfrey was set up to review the progress of the randomised badger culling trial. It reported in 2004 that, while more evidence on the precise role the badgers played in the spreading of bovine TB was strongly desirable, it believed that the weight of evidence currently justified making the assumption that badgers did indeed play a role. But the culling trials had been suspended by the independent scientific group which was overseeing the trial. It now agreed that the trial had been suspended prematurely because the sequence of events and analyses leading to the suspension had not been fully understood by the review group.[14]

Bourne's group published its fourth report in February 2005. It drew attention to difficulties and delays in implementing the results of the survey held five years previously. He blamed the government (i.e. DEFRA) for a situation which had led to 'an unfortunate waste of resources' and had resulted in a lost possibility for his independent scientific group to carry out a robust enough analysis to 'more usefully inform interim control policies'. For its part, DEFRA pointed out that dealing with the massively devastating foot-and-mouth disease outbreaks in 2001 had absorbed nearly all the resources of the State Veterinary Service.

Bourne's group discussed the shortcomings of the tuberculin skin test for diagnosing TB in individual cattle and said that the development of improved diagnostic techniques was a priority. As far as badger culling was concerned they concluded that there was convincing evidence that reactive culling of badgers did 'not offer a beneficial effect large enough to make it useful as a practical policy option'. In fact, there was 'substantial but not overwhelming' evidence of an adverse effect. However, the effect of proactive badger culling in the control of cattle TB had still to be determined.[15]

Then, on 1 March 2005, the government published a new strategy for cattle TB control. The *Record* commented that to describe the strategy as 'new' might be to overstate the case. Like the animal health and welfare strategy, of which the TB strategy would form part, the government's policy document was 'strong on aspirations but weak in terms of how they would be met'.[16] The BVA president Dr Bob McCracken welcomed the strategy's commitment to developing a stronger regional approach. He said the current bovine TB control programme had been ineffective in reducing the incidence of the disease in 'hotspot' areas and in preventing its spread from those areas. Vets had no doubt that specific control policies needed to be tailored to reflect regional variations in disease risk.

McCracken also welcomed the government's acknowledgement of the role that vets had in delivering effective surveillance for bovine TB and control, and in testing, as well as in offering essential advice to farmers. But he noted that the viability of farm animal practice in many parts of the country 'remained perilous'. The government itself had pointed out in that in some areas of the country bovine TB testing, and the income it generated played a significant role in maintaining the presence of large animal practices. In view of that acknowledgement of the vets' professional and financial stake in the testing procedure, the BVA, he said, was at a loss to see how it equated with the view that legal recognition of lay TB testers might provide a more flexible and larger pool of testing personnel.[17]

The BVA stuck to its view that there was sound scientific evidence that the infected badger was a major source of TB for uninfected cattle. It also believed that eradication and more effective control could not be achieved without addressing the infected badger reservoir. The Association felt 'the veterinary and farming professions had a responsibility to ensure that the government addressed the problem in an effective manner'.[18]

Bourne's report and the resulting government response brought 'incredulity and disappointment' among vets in those parts of the country – mainly the West Country – most heavily affected by bovine TB. Some 400 of them had written to the Secretary of State requesting action – 'action that must address the serious disease situation in the badger'. A group of eight West Country practitioners, writing from the heart of the TB-affected districts, said that over many years the role of the badger as a maintenance host for bovine TB, and the effect this disease was having on the badgers themselves, had been recognised. Culling of infected badger communities was, said the vets, unfortunately necessary to stop the 'remorseless spread' of TB. They urged wide scale field trials of badger vaccination to protect the species as far as possible. The alternative would be 'to continue with the current policy and watch the problem become completely out of control'. The policy advocated by Bourne's independent scientific group, that of control measures directed against cattle alone, was 'certain to fail'. The vets who signed the letter to the Secretary of State expressed no confidence in the 'hopelessly flawed' Krebs trials. They believed that results were likely to be both inconclusive and unreliable despite an expenditure of £31 million.[19]

The letter produced a response from Bourne and his group reiterating their opinion that cattle-based control measures, if more rigorously applied, could be expected to reduce the incidence of TB, whether or not badgers were culled. The argument between Bourne's group and the practitioners continued in the pages of the *Record* with both sides maintaining their respective positions.

While the pro- and anti- badger culling supporters continued their debate, a paper published in *Nature* said that movements of cattle from infected areas were the dominant factor in introducing bovine TB in new areas. By analysing data in the cattle tracking system archive of the British cattle movement service, the authors had found that recording movements of cattle from infected areas was the best main predictor of TB occurrence. The study was 'equivocal' in the role of badgers in the epidemiology of the disease incidence.[20] Another paper stated that badger culling reduced the incidence of TB in the areas where culling took place but increased it in adjoining areas.[21]

A policy of pre-movement testing of cattle (testing cattle for TB before they could be moved from the farm on which they were based) was recommended in 2005 by a DEFRA-sponsored group including BVA and farming interests. The recommendation was accepted and testing began to be introduced the following year.[22] For its part, the BVA urged the more rapid implementation of the scheme – even though such testing was only 'one tool in our armoury for the control of bovine TB'. This would, of course, mean more work for practitioners; the Association used the opportunity to advocate revised fees for the local veterinary inspectors who would carry out the tests.[23]

The final report of the Bourne group contained the perhaps puzzling statement that 'badgers are clearly a source of bovine tuberculosis but culling can make no meaningful contribution' to control of the problem. The group advocated a policy of vaccination, once vaccines became available, but commented that there was no evidence that the government had a plan for how it was going to implement such a measure. It also pointed out that current controls on cattle were not stringent enough.[24]

The bovine TB problem proved intractable. The opponents of badger culling still denied its role in spreading disease: cattle-to-cattle transmission had been under-estimated compared with transmission from badgers, they argued, and produced evidence in support of their case.[25] By 2010, the disease was costing the UK £87 million a year.[26] The Minister of Agriculture, Jim Paice, admitted that the approach to the disease so far had failed. In the South West of England over 14 per cent of herds were under movement restriction.

Farmers in affected areas would be given licences to cull badgers and to vaccinate them – at their own expense – and a new policy for controlling TB would be developed in consultation with stakeholders. The BVA welcomed the minister's 'across the board' approach to the TB question and, in due course, made its own response to the consultation. And no one disagreed with Paice's possibly exasperated comment on the situation: 'We can't go on like this.'[27]

AUJESZKY'S DISEASE ERADICATION; A CASE HISTORY

In 1983, MAFF decided to introduce a scheme to eradicate Aujeszky's disease in pigs. Also known as pseudorabies, Aujeszky's disease is so called after the Hungarian vet who first identified the condition and the virus responsible, *Suid herpesvirus 1.* The disease is a seriously debilitating viral infection, with profound economic consequences for the pig industry. At the time, Aujeszky's disease had been diagnosed in 224 herds spread across twenty counties in England and Wales, accounting for 300,000 pigs. The infected herds were mainly located in East Anglia, Humberside and north Yorkshire.

The disease was first recorded in Britain in 1953, in pigs in Somerset. By 1974 it had become endemic among swine herds in north Suffolk, followed by widening incidence in other areas including Yorkshire by 1982. Meanwhile, a working party had been set up by MAFF to ascertain the true incidence of the disease, and whether eradication was feasible and cost-effective. The working party, set up in 1975 and reporting in 1980, confirmed the latter points and strongly recommended immediate implementation of an eradication policy while the incidence of Aujeszky's was still low. Further, it was predicted that if eradication was not introduced, the disease would escalate.[28] The working party's recommendations (supported by the BVA) were rejected by MAFF: it was judged to be 'politically unacceptable'.

Pressure from elements in the farming industry and the Association for a control scheme continued: the disease was made notifiable in 1979 and, in 1980, pig producers were told a slaughter policy would be introduced, provided the producers themselves agreed to pay for it. In spite of a poll showing a majority in favour of such a scheme, the policy was not taken up by government. However, lobbying from industry and the BVA resulted in a second poll of producers, in 1982. The vote in favour of eradication was even more positive – 85 per cent in favour – and this time the government agreed to introduce eradication.[29]

When Howard Rees, chief veterinary officer, announced details of the eradication campaign on 4 March of that year he said it would be a unique operation. It would be the first time that the industry involved would be contributing towards the cost of a health programme by providing compensation to farmers whose pig herds were slaughtered. This set an important precedent: previous official schemes for disease compensation had been funded by the state. The money would be raised by a levy on slaughtered pigs of 30 pence a head. It was also the first time many of the animals killed in an eradication campaign would be salvaged for human consumption, thereby offsetting to some extent the cost of compensation.[30]

Although favouring the scheme, which it had been advocating for some years, the Association pointed out that its implementation would not be without problems. The campaign was to be controlled by the State Veterinary Service, which proposed to use lay personnel in the blood testing procedures involved. The BVA was unhappy about that proposal, as it always was at suggestions of lay involvement in activities seen as a vet's prerogative. Terry Heard, the BVA negotiator on the scheme, pointed out that the blood testing of pigs was an involved procedure – and as half the adult breeding stock of each herd would need to be tested it was likely to be a slow process. The use of lay staff, it was argued, might prove 'contentious' not only because local practitioners would wish to do the work themselves but also because 'many of the herds to be tested would be of high health status' and veterinary practitioners might not be happy that they should be subjected to lay – that is, non-veterinary – tests. That argument was not pursued.

Another reason for the initial concerns among LVIs was that the scheme was driven by the pig farming industry and supported by MAFF, rather than the other way round, as had been the case with previous eradication schemes. It seemed that, as had been the case when vets had wanted the support of advertisers to promote certain animal medicines, the profession wanted someone else – in this case the government – to take the initiative. Historically, vets had relied on government support in dealing with farmers' major (i.e. officially notifiable) disease problems. The Aujeszky's scheme represented a unique shift in the *modus operandi* between farmers and the veterinary profession.

There were, too, doubts about the ability of the State Veterinary Service, which was suffering one of its periodic shortages of staff, to cope with the eradication scheme. In the House of Commons on 17 February 1983, MP Tom Torney asked whether the minister of agriculture was satisfied that SVS resources were sufficient to implement the control programme. The parliamentary secretary, Mrs Peggy Fenner, sidestepped the question, saying that the government intended to support the eradication policy fully through the State Veterinary Service.[31]

However, once operational the scheme soon earned the positive support of the practitioners, who agreed the scheme's test and slaughter technique could be successful. The initial requirement to sample the blood of every pig was modified to a test (using virus neutralisation, latex agglutination or ELISA) on a statistical sample of animals – about thirty-five per herd. A side benefit was that the blood tests brought the vet on to the farms, giving the opportunity to offer additional advice on the herds.[32]

Although a target of six months had been set in which the operation should be completed, it was recognised that the herpesvirus causing Aujeszky's disease was a 'difficult' virus and it would not be until the a year or two had passed before it was known if total eradication would be possible or whether the pig industry would ultimately have to settle for a control policy instead.[33]

In a progress report in June, it was announced that while the first phase of the eradication scheme (herds diagnosed after 2 May 1982) had been completed and the second phase (herds infected between August 1979 and May 1982) was proceeding satisfactorily, many more herds not previously thought to have been infected had been picked up. The original figure of 224 herds was likely to be exceeded by quite a large margin.[34] Then concerns began to be felt that the costs of the scheme, administered by a company specially setup for the purpose, the Pig Disease Eradication Fund (PDEF), were exceeding the income from the levy of 30p a head. Valuations of pigs sent for slaughter may have been 'overgenerous'.[35]

By June 1985, charges of mismanagement of the scheme by MAFF had been made. They were rejected by the then minister, Michael Jopling. Ministry officials commented on a lack of complete information about the incidence and location of the disease and the impossibility of making firm estimates of costs. While the government regretted that expenditure had been substantially greater than anticipated, they said, the scheme had been undertaken on the understanding that the industry would bear the costs of compensation and related expenses. The PDEF said it was 'extremely disappointed by the minister's refusal to make any further contribution to the Aujeszky's disease scheme'.

The fund's overdraft was £13.8 million; producers had paid £8.3 million towards the cost of the scheme.[36]

Commenting on the situation, the *Record* said: 'What the Aujeszky's exercise does perhaps indicate is that when it comes to protecting the health of the nation's livestock against potentially crippling endemic disease, short term economic factors should not be allowed to predominate. It may also indicate that if the government and [pig] industry had responded a decade earlier when the BVA first called for Aujeszky's disease to be eradicated, the exercise would have been completed more quickly and at much less cost.'[37]

By 1987 it was reported that 'encouraging progress' had been made in eradicating Aujeszky's disease in Britain. Following a meeting between the MAFF parliamentary secretary Donald Thompson and the chairman of the PDEF it was agreed that the compulsory slaughter programme had greatly reduced disease outbreaks, although it was still too early to predict when the disease would be finally eradicated.[38]

In late March 1989 the first outbreaks of Aujeszky's disease for thirteen months were reported; one in Devon and two, linked, outbreaks in Norfolk.[39] Those were the last cases before the UK was declared officially free from the disease in 1991. The 'six months' estimate had become six years and the costs, £28 million, had exceeded estimates. But if eradication had not been introduced, it is estimated the cost of Aujeszky's disease would have exceeded £95 million. Importantly, the scheme had demonstrated a successful collaboration between MAFF, the veterinary profession and the pig industry.

NEWCASTLE DISEASE

By the 1960s, poultry meat was no longer a once a week treat for the family; chicken had become a routine staple of the diet. Consequently, the rapid expansion of flocks from farmyard hen runs to industrial levels of poultry production to satisfy the demands of the consumer brought a renewed focus on poultry health. This, in turn, necessitated an unprecedented amount of veterinary involvement in health maintenance and disease eradication schemes for the vast numbers of housed poultry involved. Large producers appointed their own veterinary advisers.

Newcastle disease (fowl pest), an official 'notifiable disease' was a recurrent scourge of the industry. Caused by a paramoxyvirus, it can result in breathing problems, diarrhoea, loss of egg production and death. In 1962 a government inquiry, to which the BVA provided evidence,[40] looked at the situation and made recommendations which accepted many of the Association's suggestions. A policy of slaughter of infected flocks and attempted eradication proved unworkable because of the scale of the problem and the expense incurred.

The chief veterinary officer, A. G. Beynon (then the Association's president), told the 1962 congress that the government had decided that a policy of vaccination was to replace one of slaughter. MAFF was to arrange a subsidised supply of vaccine to farmers; at that time, the vaccine would have to be administered individually to each bird. Beynon told the congress that it had been said with some justification that the veterinary profession had neglected the poultry industry in the past: 'Here is a new chance in the control of a major disease which should frequently bring the practising veterinary surgeon to apply his experience and competence in dealing with flock problems,' he said. The BVA arranged courses on poultry diseases to prepare members for the anticipated demand.[41] The programme was effective but the laborious process of individual vaccination was replaced by the use of live vaccines administered by aerosol or in the birds' drinking water.

The supply of subsidised vaccines ended in March 1964 but the sales through normal commercial channels actually increased, demonstrating that the vaccination programme had proved its economic effectiveness.[42] Since then, only sporadic outbreaks had occurred.[43]

BRUCELLOSIS

Brucellosis, a cause of contagious abortion in cattle and sheep (among other species), was finally eradicated in 1981. The practical possibility of eradication of this destructive disease, responsible for losses in livestock production and the cause of undulant fever in man, was established in 1944 when *Brucella abortus* Strain 19 vaccine became available; a government subsidised calf vaccination scheme was introduced in the same year.[44] This live vaccine was the basis of attempts to limit brucellosis for the next thirty-five years. Free vaccination of calves was introduced in 1962 to control the disease and control was expanded to encompass eradication when the Brucellosis (Accredited Herds) Scheme was introduced in 1967. This enabled the establishment of brucella-free ('accredited') herds which in turn led to the introduction of a policy of slaughter (with compensation) and replacement with disease-free stock when eradication areas were introduced in 1971. Areas which had been disease free, defined as a 'breakdown' rate of less than 0.5 per cent for at least two years, were designated 'attested' areas. With the declaration of the first attested areas in 1979, eradication was nearing completion; this was attained in 1981.[45]

The use of Strain 19 vaccine was supplemented in 1976 by a killed vaccine, Strain 45/20. The new vaccine did not, however, entirely supplant Strain 19, although an effective replacement had been sought for some time as many vets suffered years of ill health after contracting undulant fever from accidental contact with the live product. When the risks of human infection from the vaccine were realised, there were moves to have brucellosis classified as an industrial injury for those handling livestock. In 1976, the BVA organised a seminar on the hazards arising from unsafe handling of S19 vaccine[46] at which it became apparent that those administering the inoculation often ignored the most elementary hygienic precautions.

Eventually, human brucellosis became a disease reportable under the Zoonosis Order 1989 and entitling the sufferer to Industrial Disease Disablement Benefit.

Completion of the brucellosis eradication scheme was a tremendous step forward in the health and productivity of cattle, with concomitant benefits for public health. But ending of routine testing added to the problems of many veterinarians with farm practices. There were not a few of those in areas of low livestock density whose economic viability depended on the financial input from LVI work. Loss of that work made it more difficult to provide the 'fire brigade' veterinary service at an economic level acceptable to both farmer and practitioner. But equally importantly, the eradication schemes provided for subsidised farm visits which were often the occasion for further consultation and advice; and, of course, veterinary surveillance. How to maintain this watchdog capability, which required regular attendance on the farm, would cause increasing concern as farm practices became fewer over the ensuing years.

BSE: A DEVASTATING NEW DISEASE

In the 1980s reports of odd behaviour in cattle noted by veterinary surgeons were picked up by the veterinary investigation centres. By 1988 it was clear that there was a widespread disease problem developing. The new disease was bovine spongiform encephalopathy (BSE). This was to become a major long-standing problem with devastating implications for the British beef industry – and for public health.

As the incidence of BSE increased, concern grew. In June 1988 A. H. Andrews suggested that the disease should be made notifiable; he also suggested that its transmission seemed to have been by ingestion.[47] Almost as if acting on Andrews's prompting, BSE was made notifiable. The Order enacting this also imposed a ban on cattle rations containing animal protein (specified bovine offal) following an investigation 'which suggests an environmental agent as well as some genetic factor' was involved.

The Association used the occasion to emphasise its advocation of an effective State Veterinary Service. The arrival of BSE, it argued, highlighted yet again the vital importance of the 'state veterinary investigation service in leading and coordinating the nationwide collaboration of effort that is necessary for a satisfactory solution to the problem of BSE'.[48]

A whole new dimension was added to the already serious problem when on 20 March 1996 the Health Secretary, Stephen Dorrell, announced that a new form of Creutzfeld-Jakob disease, a spongiform encephalopathy found in people who habitually eat sheep brains, had been identified in ten individuals who had recently died. Suddenly, the official policies, which maintained that it was impossible for BSE-contaminated food to cause the disease in humans, were no longer to be trusted. The well-publicised 1990 incident when the agriculture minister, John Gummer, fed his young daughter a beef burger to demonstrate the product's safety from BSE was seen to have been a serious error of judgement. Decisions said to have been made on a sound scientific basis were found to have been misrepresented.[49]

The announcement brought the British beef industry to a standstill. A total ban on the export of British beef and beef products was imposed. There were panic reactions. The most likely explanation for the new disease was that cases in humans were linked to exposure to BSE before control of specified bovine offal (virtually all non-meat products such as thymus, kidney, lung, etc.) to prevent BSE-contaminated meat from entering the food chain had been announced in 1989. From that date the use of meat and bone meal from mammals had been banned from incorporation in animal feeds.

As always happens in a massive disease outbreak, the veterinary profession was thrust into the limelight. The BVA council meeting on 10 April 1990 was entirely devoted to a discussion of the BSE crisis. The president, Bob Stevenson, said that in the past month he and other BVA spokesmen had given more than 100 press, radio and television interviews and the Association's staff had dealt with three times that number of inquiries and press briefings. There had been several meetings with MAFF and more would be held when the ministry had developed a plan for dealing with BSE to present to the European Commission.

The president of the RCVS, Des Thompson, said it was essential that the veterinary profession should speak with one voice when dealing with BSE and by a joint decision the BVA was leading on the subject. The profession, he said, had a major role to play in restoring public confidence in the proper resourcing and adequate supervision of the meat hygiene service. But the problem was not only a British one; it involved the whole of Europe

Seventy per cent of British dairy cattle were in infected herds and a mass slaughter campaign would decimate the dairy industry. Those who had suggested wholesale slaughter as a solution were said to have misunderstood how the disease worked. On the other hand, more than three-quarters of dedicated beef herds were unaffected by BSE (as they had not been fed potentially infected rations). Although there was pressure from farmers with dedicated beef herds to establish a BSE-free herd policy, that was opposed by the Association's specialist division, the British Cattle Veterinary Association, on the grounds that it would be impossible to enforce.

As a result of the BSE crisis, however, the concept of health control 'from birth to table', based on positive identification and tracking of animals throughout their lives, would, it was felt, become a reality.[50] And the government decided to reinforce the Meat Hygiene Service to ensure that identification and inspection services were fully effective. The agriculture minister, Douglas Hogg, on 4 April 1990 acknowledged in the House of Commons that the Meat Hygiene Service had a crucial part to play in action against BSE.

While the BVA would have accepted a carefully targeted cull of British cattle it maintained its fundamental opposition to the mass slaughter of cattle, as had been suggested: Identification, eradication, protection and authentication should be the cornerstones of any policy to eradicate BSE in beef herds, said Stevenson. 'Proper, foolproof, identification of animals is now here to stay and we should get on with it.' He emphasised that the 'absolute control for the protection of public health … was at the abattoir. There could be no excuse whatever to downgrade inspection and veterinary supervision in all abattoirs.'[51] With the introduction of the Cattle Identification Regulations 1998 on 15 April of that year, identification of livestock and lifetime tracking of their location, and dealing with the bureaucracy involved, became an essential part of the farming industry.

By 1997, BSE had cost the country £2.5 billion – and that was not the end of the matter. The official inquiry into the disease noted that more than 170,000 cattle had died or been destroyed in the epidemic, for which the intensive farming practice of recycling animal protein into ruminant feed was blamed. That practice, unchallenged over decades, proved a recipe for disaster, said the inquiry's report, which ran to 16 volumes.[52] But, said the report, 'the government did not lie to the public about BSE'. It had believed the risk posed to humans was remote and did not want to cause 'alarmist over-reaction'. Consequently, when the 1996 announcement was made, that BSE had probably been transmitted to humans, the public felt that they had been betrayed. Confidence in government pronouncements was a casualty.

The ramifications of the disease would be felt for years; they led to permanent changes in attitudes to food health and safety. An important one was the setting up of the Food Standards Agency, following a report by Professor Phillip James in 1997. The agency, a non-ministerial government department established in 2000, was charged with responsibility for food safety and hygiene across the UK.

Although the BVA was consulted on the report, it was disappointed that the veterinary profession's part in the production of safe food was largely ignored in its proposals. Its main reaction was to complain of the lack of emphasis on the importance of veterinary surveillance in maintaining disease prevention.[53] Although there was little official Association comment, the vital part the practising arm of the profession had played in identifying and reporting the disease was integral in its eventual successful outcome.

CHAPTER FOURTEEN

VETERINARY PHARMACEUTICAL PRODUCTS

The post-war decades saw a tremendous surge in the output of the veterinary medicines industry, from £2.3 million in 1948 to £42.7 million in 1968.[1] Vaccines against the common sheep diseases, novel anthelmintic formulations to control parasitic worms, and, particularly, the advent of potent antibiotics had revolutionised the conventional prescribing habits of many vets. Under the 1947 Penicillin Act, and the 'ethical' agreement forged between pharmaceutical companies and the BVA, farmers could only purchase antibiotics (except those used as feed additives) and certain vaccines and sera through their vets. Additional controls over drug licensing were introduced by the Medicines Commission, set up under the 1968 Medicines Act. Nevertheless, there was mounting concern about the increasingly extensive use of antibiotics in agriculture, and its potential implications for the public's health.[2] This matter was investigated by a government-appointed committee chaired by University of Bristol vice-chancellor, Professor Swann.[3] Its report concluded that the administration of antibiotics to farm livestock, particularly at sub-therapeutic levels, posed 'certain hazards' to human and animal health. Enteric bacteria of animal origin had developed resistance to antibiotics, which was transmissible to other bacteria that infected animals and man. To manage this problem, stricter controls on the inclusion of antibiotics in animal feed were required.

The Association issued a statement on 'Antibiotics in animal feedingstuffs' in 1971[4] which reflected its views on how the Swann committee's recommendations should be implemented. The statement said that a written order for medicated feed must be supplied by the veterinarian and should apply to specified animals under the vet's care; each order should be used once only. The BVA's statement closely matched the wording in subsequent legislation under amendments to the Therapeutic Substances Act 1956. This action by the Association was the start of its increasing involvement with medicines legislation and the provision of information and courses to help ensure the correct handling of animal medicines.

In 1973, the Medicines Commission set out its proposals for regulating the sale and distribution of veterinary medicines. It proposed the creation of three categories of control: a general sale list for veterinary medicines (GSL) available for purchase by anyone; a list of prescription-only medicines (POM) restricted to veterinary surgeons (and doctors and dentists; and on prescription, by pharmacists); and a third category for the retail sale of certain veterinary medicines to farmers, which would be subject to some control by being sold only through licensed outlets; this became the pharmacy and merchants list (PML), or 'farmers list'.

It was the last of those that caused concern to the Association and the RCVS. They set up a joint working party to consider the matter. While accepting that farmers had to be able to buy freely animal medicines that were 'safe' and could be used without veterinary diagnosis, it believed that the proposed 'farmers list' [PML] contained veterinary medicines that were unsuitable for general sale. These included oestrogen implants, many vaccines, anthelmintics and coccidiostats. 'Protracted negotiations' gave hope, albeit slender, that the profession's views would be considered. But the Commission's final proposals were – from the profession's perspective – even worse than its original ones. Further evidence was submitted in support of the veterinary case, without success. According to the profession's working party, this 'very serious state of affairs ... seems to show that commercial interests have prevailed'.[5] The *Record* commented that the BVA's 1971 statement, which aimed to bring antibiotics under effective professional control, and offer proper service to the farmer and protect the public, had been reduced by the Commission to a derisory level. There would be no control over merchants (including market traders and van salesmen) – and the opportunity to develop a model for European Community legislation had been lost.[6]

Meanwhile, legal restrictions on the use of therapeutic antibiotics were evaded regularly by farmers, who used them as a cure-all, unaware of the risk of creating antibiotic-resistant bacteria. The BVA cooperated with the Royal Pharmaceutical Society (responsible for policing illegal sales) in combating the problem. One difficulty in bringing successful prosecutions was the reluctance of vets to give evidence against clients whom they knew had been buying in the black market. An article by the Society's law department published in the *Record* included the statement: 'Experience shows that the casual attitude toward therapeutic substances by farmers who buy them ... is a result of the casual way in which some veterinary surgeons have acted when supplying antibiotics.'[7] The problem of illegal sales of antibiotics did not diminish. Six years later, infection by resistant bacteria, linked to illegal sales of antimicrobials, was reported as the cause of death in calves. The *Record* commented that the case reported was only one instance of 'what is increasingly clear is a large scale black market'.[8]

ANIMAL MEDICINES AND ADVERTISING

While veterinary concerns about antibiotics focused on their overuse, they were also concerned about farmers' underuse of less conventional drugs, which pharmaceutical companies released onto the market in the 1970s. These fell into a category defined by vets as 'management tools' – drugs 'used to modify [an animal's] physiological function as an aid to animal husbandry'. One example was prostaglandin, which could be used to control ovulation and therefore fertility, as an aid to breeding and livestock management. As prescription only medicines (POMs), such products were normally advertised and promoted only to the profession. Some practitioners believed that if, instead, they were promoted directly to clients, demand would increase, making it easier for the vet to introduce them in practice.

The BVA general purposes committee accordingly recommended that 'management tool' drugs such as prostaglandins should be allowed to be advertised in the farming press, 'as requests for their use normally came from the farmer, who must be made aware of their existence'.[9] At its next meeting the committee reaffirmed this decision. Advertising would ensure that farmers were aware that such aids were available with veterinary advice.[10] However, at the subsequent council meeting the recommendation was rejected by a large majority after such members as Alastair Steele-Bodger argued very strongly that it was up to the veterinary surgeon to educate the farmer about the potential of new medical products, not the lay press.[11]

The matter did not end there. After a long debate at its June 1978 meeting, council reversed its earlier decision and voted to accept advertising in the lay press of 'prescription only' animal medicines used as 'management tools'. It should be the responsibility of the government's Veterinary Products Committee (VPC) to decide which drugs fell into this category. In proposing the motion, council member James Allcock argued that management tools (such as worming remedies) 'were already being advertised and no one was suffering as a result'.[12] The Association, or at least its council, would come to regret that decision.

The VPC duly recommended that under the Medicines (Advertising of Veterinary Drugs) Regulations, which set out controls on their authorisation, manufacture and advertising, the promotion of certain 'management tool' drugs would be allowed [to lay persons]. They included antisera, antitoxins and vaccines; substances for the control of ovulation (e.g. prostaglandins); vitamin and mineral substances for administration by injection; coccidiostats; implants to improve beef production (growth promoters); and calcium borogluconate injection against–milk fever.[13] One consequence, of course, not mentioned in the debate, was that the advertising for those products, gained by the lay press, would be lost to the *Record.*

The pharmaceutical industry – which had always played a role in educating veterinary clients about drug applications – needed little encouragement to take advantage of the BVA's relaxed attitude to the direct promotion of medicines to the farmer. By March 1982 the *Record* was asking: Are the drug companies advertising too widely to the client? It recalled that that when the BVA council gave its blessing to their advertising, it had believed that farmers needed to be informed about the applications and usefulness of new drugs used in the management of healthy animals as opposed to treatment when sick. The majority view was that it was helpful for veterinarians to have the ground prepared for them so that when such matters came to be discussed the farmer was acquainted with them. Now, however, vets felt that the original concept of management tool advertising had become distorted. The definition of a management tool drug was being widened to cover any veterinary therapeutic product. Anthelmintics were advertised not only in the farming press but on television.. The widening of media promotion had also spread to small animal products, with dog and cat vaccines advertised in the lay press. The result was that vets could be pressured by clients to prescribe what they had seen advertised rather than what might be most effective in dealing with a specific health or management problem. While legally there was nothing to stop pharmaceutical companies from advertising to farmers, the *Record* argued that they should not do so to the extent that the profession was hampered in the execution of its duty.[14]

The Yorkshire Veterinary Society called on the Association to reconsider its attitude towards advertising. Although it had originally supported advertisements in the lay press, it felt that the 'abuse of such advertising by some companies' was pressurizing farmers to use a specific prescription-only product, 'which might not be the appropriate one in the case'. It asked BVA council to resolve: 'That the BVA is opposed to the advertising of named POM products in the lay press.'[15] There was a long discussion at the meeting on 10 March 1982, at which most speakers were in favour of seeking a ban on POM advertising. However, it was not clear that the BVA had any authority to impose one; advertising to the public of 'professional' products supplied on medical prescription was not permitted by the National Health Service and there seemed to be a tacit assumption by the pharmaceutical manufacturers (the Association of the British Pharmaceutical Industry) that a similar ruling applied to 'ethical' animal medicines.

The honorary secretary, James Allcock, again opposed any restriction on advertising. He said that practitioners should have the confidence to deal with clients who demanded particular products. Allcock maintained that many owners of small animals did not have a regular vet and relied on advertising for their information on what was available. Although, on this occasion, his forceful advocacy won the argument,[16] the matter continued to rankle. Another motion opposing lay advertising was promoted at the March 1983 meeting of council by the Midwest Veterinary Association. Past president John Tandy felt that rather than trying to seek official regulation of such advertising they should try to persuade the Association of British Pharmaceutical Industry to ask its members to refrain from advertising antibiotics in the lay press. However, this view was not widely supported, and the Midwest's motion was carried 'almost unanimously': advertising of veterinary POMs should be banned.[17] The motion had no effect whatever: the stable door might be closed but the horse was gone.

It was eventually decided to set up a working party to review the whole matter of how animal medicines should be sold. Subsequently the matter was allowed to drop; the anti-advertisement lobby was overwhelmed by the tide of promotional activity from the pharmaceutical industry, and in the free-market, consumerist context of the 1980s, its desire to regulate industry practices was clearly swimming against the tide. The matter resurfaced briefly in 2010 when the BVA supported a move by the Veterinary Medicines Directorate to remove permission for antimicrobials to be advertised to farmers, on the grounds that advertising was a potential obstacle to their responsible use. The proposal, not surprisingly, was strongly resisted by the farming community and, of course, the agricultural press which gained substantial revenue from antimicrobials advertising. The resulting pressure on ministers caused the proposal to be dropped.[18]

MEDICINES SUPPLY INVESTIGATION

One of the reasons why the profession was keen to control drug sales, and to promote the use of new drugs was that practising vets were heavily reliant on the income that resulted. In spite of repeated urgings from vets such as Alastair Steele-Bodger, who felt that fees should be the basis of practice income, it was common custom to use the mark-up on medicines to subsidise a low fee structure. Consequently, the announcement on 9 October 2001, that the Office of Fair Trading was to investigate the supply of prescription-only veterinary medicines (POMs), caused some consternation at the BVA. The president, Andrew Scott, said, perhaps mildly in the circumstances, that the timing of the announcement was 'somewhat strange, given that the government had yet to respond to the report of its own independent review group on [veterinary] dispensing'.

Scott was referring to the report of the group, chaired by Sir John Marsh, on the dispensing of medicines by veterinary surgeons, published in May of that year. Marsh had made comprehensive recommendations affecting all aspects of animal medicine supply by vets and other sources, including the issue of prescriptions to clients for dispensing elsewhere (including by pharmacists), the keeping of records, and continuing professional development for the practising veterinarian. It even urged the adoption of improved business practices.[19]

This new investigation was to be weightier, and carried out by the Competition Commission after referral by the Office of Fair Trading (OFT). The market in veterinary prescription medicines was worth £200 million a year; the OFT asked the commission to examine evidence that prices of such medicines in the UK were substantially higher than in other European countries. There was also concern about a 'lack of transparency' in prices: medicines were often dispensed in the course of treatment and might not be itemised and charged for separately. Further, according to the OFT, there was a reluctance by some manufacturers to supply veterinary medicines to pharmacies; increased supply through pharmacies, it was believed, would allow price competition.

The Veterinary Medicines Directorate had briefed the review group, noting that the use of animal antibiotics had fallen in Denmark after vets had been restricted from dispensing except in emergency. It also pointed out that price differentials between UK and other EU countries might encourage the (illegal) import of unauthorised medicines (in fact, illegal imports from Ireland and elsewhere were a continuing problem).[20]

The Competition Commission found that there was indeed a complex monopoly situation existing in relation to the supply of veterinary prescription medicines; the chain of supply not only involved vets, but also manufacturers and wholesalers. The main factors creating this 'inter-related complex monopoly' included 'one or more' of the following practices: failure to tell clients that they could ask for prescriptions, or discouraging or refusing requests for them; or charging excessive prices to provide them; not telling clients of the price of prescription medicines before dispensing them; pricing them in a way that did not reflect the price the practice had paid; and pricing medicines so as to subsidise professional fees. Manufacturers, for their part, were said to operate rebate schemes that made it difficult for the vet to know precisely what they were paying. They were also criticised for refusing to supply pharmacies or to do so on terms that enabled them to compete with vets.[21]

The final report, when it appeared in April 2003, confirmed those conclusions and also made recommendations on the regulation and supply of veterinary medicines intended to make them more generally available. The BVA was deeply antagonistic to the proposals, so far as they affected veterinary practice. The president, Peter Jinman, accused the commission of failing to understand how veterinary practice worked. He said the recommendations appeared to undermine everything that had been done to put in place a system that ensured the responsible use of veterinary medicines. The BVA was particularly concerned that 'competition theory should not be prejudicial to animal health and welfare and public health.' The Association, he said, would respond vigorously to the commission's report. 'What we are dispensing are medicines – biologically active substances – not, as some of the recommendations might lead one to believe, sweets.'

The *Record* commented that in its zeal to increase competition in the supply of veterinary medicines the commission had overlooked the 'totality' of the medicines regulatory and supply chain. It seemed to neglect the fact that, overall, the effect of the measures it proposed would be to increase the cost of treating animals[22] because fees charged to clients would have to increase to replace the income lost from the sale of medicines. The government, on the other hand, in the shape of agriculture minister Elliott Morley, welcomed the report. It would, he hoped, lead to improvements in the regulation of medicines. DEFRA would carefully consider the recommendations.[23]

Of the many recommendations, the one that seemed to rankle most with practitioners was that prescriptions should, for an initial period, be offered free of charge to clients so that they could, if they chose, have the medicines dispensed elsewhere. Andrew Scott, in his presidential address to the 2002 congress, argued for the advantages of the existing situation where vets themselves supplied the products they prescribed. 'If this one-stop service is efficient, and diagnosis and dispensing are taken together, there must be a sound economic benefit for the client.'[24] The same argument (with the omission of the 'economic' factor, as the NHS was the paymaster) had succeeded in the case of some dispensing doctors in rural areas when the right of NHS physicians to dispense their own prescriptions had been removed. A telling factor in that case had been that delegating dispensing to pharmacists interposed an independent check between prescriber and patient.

And not all vets were against a move to pharmacists dispensing their prescriptions. One, J. S. Brodie, wrote: 'It is very comforting as a practitioner to know that you have a well qualified expert dispensing the medicines you have prescribed, allowing you to concentrate on clinical issues and the prescribing process.' Brodie's practice was, however, not typical: it operated a registered pharmacy.[25]

Even a government body, DEFRA, in its evidence to the commission, had expressed concern that its recommendations should not affect the viability of rural practice.[26] Although the BVA was, of course, overwhelmingly concerned with those recommendations that directly affected its members, other measures, such as revising existing regulations so as to make more widely available some products such as flea killers, were more likely to be of immediate relevance to members of the public.[27]

While the existence of a black market in illegally imported medicines was widely acknowledged as already affecting the vets' sales, what had not been foreseen was the emergence of a 'gray' market: the availability of drugs via the internet. The internet pharmacy, which could often supply medicines more cheaply than other sources, was one factor that persuaded some clients to ask for veterinary prescriptions. Some, particularly those whose animals were on long-term medication, tended to shop around for their medicines. They were usually pet owners whose cat or dog was on long term medication.[28]

ADVERTISING VETERINARY SERVICES

In the late twentieth and early twenty-first centuries, controversy surrounding the advertising and sale of veterinary medicines extended also to the advertising of vets and their services. Traditionally, veterinary advertising had been strictly regulated by the Royal College through its Guide to Professional Conduct. In the 1960s, the official advice was that the only form of publicity allowed to a practice was the name and qualifications of a veterinary surgeon on a plaque of specified size (about 8 inches by 10 inches) affixed to the front of the practice premises. Such restrictions reflected the College's views of the sorts of behaviour and ethical standards expected of professional – as opposed to commercial – enterprises.[29] Those who did not comply risked being struck from the RCVS register.

This restriction had been the subject of complaints from practitioners for many years; the animal charities' free veterinary clinics were not so constrained.[30] One young vet from St Helens, John Tandy, had established a new practice in 1961 and invested in fitting it out to a high standard. Tandy was one of those vets determined to modernise his profession. He had been greatly influenced by a visit to the United States, where he saw veterinary practice premises equipped to offer standards of service far in advance of what was generally available in Britain at the time.[31]

Tandy's premises were entered from a side street and a plaque by the door would not have been visible to passers-by. Tandy therefore put up a modest sign facing the main road with the name of the practice, illuminated so as to be visible to the passing public. He wrote to the Royal College enclosing a photograph of the sign and its location. The College called him down to London and told him that what he had done was not acceptable and suggested amendments, to include illumination no greater that that given by a 40 watt bulb and letters no more than two inches high. Tandy argued his case and, eventually, the objection was withdrawn. But there was further trouble with the RCVS when Tandy produced an illustrated brochure describing the facilities of his practice. The brochure was intended for distribution to the practice's clients; the text would have been acceptable but the College objected that the brochure might be seen by people who were not existing clients and thus constituted unacceptable advertising: again, the objection was eventually withdrawn.[32]A 1976 report by the Monopolies Commission spelt an end to such disputes. One of a raft of government-commissioned enquiries into the professions, it recommended that vets should be allowed to advertise in any way they chose, and to canvass for custom if they so wished. There were some provisos: no publicity should claim superiority over other veterinary practices; it should not contain any inaccuracies; it should not include claims to specialisation in particular areas of veterinary treatment except where the vet's academic qualifications justified the claim; and it should not be of a character likely to bring the profession into disrepute.[33] The *Record* commented that the actual form of the new advertising rules would be decided after discussions between the profession and the authorities under the Fair Trading Act. What would ultimately emerge, it pointed out, 'may be something not vastly different . . . from the type of media advertising now permitted'.[34]

Following the Monopolies Commission report the RCVS issued a statement on veterinary practice titles and names for practice premises.[35]

The RCVS summed up its guidance in a leading article:

'Aren't you Jones, the Blanktown vet?'
'Well, I'm Jones, I am a veterinary surgeon and I do practice in Blanktown. But I must not be known as the Blanktown vet because that would create an invidious distinction between my practice and that of any other veterinary surgeons in the town.'
'I thought yours was the only practice in Blanktown'
'Well it is – at the present time, anyway. But there may be more than one practice at some time in the future and a title

including the name of the town might give the impression that one practice was pre-eminent; it would not be acceptable to the Royal College.'

'What do you do, then, if your partners wanted to carry on the practice after you've retired? They can't use your name indefinitely, can they?'

'No, they can't. What we can do is to decide on a neutral name – perhaps that of the house the practice is sited in – and call it the High Oaks Veterinary Clinic or some other name. The Royal College would accept that. We could keep the title "practice" in the name by using a description such as the Beech Crescent Veterinary Practice, for example.'

'What do you do if another veterinary practice sets up in Beech Crescent?'

'Ah . . .'[36]

In fact, the majority of the profession was firmly against any liberalisation of the rules governing advertising by individual veterinary surgeons. It was agreed not to pursue proposals to allow individual practice advertising in local newspapers. It was also confirmed that the Association was not in favour of practices being allowed to state which species they did or did not normally deal with.[37]

The Office of Fair Trading (OFT), the government department charged with implementing the Monopolies Commission recommendations, thought that was nowhere near good enough. It sent a letter to the Royal College asking it to conform to *all* the recommendations on advertising of the Monopolies Commission as they had been set out in 1976. Council was deeply divided as to the best course of action. In the event council member Henry Carter moved a resolution that: 'This council accepts the principle that veterinary surgeons should be allowed to advertise subject to certain restraints.' The motion was carried by 18 votes to 15. The BVA council discussed this outcome at its meeting later that month. There was not a single voice raised in favour of advertising. On the contrary, many spoke of their unhappiness at the prospect. Paradoxically, however, on a show of hands a substantial majority supported the resolution. It was felt that, as one member put it, that the change had to be accepted; otherwise worse changes would be forced upon them.[38]

The profession was supported in its opposition to canvassing by the knowledge that both the Law Society and the Institute of Chartered Accountants also viewed the practice as objectionable and not a proper way to make known the availability of professional services. The OFT argued that there was a distinction between canvassing by personal telephone approaches on the one hand, and the distribution of leaflets and written material on the other; they suggested that the latter need not be an objectionable form of approach. The College countered that once one departed from strict adherence to the principle it became increasingly difficult to draw a line and accordingly it stood fast against canvassing in any form. There was not a single voice raised in favour of advertising.

The Association discussed the advertising quandary in more detail at its next meeting. The president, Trevor Blackburn, noted that the OFT Minister, Alex Fletcher, had indicated that advertising by radio and television, canvassing and advertising of fees should all be permitted. Members urged both the Royal College and the BVA in dealing with the OFT to press for the 'best possible settlement for the benefit of the public, the profession and the animals for which they all cared'. Several members said that while some advertising was acceptable they were 'appalled' at the suggestion that they should advertise fees and that there should be any form of canvassing. Bernard Wells warned that 'as time went on things changed'. He noted that very recently two vets had been taken to court for charging 'unreasonable' fees. Legal experts had, he said, advised the profession to display its fees as a defence against the charge of unreasonable fees. The president reiterated the view of the Royal College: 'One thing was sure; that was, that the recommendations of the Monopolies Commission were going to be implemented in one form or another; and if they were going to be forced on the profession, they would prefer to have some say in it.'

Eventually, a motion proposed by Nigel Snodgrass to the effect that the BVA supported the RCVS position, i.e. that advertising on television and radio would be tolerated, but they were strongly opposed to the advertising of fees and canvassing, was carried without dissent. On a show of hands not a single member of the College was in favour of TV and radio advertising, endorsing the Association's view.[39]

Nevertheless, the OFT continued to press for acceptance of advertising of competitive fees and canvassing. They had emphasised this point at a meeting with the Royal College in which BVA president Trevor Blackburn had also been involved. The veterinary side pointed out why fee advertising would be very difficult without there being any danger of the public being misled: the fee had to take into account such factors as the health, weight and age of an individual animal and other factors in relation to a flock or herd as well as the complexity of the particular procedure. The director-general, Sir Gordon Borrie, and the Minister, Alex Fletcher, had apparently appreciated this but made the point that ranges of fees might be suggested. The College view was that the preferable approach would be that a practice should indicate that it would always be prepared to make a preliminary assessment of the likely cost of the procedure or service based on the facts of the particular case. The profession was supported in its opposition to canvassing by the knowledge that both the Law Society and the Institute of Chartered Accountants also viewed the practice as objectionable and not a proper way to make known the availability of professional services.

The OFT argued that there was a distinction between canvassing by personal telephone approaches on the one hand and the distribution of leaflets and written material on the other; they suggested that the latter need not be an objectionable form of approach. The College countered that once one departed from strict adherence to the principle it became increasingly difficult to draw a line and accordingly it stood fast against canvassing in any form.[40] The British Veterinary Association fully supported that stand, believing that to give way to all the OFT's demands would be inimical to the interests of animal patients, which was the profession's prime concern.[41]

The OFT finally agreed to accept the profession's decision not to approve the advertising of fees or canvassing. It appreciated that the College had significantly changed its position, as represented by a new code of advertising practice and the revision of the Guide to Professional Conduct. However, it expected the profession to keep the matter under review and re-examine the issue in two years.[42] The Association, in a *Record* comment, expressed relief that the long drawn out negotiations on advertising of veterinary professional services had at last reached a reasonable conclusion – some eight years since the matter had been first referred to the Monopolies Commission. It believed that each side in the negotiations could take some satisfaction in the outcome The OFT had gained acceptance of the principle of advertising and had seen the RCVS and the BVA accept most of the practical points it had urged upon the profession. The profession, as the reluctant partner in the discussions, retained some control over professional advertising and would be able to prevent excesses. But at the end of the day no one would be compelled to advertise and how many would take advantage of the situation remained to be seen.[43]

Initially, there was a very cautious response to the freedom to advertise. However, the BVA sought to seize the initiative by investigating the possibility of having professionally designed advertisement layouts to which practice names and addresses could be added made available for use in local newspapers. It also participated in roadshow meetings with farmers 'up and down the country' at which the benefits deriving from utilisation of veterinary advice were discussed in practical terms. In addition, it helped to develop a new publication for practice clients, *You and Your Vet*.[44] This popular magazine-style presentation, was designed to educate clients about looking after their pets and inform them about the services available from their veterinary practice.

Chapter 14

THE QUESTION OF GENDER

In addition to these changes imposed from without, the profession was also changing within, a result of a radical shift in its gender balance. At the turn of the nineteenth century, the notion that women had a place in the veterinary profession was widely resisted. According to one correspondent in the *Veterinary Record*:

> Veterinary surgery is of all learned professions the one least adapted for women . . . even if the female practitioner were to confine herself entirely to canine and feline practice, yet she is bound to meet with certain operations in the pursuit of her calling which must be utterly repugnant to anyone possessing what is the greatest charm of any true woman, namely, modesty.
>
> No lady (using the word in its true sense) would like to perform those operations which are the almost daily work of the veterinary practitioner, especially when we take into consideration the fact that male assistance in securing the patient is practically indispensable.
>
> Of course, if a woman is prepared to unsex herself completely and to throw to the four winds all feelings of modesty and delicacy there is no reason why she should not become a successful practitioner of veterinary surgery even among the larger animals; but all who know what the nature of veterinary practices is will, I am sure, agree that unless prepared to do this no woman can hope to practice with any degree of pleasure, to say nothing of success.
>
> Another point which from a business point of view women would do well to consider, is this. Whether the general public would place confidence sufficient in them to employ them to such an extent as to make the profession a remunerative one to them.[45]

It was not until twenty-five years later that Aileen Cust, the first woman to be officially recognised as a vet in Britain, won her battle to become registered as MRCVS. She had

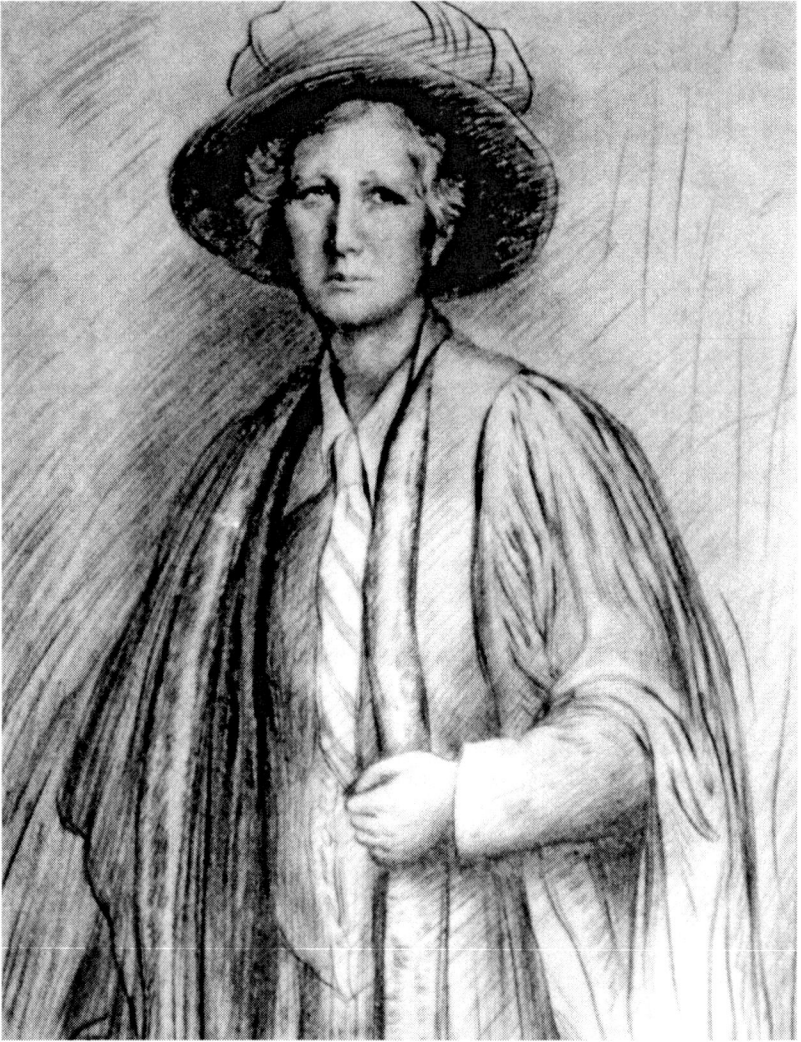

Figure 18. Aileen Cust, the first woman to be become a Member of the Royal College of Veterinary Surgeons in 1922, and of the NVMA, 1923.

actually been practising, mainly in Ireland, after successfully completing a course at the New Veterinary College, Edinburgh, in 1900. Cust was also one of the very first women to become a member of the NVMA, enrolling in 1923.

Her admittance resulted from the Sex Disqualification (Removal) Act 1919 which forced the professions to open their doors to women. The veterinary profession was one of the last to do so, over forty years after human medicine had taken a similar step.[46] One of the few RCVS council members in the 1920s who supported the admittance of women was Major Frederick Hobday. When he became principal of the Royal Veterinary College in 1927, he encouraged the enrolment of women students. One former student reckoned that part of Hobday's motive was that the publicity generated by such an unusual occurrence as a female veterinary student helped raise funds for the cash-strapped RVC.[47]

Once the College had, with reluctance, accepted the valid claims of females to be allowed to practise, more veterinary schools opened their doors to women. By 1934, of the UK veterinary colleges then in existence (the RVC in London, Glasgow, Liverpool, and 'The Dick' in Edinburgh), only Edinburgh still refused to enrol women.[48] A possibly apocryphal story once current in the after-hours chat in the Association members' room concerns a complaint made by an old-fashioned vet to the principal of a veterinary school that had decided to admit women. The vet said that letting women in would deprive men of jobs. 'Not at all,' replied the principal. 'Women only work a short time before retiring to have a family; besides, a man would always be hired in preference to a woman.'

The new generation of women vets soon began to take a full part in the affairs of the Association, participating in its debates and filling leading roles on its committees. By 1934, at which time there were still only about thirty female vets, the *Veterinary Record* was able to devote most of one issue to a seminar, 'Women in the Profession' held by the Central Veterinary Society. Three papers and thirteen short communications were presented by women, with a memoir by Aileen Cust herself.[49]

Those early female veterinarians did, however, face prejudice from a considerable minority of male practitioners. Some had to pay large premiums to obtain places to 'see practice' with established vets. And rates of pay for female assistants were often lower than those for male colleagues.[50] That situation was the norm for very many years: a survey by the Society of Practising Veterinary Surgeons in 1993 found a similar situation among young graduates.[51]

Women vets in those days had to be rather special to make their mark. And among their small number were some who became important figures in the profession. One of those was Olga (later Dame Olga) Uvarov, who qualified in 1934. She came of a distinguished Russian family dispossessed during the 1917 Bolshevik revolution –.she recalled: 'We set off in a coach with four horses; we ended up trudging through the snow.' Both parents died; her father was shot. An undernourished Olga, aged seven, labelled 'Orphan Uvarov', eventually arrived in London, one of a group rescued from a refugee camp by an American benefactor. She was taken into the home of her uncle, Dr Boris Uvarov, a distinguished entomologist who was working at the Natural History Museum. A love of animals, nurtured in the scientific background of her new home, directed Olga Uvarov towards a veterinary career.

After qualifying, she opened a practice; twenty successful years later she joined the pharmaceutical industry – a career move previously unheard of for a woman – with Glaxo Animal Health, a major manufacturer of animal medicines. She eventually rose to head the firm's veterinary advisory department, becoming widely known throughout the profession. A prominent member of the Association's council, Olga was a notably effective contributor to discussions; fellow members soon learned to be sure of their facts if they challenged her in debate. Upon retirement from Glaxo, she joined the BVA staff as technical information officer. She later became a member of the government's Veterinary Products Committee, secretary of the Research Defence Society and president of the Royal Society of Medicine's section of comparative medicine. At the same time she devoted more time to veterinary politics and in 1976 became the first woman president of the RCVS. A keen intellect complemented by an aristocratic elegance enabled

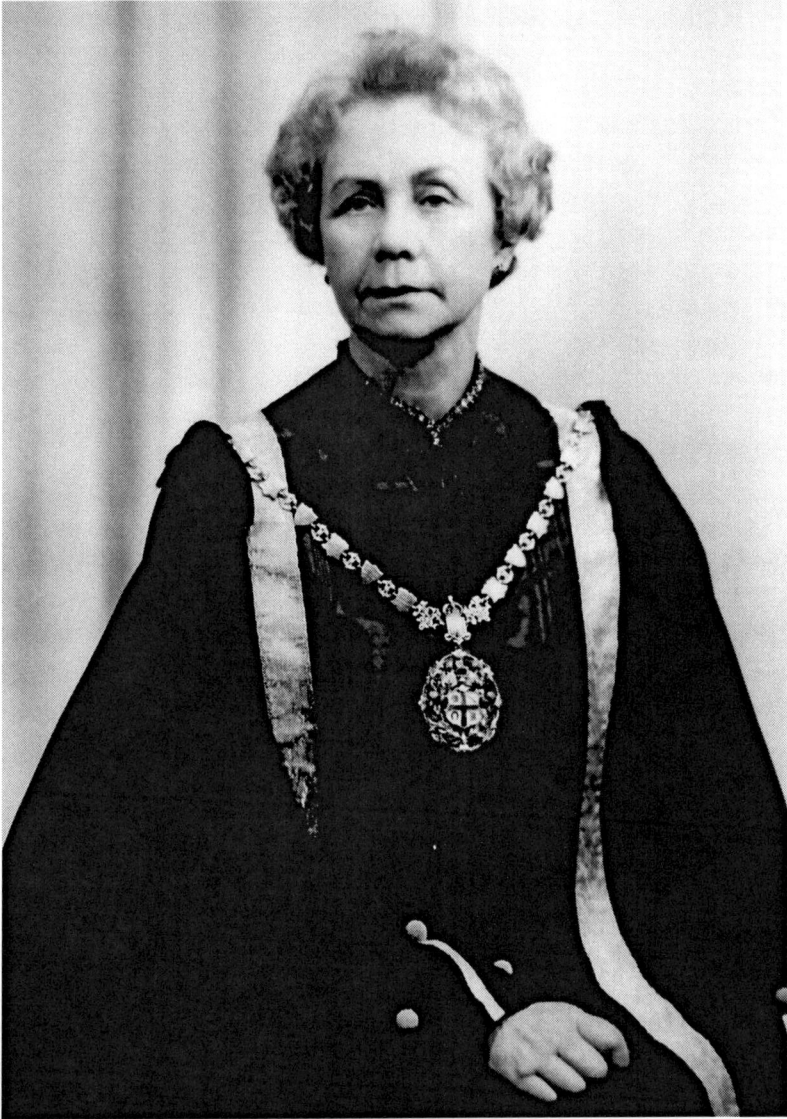

Figure 19. Dame Olga Uvarov, in 1976 the first female president of the RCVS; she was a prominent member of the BVA council, the first woman to have been head of a pharmaceutical company's veterinary advisory department, and a member of the government's Veterinary Products Committee.

her to bring considerable distinction to the presidential chair. Olga Uvarov was appointed DBE in 1983.[52]

Slightly younger than Uvarov, Mary Brancker qualified, also from the RVC, in 1937. She then joined the Lichfield practice of that remarkable man, Harry Steele-Bodger. There, as has been recounted earlier, she was soon thrust into the centre of veterinary politics. Her clarity of expression, easy self confidence and engaging personality, not to mention hard work and acute political awareness, made her many friends among the profession and outside it. A member of BVA council since 1952, she combined running a busy mixed practice with an increasing involvement in the Association's affairs. Then, in 1967, she became the BVA's first female president. She was to be the sole woman to hold that office for almost 40 years.

A year after Mary Brancker, Joan Joshua qualified. She was another doughty champion of the rights of women vets. Coming from an impecunious background, her first battle was to find the funds to support her studies. As a new, young veterinary surgeon she set herself up in practice in her mother's front room. Limited facilities did not hinder her scientific investigations, inspired by the patients she treated. One such study led to her becoming the first woman Fellow of the RCVS in 1950.

In 1941, Joshua was one of the founders, and the first president, of the Society of Women Veterinary Surgeons; Mary Brancker was among the other founder members.[53] As a division of the Association with eighty members, in 1949 SWVS had four members on council. Joshua, as one of those councillors, served on several committees and was a long serving chairman of the publications committee. In 1966, at the age of fifty-four, Joan Joshua's career took an unexpected turn. She was invited to take up the post of reader in clinical studies at Liverpool veterinary school. Known affectionately as 'Auntie' by her students, her years of experience in practice made her an effective, if somewhat authoritarian, lecturer. Retiring in 1973, she remained active as a lecturer, breeder and judge of chow-chows and a popular figure at Association gatherings until she died aged eighty-one.[54]

There were many other women, less prominent in the public areas of their profession, who demonstrated by the quality of their performance in all branches of practice, that females were a worthy match for their male colleagues. As it happens, the three women noted above were all single. But as time went on the additional responsibilities of marriage and children – often quoted as being incompatible with a woman's full participation in a career – did not prove a bar to success both in practice and in veterinary politics. For example, in 2005, Dr Freda Scott-Park was elected president of the BVA after heading its largest division, the BSAVA. Dr Scott-Park was not only the first woman to head the Association for four decades, she was the only one to have come from a background mainly of small animal experience. And in 2008 Nicky Paull, a farm animal vet, principal of a considerable mixed practice, succeeded to the presidency.

There was, however, still some way to go in the equality stakes.

When the Duke of Devonshire opened the BVA congress in 1956 he devoted a major part of his address to the burgeoning part that women were playing in veterinary matters. Referring to the great increase in the number of women vets, he said: 'Twenty-five years ago there were only two ladies in the profession and at that time ladies were advised not to deal with calving cases and such work; but there were excellent opportunities for women in private practice on small animals.' Now, he said, there were no fewer than 387 women veterinary surgeons on the register, quite a number of them in full-time appointments including senior scientific posts: their influence had spread right through the profession.[55] Even then, there was just a hint of patronising.

At the start of the 1950s, although 70 per cent of applications to veterinary schools were from women, the intake was limited 'by agreement' to 12 per cent.[56] The number of women increased, but only slowly. It was in the early 1970s that there was a surge in the number of female veterinary students. Equal opportunities legislation ensured entry to veterinary courses on merit. At the same time, the enormous popularity of the books, TV series and films of James Herriot's romanticised stories about the life of a pre-war country vet brought an embarrassing flood of applications from young people of both sexes entranced by the fictionalised version of veterinary life.[57] Applicants for acceptance at veterinary schools now found that the academic grades required to stand a chance of a place were higher than for almost any other course.

The number of women veterinary students started to rise dramatically. In the ten years 1962 to 1972, their number rose from twenty-four (10 per cent) to sixty-five (25 per cent).[58] Thereafter, the increase accelerated yearly. By 2010, 76 per cent of veterinary students were female; by that time, there were already more women (53 per cent) than men on the register.[59] The old order, by which membership of the veterinary profession was a male prerogative, had been swept away.

However, old prejudices lingered on. As late as 1988 the controversy over women vets had not entirely died away. Oddly enough, the practitioner who raised the issue was female. Wiltshire vet Beatrice Williams complained of a shortage of permanent assistants; she had advertised for an assistant but had not been successful in engaging anyone. She attributed the difficulty to the number of women qualifying. A very high percentage of women vets, she said, only worked for a short time before marrying and having a family. And thereafter a 'fairly high percentage' did no further work.

She argued that the intake of women veterinary students should take account of this fact. She concluded: 'If women do not want to make the profession a full-time job . . . they must accept the fact that more students who wish to do so should be taken into the profession – namely, men.'[60] She was herself an exception to her own rule: a married woman, with a family, and working full-time. Mrs Williams found little support for her view. Correspondence which followed her letter to the *Record* included replies from Ms E. K. Shepherd, who pointed out that the situation was not a problem facing the veterinary profession alone: was Mrs

Williams really suggesting that the entrance of women into other professional areas should be restricted? She advocated that the solution was to attract back to work qualified women who had taken time out to have children and to create an environment in which family ties, the needs of flexible hours and occasional time off at short notice was seen as part of a mutual benefit instead of unavoidable nuisance. She also pointed out that instead of the usual perks offered to job applicants of a house and car, only really helpful to 'unencumbered' vets, a salary fully comparable with that of others of similar age and experience would be helpful.

Another female correspondent pointed to the advantages of working as a locum rather than as an assistant 'working often ten hours a day and some weekends, finishing late, of never having a social life, all on relatively low wages'.

The only letter with a modicum of support for Mrs Williams concentrated on a general shortage of veterinarians rather than any bias due to gender. A. M. Edwards blamed a general dearth of assistants on the conditions of work – late hours, routine surgery, half-days starting at 18.30 and employers devoid of feeling for staff.[61] That theme was taken up by Mrs H. M. Bentley, who commented that it was not surprising that many assistants had become disillusioned by practice and entered industry or even left the profession: many of those determined not to 'waste their hard earned qualifications' set up their own practices. However, she continued, this led to numerous small and often poorly equipped practices offering 'a poor service from one exhausted vet' which did nothing to promote the professional image.

'Too many practices,' she said, 'expect assistants to work under poor conditions for a poor salary and expect utter commitment to the practice.' Having to devote one's entire life to one's job was neither healthy nor productive. 'Practice bosses must wake up to 1989 and realise that veterinary graduates are human beings with human needs. They need rest and time to enjoy family life as well as having a fulfilling job in a well-equipped practice enabling them to expand the knowledge and expertise gained at college with appropriate financial rewards.'

In the same issue, D. A. MacArthur said he could see no justification for increasing veterinary school intakes until the veterinary fees and salaries had risen enough to attract those who had left [the practising arm of] the profession back to active working in it.[62] Another take on the perceived shortage of practice assistants at the time was that it was at least in part due to a wider variety of careers becoming available to veterinary graduates.

In a move to encourage those who had given up professional work for family or other reasons, retraining courses for women returning to practice were soon available.

In 1990, the Society of Women Veterinary Surgeons had been disbanded. It was no longer considered necessary, in the confident expectation, soon to be fulfilled, that women would become the majority in the profession.[63] By that time, the SWVS representative on BVA council was just one of many women representatives of specialist and territorial divisions. Twenty years later, in 2010, the RCVS register showed that there were twice as many female as male vets in the age group twenty-six to thirty and there were only one-quarter as many men as women veterinary students.[64] The 'confident expectation' had been realised.

What are the reasons for this radical change in the gender demographic? An obvious one is that the law changed to eliminate a gender bias in the selection of students. A corollary of that was, presumably, a previously unfulfilled demand from females who wished to join the profession aided by the fact that their academic ability at entry level was high. Was there another reason: did the number of men seeking to become vets decline? A study in the USA suggested that a number of men interested in joining a veterinary course were put off when they visited a college by the preponderance of women students on the course; men were also negatively influenced by the need to gain a first degree before they could be accepted on a veterinary course (veterinary medicine is a postgraduate course in the United States).[65]

On the other hand, similar swings to a predominantly female profession prevail in the UK, and in the medical and pharmaceutical professions. Another American study showed that, in the small animal sector, neither vets nor their clients seem concerned about the gender of the practitioner; the important thing was that they were given a professional service.[66] So the gender shift seems permanent and must be accommodated as a permanent factor in working and in social life.

There is no doubt that this change has affected practice. The recognition that there is a life outside practice is now fully accepted; many posts are advertised with descriptions of the attractive leisure opportunities available as part of the package. Nor is this by any means entirely, or perhaps even mainly, because of the change in the balance of the genders – although the needs of employees with family responsibilities are recognised. Part-time working is common. Twenty-four hour on-call duties are often delegated. The days of the old-time vet, whose house was his practice premises, and whose working hours were elastic, may be no more. But, at least in the opinion of one senior vet, R. M. Stevenson (a past-president of the BVA with a successful practice employing 35 people) what he called the 'tingle factor' has largely gone from practice.[67]

The opinion quoted at the beginning of this chapter, 'that veterinary surgery is of all learned professions the one least adapted for women', could hardly have been more wrong. Like pharmacy (and to a lesser extent medicine), the veterinary profession has become predominantly a female calling. The implications for the BVA membership are considerable. Many women are likely to opt for working part-time or as locums: how many will wish to continue including membership of the Association among their involvements?[68]

What would be the ambitions and aspirations of this new mixture of vets? In 2010, a survey sought to gauge the differing reasons of male and female veterinary students for choosing a veterinary course. When asked what were the top three reasons for wanting to be become a vet, men were almost ten times as likely as women to select 'want to train as a scientist' as a reason than were women, and five times more likely to say it was because they wanted to join a profession. Men were also more likely – thirteen times more likely – than women to have chosen to select a veterinary course as their choice because it was the 'hardest course to get into'. Overall, women's choice of a veterinary course was most strongly influenced by their ownership of animals; men's by the challenging reputation of the course.[69]

Those choices indicate only the way one group of young people felt about their chosen vocation at a particular time. How, if at all, those impressions will be reflected in the careers of those aspirants will, of course, depend on what mature influences, and opportunities, dictate.

CHAPTER FIFTEEN

DECLINE OF FARM PRACTICE

One factor commonly advanced as an explanation for the changing gender balance of the profession is the rise of small animal practice and the corresponding decline of farm animal work. While the wartime and post-war food production campaigns translated into plentiful employment for vets on farms, by the 1960s and 1970s, anxiety about the future had begun to arise. As farmers' profit margins narrowed, they cut back on veterinary services, stockpiled drugs, and sought help preferentially from free farming advisers supplied by the state and by feed and drug companies. Part-time work as local veterinary inspectors involved in disease control campaigns was also threatened as swine fever was eliminated and tuberculosis brought under control. The promotion of a more preventive approach to veterinary practice was one solution advocated, but this made little headway.[1] By the 1980s, BVA president Neal King was advocating a new (and perhaps more realistic) approach which recognised the importance of drug sales to veterinary practice budgets. The profession, he said, should aim to provide traditional 'fire brigade' services, integrated with whole-unit preventive medicine schemes and with the provision of pharmaceutical products at competitive prices.[2]

King also argued that society required services from the profession 'other than those suited to privatisation'. He was referring to the vets' role in disease control and surveillance, animal welfare and food hygiene. In that area, he said, 'central government should seek to provide the optimum framework within which the benefits of that work could be maximised' – presumably by providing financial support. However, the Parliamentary Secretary, MAFF (Mrs Peggy Fenner), opening the congress, said it was 'highly unlikely' that government funds would be available to finance compensation in any future disease eradication schemes.[3] King was not talking about emergency situations, however. He was concerned with the quotidian routines of farm practice. The continuing strength of small animal practice meant that more mixed practices were opting out of farm work or closing: small animal work, with the convenience of operating mainly from a single location had proved more attractive than farm work, where clients could be scattered over a relatively wide area, with expensive travelling time between visits. At the same time the nature of farming was changing. Livestock numbers fell significantly; dairy cow numbers dropped by almost a third between 1995 and 2008, from 2.3 million to 1.6 million; in the same period there were almost 4.5 million fewer sheep, a fall of 23.5 per cent.[4] Between 1995 and 2005 the average dairy herd size rose from sixty-seven to eighty-four and the proportion of those herds with one hundred or more cattle rose from 45 per cent to 58 per cent; smaller but still significant changes affected beef cattle and sheep.[5] Those smaller numbers were accommodated in fewer, larger dairy and beef enterprises, further reducing the demand for veterinarians.

Particularly for clients in areas distant from a practice, the BVA was also concerned about a potential loss of farming expertise and a decline in ancillary services such as disease surveillance. For years, it had noted that, particularly in mixed practices, farm veterinary services were less rewarding than was companion animal work, particularly canine, feline and equine. In some areas, LVI work, for so long the mainstay of many practices, was becoming less attractive. Some practices had refused to take on more LVI appointments; there were fears that farmers would be left without veterinary cover.[6] The government, too, was concerned about what might happen. In 2003 its Environment, Farm and Rural Affairs Committee (EFRACom), in the light of such concerns, issued a report on vets and veterinary services.[7] The report found that there was not an overall shortage of veterinarians but some concern as to whether there were enough of them experienced in farm practice to cope with all that was expected of them. That included services in such areas as disease surveillance and health and welfare. More large-animal vets would be needed if DEFRA was to fulfil its own strategies for those functions.

EFRACom cast its net wide: as well as the actual number of vets for on-farm services, it considered the needs for research, education – retracing the tracks of earlier veterinary surveys – and even extended its remit to the potential impact of the Competition Commission's impact on the supply of veterinary medicines and of the Common Agricultural Policy. The committee urged DEFRA and the profession to make projections of the number of practising veterinary surgeons and to conduct a risk analysis of the consequence of not having enough large-animal vets. It recommended that greater attention be paid in the veterinary schools to teaching and research on farm animal topics, topics which were slewed towards companion animal studies. Relations with the State Veterinary Service should be reviewed and the important links with the private veterinary providing LVI services (at that time under review) strengthened. The Association was, of course, in favour of those recommendations that benefited its members.

The EFRACom report was detailed; so was the BVA response to the recommendations. It said the extent of the shortage of vets in the livestock sector should be examined jointly by the BVA and the NFU with the Royal College and DEFRA producing its own projections for the sector. The Association reiterated its claim that there was strong evidence that (other than in areas remote and marginal) the future for veterinary practice would be bleak without some sort of intervention; the 'strong evidence' was not specified.

A system of farm licensing, incorporating regular veterinary inspections for livestock would be beneficial for animal health, welfare and surveillance; the government's agreement to the establishment of a database of farm holdings and number of livestock was welcomed. Collaboration between DEFRA and the National Disease Information Service (NADIS), a network of sixty veterinary practices and the veterinary schools, monitoring diseases in cattle, sheep and pigs, would also be beneficial.

As for herd health planning schemes, whose establishment was recommended by the committee, the Association said there was a need to convince livestock keepers of their real benefits and of the willingness and ability of the veterinary profession to deliver them. The nub of the matter was that the farmer had to be persuaded that the benefits of farm health planning would outweigh his costs and that the call on the vets' services would be sufficient to justify the costs of the training involved. Pump-priming finance from the government to encourage uptake of the plans was called for

In the implementation of veterinary surveillance strategy the BVA was in favour of a partnership approach between vets and livestock farmers, with DEFRA and other stakeholders being involved to ensure maximum integration. DEFRA was simultaneously launching 'A strategy for veterinary surveillance in the UK'[8] with those same aims.

The BVA was adamant that veterinarians should be enabled to regularly inspect animals on the farm either by random checks, pre-announced visits or in the course of routine clinical work. Costs for such work 'should be borne by all the beneficiaries including the government'. The Association was disappointed that the government wanted such costs to be born in the main by the farmer. It was also pointed out that vets were asked to include surveillance information on submissions to the Veterinary Laboratories Agency at their own expense. It felt that private vets should not do this unpaid work for the government without recognition.

Chapter 15

Unsurprisingly, the BVA was disappointed that the EFRACom recommendation that it might intervene directly in the market to ensure that vets were paid appropriately for the services they provided had been 'flatly rejected'. Overall, the Association was massively critical of the way the government had responded to the committee's recommendations. Apart from criticising a lack of clarity in the wording of DEFRA's reply, the BVA said that, although the government had repeatedly emphasised the central role of the veterinarian in its strategies on animal health and welfare and surveillance, its response to the EFRACom report indicated a lack of interest in the viability of practices and the continuing failure to recognise the importance of getting vets onto farms.

The net effect of the response, said the BVA, would be to reinforce the views of those who suggested that valuable time was being wasted as agriculture and services that surrounded it declined through lack of positive action. Further, it was critical of the quality of the response: it indicated a lack of respect for the select committee and the report it had produced, and was poor reward for those vets who had been involved in the discussions.[9]

The animal health minister, Ben Bradshaw, replied that: 'The veterinary profession must be prepared to evolve with its customers. Like any other service industry it must renew and refresh the services it provides and the way it provides them.' This did nothing to assuage matters.

There were others who thought the profession should, as it were, clear out the attics.[10] One of those was Professor Philip Lowe, director of the UK Research Council's Rural Economy and Land Use Programme. In the wake of the EFRACom report Lowe, on behalf of the Vets and Veterinary Services Steering Group, took a fresh approach to how food animal veterinary practice should be run. Like the EFRACom committee, it cast its net wide but Lowe's approach was more radical: broadly, he asked, what did the food animal client ('customer') expect from his vet services? This latest report was, in part, prompted by the publication of DEFRA's animal health and welfare strategy for Great

301

Britain, which supported a stronger partnership approach, with greater clarity given to the roles and responsibilities of all those with an interest in animal health and welfare. Lowe felt there was a leadership vacuum in this area into which the veterinary profession should step and assume greater responsibility for shaping the future structure of farm animal veterinary services. A unified voice for the veterinary profession would, he felt, stand a far greater chance of encouraging partners in the farming and food industries, and government agencies, to collaborate in joint initiatives.

Such partnerships should include the private sector for clients of veterinary services, which were felt to have been sidelined by squabbles between government and the veterinary profession. The narrow regulatory and task-based roles into which the profession had been pressed by government, and a failure to engage strategically with other major customers, had led to a 'certain conservatism' in farmer-vet relationships. The vets' heavy reliance on emergency 'fire fighting' services and routine clinical work should give place to a knowledge-based approach in which vets advised clients in risk management, he said. Lowe also considered that the veterinary profession had lagged behind other health professionals in the involvement of paraprofessionals and in the provision of ancillary technical services. From the available data, however, he was clear that there was no absolute shortfall in the supply of vets who might be available for farm animal work.

Lowe spoke of the differences between the traditional business structure of practices with their focus on reactive services and the new and evolving business model used by those, usually larger, practices offering herd health planning and advisory services. The BVA, looking at the relative strengths and weaknesses of both types of practice, considered that the strengths of the traditional business structure derived from the relatively small localised nature which allowed them to maintain close working relationships with customers and provide continuity of care. Smaller practices were likely to have good local knowledge and also to have maintained a veterinary presence on smaller farms.

That enabled them to make a significant contribution to animal welfare, disease surveillance and emergency response. That model's potential weaknesses included their more limited degree and range of specialist expertise, which was compounded by their reluctance to call in outside specialists for fear of losing business.

On the other hand, practices based on the newer business model might pay less attention to the individual animal, lack local knowledge and, according to the BVA, were more likely to focus on high product sales than on good health outcomes. But they could make more effective use of external and in-house specialist advice and were better placed to develop new approaches by maintaining a clear focus on the market and adopting a progressive approach to business management. However, the Association said the extensive animal population knowledge offered by the new, larger, practices put them in a strong position to promote preventive medicine, conduct strategic surveillance and assess public health risks from animals and animal products.

Lowe's report also described how the government's position had changed over the years from a situation in which it acted as patron and sponsor to the veterinary profession, mainly through its LVI services, to the quite different circumstances in which responsibilities were devolved and the industry had a much greater role. Nevertheless, it argued, the government must not relinquish its responsibilities for animal health and the profession must renew its relationship with government to reflect the changing circumstances. To cater for his ideas on developing food animal veterinary services Lowe proposed that a Veterinary Development Council (VDC) should be established 'to provide a structure in which the veterinary profession could work with its customers/partners'.

This proposal, it is probably fair to say, came as something of a surprise to the BVA which might have thought that the Association already provided such a structure. Nevertheless, the BVA welcomed the opportunity for vets to 'take stock and take a look at where we are going'.[11]

The Association took the initiative and set up the new council under the chairmanship of Professor Richard Bennett, professor of agricultural economics at Reading University; the post is funded by DEFRA. The VDC's members included representatives from the meat industry and retail organisations as well as the veterinary profession. The point was made that while the council's focus was on veterinary engagement in the food chain, implications for companion animals would be kept in mind. It is a fact that while farm and food veterinary services are vital to the profession, to government and the wider economy, companion animal services represent 80 per cent of veterinary activities[12] and a similar proportion of its income.

COMPANY PRACTICES

Nineteen ninety-seven saw a new development in the organisation of veterinary services. Whereas veterinary professionals had carried on their practices as individuals, principals and assistants, or partners, changes in the size and complexity of practices had meant that some of them had become quite large enterprises with several vets and numerous lay personnel. That, and the consequent increased financial investment required in property and expensive surgical and diagnostic equipment, meant there had been pressure from some business-minded vets to allow veterinary practices to be operated under the umbrella of a limited company. This incorporation, it was argued, would create greater flexibility in organising the financial affairs of a practice and perhaps avoid some of the complications that could arise in practice partnerships, when a partner left or retired.

The Royal College was probably in line with the majority of the profession at the time in discouraging the idea. It did not, however, have any statutory powers to prevent any vet, or anyone else, setting up a veterinary practice company.

Long before the incorporation of practices as limited companies became acceptable, however, something close in concept and organisation to an incorporated practice had been inaugurated by John Sheridan, a vet who had involved himself in the business and management aspects of the provision of veterinary services. Sheridan had originated the concept of franchised practices in the UK. He believed that the provision of business services specifically designed for vets would enable small practices to concentrate more effectively on professional matters. This led him in the 1970s to set up a company, Anicare Group Services (Veterinary) Ltd; this was not itself operating as a practice, so there could be no objection to its establishment. In addition to offering business services to existing practices who took up the franchise, Anicare aimed to make it easier for vets who wished to set up in practice on their own to do so.

Veterinary surgeons wanting to start a new practice and wishing to take up a franchise received assistance from his company in finding suitable premises, negotiating with the vendors or landlord, seeking planning permission where necessary and drawing up plans to bring the premises up to an agreed standard. The premises would be leased to or bought by Anicare and leased or sub-leased to the franchisee. To aid the actual running of the practice Anicare provided a reference manual and staff handbook setting out business procedures, operational standards, guidance on equipment, dressings and drugs, accounting methods and so on, backed by personal advice from Sheridan. Business stationery was provided and assistance in setting up the practice and planning its development were given as well as help with recruiting and training lay staff.

Once in operation the company continued to provide management, advisory and support services while the veterinary surgeon holding the franchise developed the practice in their own way. The franchisee paid an initial 'license' fee and thereafter a fee of 8 per cent of turnover exclusive of VAT. Of the revenue raised by the levy, 10 per cent was applied to a use agreed by the franchise holders, usually funding continuing professional development courses.[13]

In 1997, the RCVS, which had still turned its face against corporate practice, accepted that such a development was inevitable. It had set up a committee to consider the matter of incorporation, no doubt responding to pressure from individuals who saw company-run practices as a necessary step forward in practice management. Also no doubt in the College's mind was the long, expensive, and ultimately unsuccessful campaign fought by the Royal Pharmaceutical Society to prevent pharmacies being run by limited companies.[14]

In due course, *RCVS News*, the College's newsletter for members, carried the following notice:

> ### Incorporation
> While accepting that the College has no legal powers to stop incorporation, Council agreed that members should be warned of the possible risks from non-veterinary surgeons who might try to compromise the professional judgement of veterinary surgeons, for example in clinical matters, choice of drugs, hours of attendance, and advice to owners.[15]

The notice concluded by stating that 'for further advice, members should write to the College professional conduct department'. Hardly a green light to go ahead: more an amber – proceed with caution.

The first corporate practice to be set up was, not unexpectedly, by John Sheridan with two colleagues. Veterinary Practice Initiatives (VPI) Ltd, as the company was called, was financed by a 'multi-million pound finance and equity deal'. Its remit was to acquire and manage small animal practices. The company, Sheridan said at the 1997 launch, was founded on the conviction that corporate ownership offered benefits to the profession and client alike, provided there was a 'strong commitment to clinical excellence, professional ethics and the delivery of high quality veterinary services'. To ensure that, a clinical advisory board had been set up; this would be chaired by

Lord Soulsby of Swaffham Prior, a distinguished academic vet who had a strong interest in veterinary ethics.

Lord Soulsby

Lawson Soulsby, who was created Lord Soulsby of Swaffham Prior in 1990, was a brilliant academic who also made an invaluable contribution to veterinary professional organisations. A graduate of the Edinburgh school, he was a scientist of international renown whose fields encompassed both animal and human parasitology. He held chairs at the University of Pennsylvania, 1963 to 1978, and, from 1978 to 1993, that of Cambridge, where he was a Fellow of Wolfson College. His interests spread from his international scientific and teaching activities to consultancies with international organisations such as the World Health Organisation, the United Nations Organisation, pharmaceutical companies and those veterinary professional associations with which he became more closely involved after his appointment as emeritus professor in 1993.

Deeply concerned in animal welfare, Soulsby was chair of the BVA's Ethics Committee (now, Ethics and Welfare Group) from 1984; a frequent speaker at the Association's congresses, he had delivered the annual Wooldridge Memorial Lecture, and received the Centaur Award, the BVA's highest accolade in 1999. He was president of the RCVS in 1984. Soulsby's interest in comparative medicine – 'one health' – was acknowledged by his election to the chair of the Royal Society of Medicine in 1998.

There are few important organisations in the fields of veterinary education, medicine, welfare or politics that have not benefited from the contributions of Lawson Soulsby. Not least among his qualities, however, was his genial and courteous manner, much appreciated by his colleagues.

According to one of the directors who owned veterinary practices in the USA, the new company had had the advantage of being able to scrutinise the development of corporate veterinary practices in that country. They were convinced that, at its best, corporate ownership of practices lay ahead for a large segment of the profession.[16]

By the time Veterinary Practice Initiatives ceased trading in 2006 (most of its practices having been acquired by a company called CVS Ltd) the corporate ownership of practices had indeed proliferated. The two main types of ownership were described at the BVA congress in 2006. In one, the practices were wholly owned, and operated by, the company. The other used a 'joint venture' approach, more like that pioneered by Sheridan almost thirty years previously.

The first model, used by CVS Ltd, owned the practices outright. They were mainly small animal practices, although it had also involvement in equine practice, referral practices, exotics and diagnostic laboratories. Practices purchased by CVS continued to operate under their existing name as the company believed that each practice should remain a local one with its own identity. Business targets were not set for the practices as the company believed in encouraging the practice members to work as a team and 'to do the right things clinically' for its clients and their animals. 'In simple terms' said the company, 'we are trying to create a world where each practice has its own identity, where the team within it feel the practice is theirs, that they can get on and do what they want to do and look after their patients in the way they want to.'

Another company, Companion Care Ltd, by contrast, utilised a 'joint venture' partnership system. It believed that vets still wanted to run practices, but 'perhaps in a different way from the traditional partnership system'. Each practice was a limited company in its own right and practice partners were employed directors and shareholders of the company. Companion Care felt it important to have a national brand (as opposed to individually named practices) as all practices then benefited from the growth and promotion of that brand.[17]

Not everyone had initially welcomed the change. One vet, Chris Walster, felt there were dangers in the increasing number of practices owned by companies. He said: 'Once corporates reach a certain size . . . they will open purpose-built practices, perhaps on greenfield sites, and they will take the heart out of our profession. Many of those involved in corporate practice are there for financial gain . . . They are investing money that comes at a high price from venture capitalists and investment banks.' However the position of vets was 'dressed up', they would become totally answerable to the real owners of the business, the financiers.[18]

Whatever the misgivings, corporate ownership did indeed take off. Many vets turned their practices, whether large or small, into limited companies, and a number of non-veterinary businessmen launched veterinary practice companies. Some of the new practices were opened within the large supermarket-style pet stores on out-of-town shopping developments. Nowadays, it is as likely as not that the local veterinary practice, large or small, will belong to a limited company. And the management of practices has itself become specialised; in common with almost every aspect of veterinary life it spawned its own representative body, the Association of Veterinary Practice Managers (AVPM), affiliated to the BVA.

THE MILLENNIUM

When the BVA entered the millennium year of 2000, it could look back on 120 years of progress – some of it, perhaps, a little unsteady. With membership standing at 10,434, of which 1,754 were students,[19] stable finances and an established position in the veterinary world, the situation seemed satisfactory in spite of the depressed state of UK agriculture in the aftermath of the BSE outbreak. But if the organisation's size and experience had increased, so had the challenges it had to face. The veterinary profession and the country were about to be faced with serious problems. In the calm before the storm, as it were, the BVA marked the millennium with one of its periodical exercises in crystal ball gazing, a joint initiative with the Royal College, 'Seminar 2000 – developing a veterinary strategy for change', held on 29 and 30 March.[20]

The event coincided with the government's announcement that it intended to review the dispensing of prescription-only medicines by vets 'to reduce costs to farmers' and also to review the scope for vets to be replaced by paraprofessionals for some tasks currently restricted to the profession. As is the norm for such occasions, speakers based their prognostications on what was current. Strengths identified included the quality of veterinary education – 'the best biomedical education there is' – and its grounding as a springboard to develop further skills in the future. Implied weaknesses included the need for farm practices to determine precisely what services livestock producers needed in the changed environment of larger stockholdings and lower farming incomes. Small animal practices had to match their skills and the services they offered to the expectations of an increasingly knowledgeable clientele.

On the economic side, much was made of the heavy reliance of practices on income from sales of medicines. Reiterating what had been said for decades, RCVS president-elect Roger Eddy pointed out that medicines contributed 60 per cent of the turnover of farm animal practices and 75 per cent of the profits. The proportion was lower, but still substantial, in small animal practice. And prices of animal medicines in the UK were the highest in the EU. A (substantial) illegal trade in medicines was 'driven by price'.

The challenge for the future, he said, 'lies in determining what services are needed by producers and how veterinarians can economically provide them'. Looking at small animal practice, the seminar heard it would continue to develop technically, with increased use of laboratory diagnosis and sophisticated surgical procedures and increasing specialisation in practices. Mixed practices would become rare, with larger practices having dedicated managers (as had happened in human medical practices). The chairman of the small animal session, Neal King, said he hoped that vets would not lose sight of animal welfare in the interests of 'turnover, transaction volume, defensive medicine, and the opportunity to use the latest diagnostic "toy" '.[21]

Chapter 15

WHAT OF THE FUTURE?

After 120 years, how does the BVA stand? The fact of its survival as a voluntary organisation indicates that it continues to serve a purpose today, but for the best part of four decades that survival was by no means assured. From its optimistic beginnings in 1882 it ended in 1919 virtually bankrupt and with a membership numbering less than 400, only one-tenth that of the profession. It had struggled to achieve a solid basis of support from the profession's local divisions, which always refused to mandate divisional support for the Association's subscription, leaving it a matter for the individual. Its administration was hampered by the governing council whose constitution and extended membership virtually ensured inefficiency. Its activities were said to have become no more than the occasion of a pleasant outing; virtually the sole activity was its annual conference.

The conference did discuss clinical matters and, presumably because influential members were involved in meat hygiene and public health, pass resolutions aimed at creating a more structured system for organising those services. The fledgling Association continually sought to persuade its members to form themselves into a more cohesive body; the members themselves, however, resisted any suggestion that they might allow the sovereignty of their strong local divisions to be diminished thereby. Without the tacit support of the Royal College and practical support of a very few dedicated members, the Association probably would not have survived as an effective body.

The events of the 1914–1918 war began to change that. The war created a demand for increasing numbers of vets to be mobilised, with a recognition by government of the essential need for their services in caring for the vast numbers of animals needed to transport the army and its equipment. The involvement of the Association in the

311

negotiations concerning deployment of veterinary personnel brought it some recognition as a negotiating body, albeit an informal one.

A fundamental change in the Association after World War II came about in two ways: the return to civilian life of veterinarians released from the constraints of life in the army, and, importantly, the acquisition in 1920 of the *Veterinary Record.* Its adoption as the official journal of the Association and, hopefully, of the whole profession, brought increased membership, subscription income and, through the associated commercial activities, a measure of financial stability. This strengthened ambitions towards greater effectiveness.

The setting up of the State Veterinary Service in 1937 was the occasion of wrangling over the involvement of private practitioners in the service. More serious disagreements over negotiations on the salary scales for employed vets in government and local authority posts led in the 1940s to a public falling out between the BVA and the Minister of Agriculture. The Association, whose negotiating power was not strong, had to give way. It had by then been accepted fully that the Association was the negotiating body for such matters although it had no official powers of action; the nearest it could come to withdrawal of labour was to refuse to carry advertisements for official posts in the *Veterinary Record.*

Political activity during the inter-war period centred largely on attempts to increase government support for some state subsidy on the lines of that enjoyed by medical practitioners under the National Insurance scheme. This was not achieved, but veterinary practitioners were able to participate as 'licensed veterinary inspectors' in the various health schemes promoted by the state. These licensed functions varied from the routine tasks prescribed by the various Diseases of Animals Acts to the emergency operations to combat outbreaks of epidemics such as foot-and-mouth disease. There were regular negotiations between government and the Association on the terms for provision of such work; these became fractious at times, as on the question of tendering for contracts for veterinary services. For the BVA, this was primarily a professional matter, while the government saw it as business transactions; there was no resolution of that dispute, which recurred at intervals up to the present day.

From the onset of World War II, political activity of a different sort centred around the notion of an official system of veterinary preventive medicine. The idea had been current since the successful animal health schemes initiated in the 1939–1945 war; various projects were launched but fizzled out over time as practices became busy with their ordinary work, buttressed by the income from official licensed duties. In fact, with the increased availability of vaccines, antibiotics and anti-helminthics, drug-dependent disease prevention became routine in both large and small animal practice.

The BVA participated fully in the discussions surrounding the passage of the Veterinary Surgeons Act 1948, which moved veterinary education into the universities, and enlarged the RCVS register to include unqualified (but not inexperienced) practitioners. These bitterly contested moves were forced on the profession by a severe shortage of vets and by the need to raise the standards of veterinary education. Subsequently, however, the BVA became a strong supporter of university veterinary education, and claimed success in its 1985 campaign against the closure of two of the existing six veterinary schools;

Changes in social and political perceptions of the professions meant that in the later twentieth century, the BVA had also, initially reluctantly, to accept the liberalisation of constraints on professional advertising and competition, although not all members opposed those changes as they represented little more than what was normal practice in other fields.

Other important influences on veterinary practice in this period were the expansion and eventual domination of small animal practice and the concomitant increase in the number of women vets. The Association was slow to recognise these changes just as, earlier, some of its members had been slow to accept that the horse was no longer the core client for the vet. The economic success of small animal practice meant that practices could afford to buy new equipment and pay for postgraduate training in the new techniques now being delivered. The dominance of small animals in the veterinary spectrum brought fears that care of farm animals – and the profession's claim to a public role – might be jeopardised; that did not happen, although practice itself was modified to accommodate a livestock industry based on intensive farming.

For a period, the Association's specialist divisions, large and small animal, tended to outrun the Association, which came to be seen as out of touch with modern developments. For some years, relations between the large divisions, particularly the British Small Animal Veterinary Association and the British Cattle Veterinary Association, were not good. Improvement came, albeit gradually, with restructuring of the BVA's internal organisation, the long desired revision of its council structure, the adoption of modern IT systems and enhanced public relations, both internal and external.

The most important development, however, was the acceptance by the divisions that while each had its role, the veterinary profession was too small to allow independent groups to be truly effective on a national scale.

Politically, the results for the Association over the years may seem mixed. In fact, it has fought its corner hard, in spite of initially very limited resources. Success may sometimes have been seen in terms of damage limitation rather than absolute victory but the BVA came to be fully accepted as speaking for the all branches of the veterinary profession.

What of the future? The nature of all professions, not least that of the veterinarian, changes with time. A century ago, it was hostile to the entry of women into the profession; now it has a majority of female members; it is increasingly made up of employees rather than the self-employed, as formerly; the economic situation is changing and guaranteed jobs less certain. Although a minority of the profession will continue to work in mixed practice or the public sector, there is unlikely to be any reversal of the historical transition from horse, to livestock, to pet-dominated veterinary work.

The Association remains a small organisation with relatively modest resources. In representing the veterinary profession it has worked with, and occasionally against, much larger bodies – government, farming, industry. But whatever developments may occur in practice, in the demography of the profession or its relations with other organisations, those who speak for its members believe the BVA will continue to adapt to whatever changes may be in store and maintain its representative role.[22]

And in fulfilling that role, the BVA and its members have always sought to punch above their weight.

NOTES

'Proceedings' in the following notes refers to the Proceedings of the National Veterinary Association and its successor from 1920, the National Veterinary Medical Association.

CHAPTER 1

1   Louise Hill Curth, 'Care of the brute beast: animals and the seventeenth-century medical market-place', *Social History of Medicine*, 15 (2002), 375–92; L. Pugh, *From farriery to veterinary medicine, 1785–1795* (Heffer: Cambridge, 1962); Ernest Cotchin, *The Royal Veterinary College* (Barracuda Books: London, 1990).
2   S. A. Hall, 'The struggle for the charter of the Royal College of Veterinary Surgeons, 1844', *Veterinary History*, 8 (1994), 2–21.
3   Iain Pattison, *The British veterinary profession 1791–1948* (J A Allen: London, 1984).
4   Michael Worboys, 'Germ theories of disease and British veterinary medicine, 1860–1890', *Medical History*, 35 (1991), 308–27; J. R. Fisher, 'Not quite a profession: the aspirations of veterinary surgeons in England in the mid 19th century', *Historical Research*, 66 (1993), 285.
5   A. Woods, S. Matthews, ' "Little, if at all, removed from the illiterate farrier or cow-leech": The English veterinary surgeon c.1860–85 and the campaign for veterinary reform', *Medical History*, 54 (2010), 32.
6   Fisher, 'Not quite a profession'.
7   P. Bartrip, *Themselves writ large: The British Medical Association 1832–1996* (BMJ Publishers: London, 1996), 21; I. Waddington, *The medical profession in the industrial revolution* (Gill and Macmillan: Dublin, 1984); I. Loudon, 'Medical education and medical reform', in V. Nutton and R. Porter (eds), *The history of medical education in Britain*, Clio Medica 30 (Rodopi: Amsterdam, 1995), 229–49.
8   Obituary, *Veterinary Record*, 13 (1901), 593.
9   Editorial, 'The practical training of veterinary students', *Veterinary Journal*, 11 (1880), 22.
10 Pattison, *The British veterinary profession*; Fisher, 'Not quite a profession'; Woods & Matthews, 'Little, if at all, removed'.
11 Woods & Matthews, 'Little, if at all, removed'.
12 T. Greaves, 'Farriers on strike, or a veterinary medical association on trial', *Veterinarian*, 37 (1864), 578.
13 A. Hardy, 'Pioneers in the Victorian provinces: Veterinarians, public health and the urban animal economy', *Urban History*, 29/3 (2002), 372–387.

Notes to Chapter 1

14 I. Pattison, *John McFadyean: A great British veterinarian* (J. A. Allen: London, 1981).
15 Graham Wilson, 'The Brown Animal Sanatory Institution', *Journal of Hygiene,* 82 (1979), 155–76, 337–52.
16 P. G. G. Jackson (2011), personal communication.
17 *Proceedings* (1886), 30.
18 *Veterinary Record,* 53 (1941), 97.
19 *Proceedings* (1882), 12.
20 Ibid.
21 P. J. Simpson, *Veterinary Record,* 11 (1931), 20.
22 *Proceedings* (1883), 7.
23 Hardy, 'Pioneers in the Victorian provinces'.
24 *Proceedings* (1884), 84.
25 'The history of veterinary ethics in Britain, c1870–2000', in C. Wathes et al. (eds), *Proceedings of the first international conference on veterinary and animal ethics, September 2011* (Wiley-Blackwell: London, 2012), 3–18.
26 Ruth D'Arcy Thompson, *The remarkable Gamgees: A story of achievement* (Ramsay Head Press: Edinburgh, 1974).
27 A. Woods, 'A scientific policy?: Contagious disease control at the British Board of Agriculture, 1890–1922.' Paper presented to European Science Foundation workshop, Paris, 2008.
28 Michael Worboys, *Spreading germs: Germs and British medicine, 1860–1900* (CUP: Cambridge, 2000).
29 *Proceedings* (1885), 102.
30 *Proceedings* (1886), 5.
31 Ibid. 13.
32 RVC quarterly meeting, *Veterinarian,* 54 (1881), 337–8; S. Snow, *Operations without pain: The practice and science of anaesthesia in Victorian Britain* (Palgrave MacMillan: Basingstoke, 2006).
33 *Proceedings* (1886), 30.
34 *Proceedings* (1887), 10–56.
35 J. Woodroff Hill, Correspondence, *Veterinary Journal,* 11 (1880), 71.
36 Woods & Matthews, 'Little if at all removed'.
37 *Proceedings* (1887).
38 Hardy, 'Pioneers in the Victorian provinces', 373.
39 Interview by A. Woods with Mrs J. Dollar, Salisbury, 2006.
40 *Veterinary Record,* 1 (1888), 1.
41 Woods & Matthews, 'Little, if at all, removed'.
42 *Proceedings* (1888), 137.
43 S. Reiser, *Medicine and the reign of technology* (CUP: Cambridge, 1978).
44 W. Hunting, *Proceedings* (1889), 70.
45 Anon, *Veterinary Record,* 3 (1890), 130.

Notes to Chapters 1–2

46 J. S. Hurndall, *Veterinary Record,* 2 (1889), 130.
47 G. A. Banham, *Veterinary Record,* 3 (1890), 204.
48 G. A. Banham, *Veterinary Journal,* 28 (1890), 146.
49 Special general meeting, *Proceedings* (1890), 2.
50 Ibid. 77.

CHAPTER 2

1   K. Waddington, 'The science of cows: Tuberculosis, research and the state in the United Kingdom, 1890–1914', *History of Science,* 39 (2001), 355–81.
2   *Proceedings* (1892), 70.
3   *Proceedings* (1893), 20.
4   Ibid. 23.
5   Ann Hardy, 'Professional advantage and public health: British veterinarians and state veterinary services, 1865–1939', *Twentieth Century British History,* 14 (2003), 1–23.
6   *Proceedings* (1893), 60.
7   Anon, *Veterinary Record,* 6 (1893), 117.
8   W. Pallin, 'Castration in horses' (RCVS fellowship thesis no 1, 1896), held in RCVS library.
9   *Proceedings* (1894), 12.
10 Hardy, 'Professional advantage and public health'; A. Woods, *A Manufactured Plague?: The history of foot and mouth disease in Britain* (Earthscan: London, 2004), chapter 5.
11 *Proceedings* (1894), 8.
12 Ibid. 22–55.
13 Interview with Mrs J. Dollar by A. Woods.
14 Richard D. French, Anti-vivisection and Medical Science in Victorian Society (Princeton University Press: Princeton, 1975); Nicolas Rupke, 'Pro-vivisection in England', in N. Rupke (ed.), *Vivisection in Historical Perspective* (Croom Helm: London, 1987).
15 *Proceedings* (1894).
16 *Proceedings* (1895), 21.
17 *Proceedings* (1895), 25.
18 *Proceedings* (1895), 45.
19 R. Perren, 'Manufacture and marketing of veterinary products from 1850 to 1914', *Veterinary History,* 6 (1979), 43.
20 *Proceedings* (1896), 15.
21 A. Woods, 'A scientific policy?: Contagious disease control at the British Board of Agriculture, 1890–1922', paper presented to the European Science Foundation workshop, Paris, 2008.

Notes to Chapter 2

22 *Report of the Departmental Committee appointed to enquire into aetiology, pathology and morbid anatomy of swine fever* (PP 1896, c.8023, xxiv, 163), 3.
23 *Proceedings* (1896), 91.
24 Woods, 'A scientific policy?'.
25 K. Waddington, ' "To stamp out so terrible a malady": Bovine tuberculosis and tuberculin tesing in Britain, 1890–1939', *Medical History*, 48 (2004), 29–48.
26 *Proceedings* (1896), 103.
27 *Proceedings* (1897), 24.
28 *Proceedings* (1898), 17.
29 *Proceedings* (1898).
30 Susan Jones, 'Mapping a zoonotic disease: Anglo-American efforts to control bovine tuberculosis before World War I', *Osiris,* 19 (2004), 133–148.
31 *Veterinary Record,* 12 (1899), 85.
32 Ibid. 179.
33 *Veterinary Record,* 13 (1900), 113.
34 *Proceedings* (1900).
35 *Proceedings* (1901).
36 *Proceedings* (1902), 146.
37 Ibid. 97.
38 Obituary, *Veterinary Record,* 2 (1922), 680.
39 *Proceedings* (1903), 23.
40 C. M. Warwick, A. M. Macdonald, 'The New Veterinary College, Edinburgh, 1873–1907', *Veterinary Record,* 153 (2003), 380.
41 *Proceedings* (1904), 131.
42 *Veterinary Record,* 16 (1904), 765.
43 *Proceedings* (1905).
44 Ibid.
45 *Proceedings* (1906).
46 *Proceedings* (1907).
47 *Proceedings* (1908).
48 C. M. Warwick, A. A. Mcdonald, 'The life of O. Charnock Bradley, 1871– 1973', *Journal of the Veterinary History Society,* pt. 2/15 (2011), 308–334.
49 *Veterinary Record,* 22 (1909), 22.
50 *Proceedings* (1909), 13 ff.
51 *Proceedings* (1910), 21.
52 *Proceedings* (1907).
53 *Proceedings* (1912).
54 *Veterinary Record,* 25 (1913), 467.
55 *Veterinary Record,* 26 (1914), 765.
56 Department of Employment and Productivity data, 1981.

57 *Proceedings* (1913), 113.
58 John Francis in *Veterinary Record,* 55 (1943), 350–352.

CHAPTER 3

1 *Veterinary Record,* 22 (1914), 381.
2 *Veterinary Record,* 26 (1914), 381.
3 *Veterinary Record,* 27 (1915), 503.
4 F. Hobday, *Fifty years a veterinary surgeon* (Hutchinson: London, 1938); *Veterinary Record,* 28 (1915),109.
5 RAVC, '200 years of history', <http://www.army.mod.uk/ documents/general/RAVC_History.pdf> accessed 30 August 2012; Frederick Smith, *A history of the Royal Army Veterinary Corps, 1796– 1919* (Baillière, Tindall & Cox: London, 1927); R. Passmore, 'The British horse in WWI: Care, development and importance on the western front', *Veterinary History* , 15 (2011), 539.
6 *Veterinary Record,* 28 (1915), 20.
7 Reprinted from *The Scotsman* in *Veterinary Record,* 28 (1915), 472.
8 F. M. L. Thompson, 'Nineteenth century horse sense', *Economic History Review,* 29 (1976), 60–81.
9 *Veterinary Record,* 29 (1916), 249.
10 F. Trentmann, 'Bread, milk and democracy: consumption and citizenship in 20th century Britain', in M. Daunton & M. Hilton (eds), *The politics of consumption: material culture and citizenship in Europe and America* (Berg: Oxford, 2001), 129–163.
11 *Veterinary Record,* 30 (1918), 420.
12 *Veterinary Record,* 31 (1918), 24.
13 A. Woods, 'A scientific policy?: Contagious disease control at the British Board of Agriculture, 1890–1922', paper presented to European Science Foundation workshop, Paris, 2008; A. Woods, ' "Partnership" in action: contagious abortion and the governance of livestock disease in Britain, 1885–1921', *Minerva,* 47 (2009), 195–217; K. Waddington, ' "To stamp out so terrible a malady": Bovine tuberculosis and tuberculin testing in Britain, 1890–1939', *Medical History,* 48 (2004).
14 *Veterinary Record,* 31 (1918), 18.
15 Ibid.
16 A. Woods, S. Matthews 'The English veterinary surgeon c.1860–1885' (in press).
17 *Veterinary Record,* 31 (1918), 18.
18 *Veterinary Record,* 31 (1919), 201.
19 Ibid. 291.
20 *Veterinary Record,* 31 (1919), 96.

Notes to Chapters 3–4

21 *Veterinary Record,* 32 (1919), 66.
22 *Proceedings* (1919), 6.
23 Ibid. 9.
24 *Veterinary Record,* NS 1 (1921), 2.
25 Hardy, 'Professional advantage and public health'.
26 J. Wacher, ' "Lessening our greatest scourge": managing the tuberculosis milk problem in Birmingham at the turn of the 20th century', *Midland History,* 33 (2008), 115–30.
27 *Veterinary Record,* NS 1 (1921), 2.
28 *Veterinary Record,* 33 (1920), 309.
29 A. Hardy, 'Professional advantage and public health: British veterinary surgeons and state veterinary services, 1865–1939', *Twentieth Century British History,* 14 (2003), 1–23.
30 *Veterinary Record,* NS 1 (1921), 123.
31 BVA press statement, 25 March 2010.
32 *Veterinary Record,* 66 (1954), 31.
33 *Veterinary Record Supplement* (3 July, 1954), 63.
34 *Veterinary Record Supplement* (18 September 1954), 115.
35 Charles Mitchell, 'The Official Journal', *Veterinary Record,* 100 (1977), 542–544.
36 BVA *Annual Report and Accounts* 1955.
37 *Veterinary Record,* 68 (1956), 778.
38 Ibid. 867.
39 *Veterinary Record,* 68 (1956), 1023.
40 *Veterinary Record,* 71 (1959), 357.
41 Entry in *Research in Veterinary Science* minute book.
42 *Veterinary Record,* 104 (1979), 42.
43 Ibid. 32.
44 BVA *Annual Report* 2008–2009, 19.

CHAPTER 4

1 *Veterinary Record,* NS 9 (1929), 8.
2 A. Woods, 'The Lowe report and its echoes from history', *Veterinary Record,* 169 (2011), 434–6.
3 F. M. L. Thompson, *Economic History Review,* 20 (1976), 80.
4 E. H. Whetham, 'The Agriculture Act, 1920 and its repeal – the "Great Betrayal" ', *Agricultural History,* 22 (1974), 36–49.
5 *Veterinary Record,* NS 1 (1921), 799.
6 See Susan Jones, *Valuing Animals: Veterinarians and their patients in modern America* (Johns Hopkins: Baltimore, 2003) for USA views on the decline of the horse.
7 Data: Office for National Statistics.

Notes to Chapter 4

8 John Martin, *The development of modern agriculture: British farming since 1931* (MacMillan: Basingstoke, 2000).
9 *Proceedings* (1919), 17.
10 *Proceedings* (1924), 17; K. Waddington, ' "To stamp out so terrible a malady": Bovine tuberculosis and tuberculin testing in Britain, 1890–1939', *Medical History,* 48 (2004), 103.
11 C. M. Warwick, A. M. Macdonald, 'The Life of Professor Orlando Charnock Bradley', *Veterinary History,* 15 (2011).
12 K. Angus, *A history of the animal diseases research association* (ADRA: Edinburgh, 1990); 'The Central Veterinary Laboratory Weybridge, 1917–67', *Veterinary Record,* 81 (1967), 62–68.
13 Iain Pattison, *The British veterinary profession 1791–1948* (J. A. Allen: London, 1984).
14 *Veterinary Record,* NS 2 (1922), 632 ff.
15 *Veterinary Record,* NS 6 (1926), 319.
16 Ibid. 313.
17 *Proceedings* (1927), 117.
18 *Proceedings* (1928), 77.
19 Ibid. 20.
20 *Veterinary Record,* 32 (1920), 47.
21 Ibid. 473.
22 A. Digby, 'The economic and medical significance of the British National Health Insurance Act', in M. Gorsky, S. Sheard (eds), *Financing Medicine* (Routledge: London, 2006).
23 *Veterinary Record,* 10 (1930), 814.
24 *Veterinary Record,* 32 (1920), 473.
25 *Veterinary Record,* 10 (1930), 81.
26 Ibid. 634.
27 *Veterinary Record,* 15 (1935), 131.
28 *Proceedings* (1934), 28.
29 *Proceedings* (1932), 33.
30 S. Wilmot, in 'From "public service" to artificial insemination: Animal breeding science and reproductive research in early twentieth-century Britain', *Studies in the history of the biological and biomedical sciences,* 38 (2007), 411–41.
31 *Proceedings* (1932), 27.
32 T. A. R. Chipperfield, in 'The Society of Practising Veterinary Surgeons, 1933–1950', <http://www.spvs.org.uk/sites/default/files/SPVS_History_0.pdf> accessed 20 August 2012.
33 *Veterinary Record,* 13 (1933), 1042.
34 Ibid. 254.
35 *Proceedings* (1934), 36.
36 *Proceedings* (1934), 31.

Notes to Chapters 4–6

37 A. Gardiner, 'Small animal practice in British veterinary medicine, 1920–1950', PhD thesis (University of Manchester, 2010).

CHAPTER 5

1   A. Woods, *A manufactured plague?: The history of foot and mouth disease in Britain* (Earthscan: London, 2004). This work provides a comprehensive survey of FMD and its control.
2   *Veterinary Record,* 4 (1924), 35.
3   *Veterinary Record,* 3 (1923), 904.
4   A. Woods, 'The 1951–1952 vaccination controversy', in *A manufactured plague?*
5   *Veterinary Record,* 64 (1952), 277.
6   *Veterinary Record Supplement* (10 January 1953), 4.
7   *Report of the Departmental Committee on FMD, 1952–1954,* 41.
8   Hansard, quoted in *Veterinary Record,* 81 (1967), 573.
9   *Veterinary Record,* 83 (1968), 297.
10 *Veterinary Record,* 81 (1967), Letters, 2 December, 16 December, 23 December.
11 *Veterinary Record,* 81 (1967), 674.
12 Ibid. 603.
13 National Audit Office: *2001 Outbreak of foot-and-mouth disease* (HMSO: London, 2002).
14 *Veterinary Record,* 148 (2001), 386.
15 Ibid. 389.
16 Ibid. 695.
17 Ibid. 417.
18 *Animal Health 2001: Report of the Chief Veterinary Officer* (DEFRA publications: London, 2001).
19 'Epidemic 2001', in Woods, *A manufactured plague?*
20 *Veterinary Record,* 148 (2001), 547, 578, 580.
21 National Audit Office: *2001 Outbreak of foot-and-mouth disease* (HMSO: London, 2002).
22 RCVS submission published in *Veterinary Record,* 150 (2002), 393.
23 Ibid. 390.
24 'Investing in innovation; a strategy for engineering, science and technology', in *Comprehensive spending review* (HM Treasury: London, 2002).

CHAPTER 6

1   *Veterinary Record,* NS 14 (1934), 102.
2   *Veterinary Record,* 49 (1937), 749–754.

Notes to Chapter 6

3   A. Hardy, *Twentieth Century British History,* 14 (2003), 18.
4   *Veterinary Record,* NS 14 (1934), 948.
5   *Veterinary Record,* NS 15 (1935), 116.
6   Ibid. 138.
7   R. C. Locke, *Veterinary Record,* NS 15 (1935), 247; H. L. Torrance Ibid. 216.
8   J. A. Dixon, Ibid. 247.
9   *Veterinary Record,* 49 (1937), 856.
10 *Veterinary Record,* 59 (1937), 1941.
11 A. Hardy, *Twentieth Century British History,* 14 (2003), 20.
12 *Veterinary Record,* 49 (1937), 1615.
13 'Centralisation of public veterinary services', *Report of the special consultative committee, NVMA, Veterinary Record,* 50 (1938), 3–12.
14 *Veterinary Record,* 50 (1938), 93.
15 Ibid. 123.
16 T. A. R. Chipperfield, in 'The Society of Practising Veterinary Surgeons, 1933–1950', <http://www.spvs.org.uk/sites/default/files/SPVS_History_0.pdf> accessed 20 August 2012.
17 *Veterinary Record,* 50 (1938), 239.
18 A. Hardy, *Twentieth Century British History,* 14 (2003), 21.
19 *Veterinary Record,* 51 (1939), 641.
20 *Veterinary Journal,* 95 (1939), 171.
21 A. Hardy, *Twentieth Century British History,* 14 (2003), 22.
22 *Veterinary Record,* NS 15 (1935), 116.
23 *Veterinary Record,* 51 (1939), 107.
24 Ibid. 1126.
25 *Veterinary Record,* 52 (1940), 707.
26 Ibid. 86.
27 Ibid. 797–798.
28 *Veterinary Record,* 54 (1942), 435–438.
29 Conversation with Mary Brancker at Veterinary History Society, 9 December 2009.
30 MAFF, *Animal health, a centenary 1865–1965: A century of endeavour to control animal disease* (HMSO: London, 1965), 231.
31 A. Woods, 'The farm as clinic: Veterinary expertise and the transformation of dairy farming, 1930–1950', *Studies in History and Philosophy of Science Part C: Studies in History and Philosophy of Biological and Biomedical Sciences,* 38 (2007), 462–487.
32 *Veterinary Record,* 54 (1942), 467.
33 *Veterinary Record,* 56 (1944), 467.
34 Ibid.
35 Beveridge report, *Social insurance and Allied Services,* Cmd 6040 (HMSO: London, 1942).
36 *Veterinary Record,* 54 (1942), 437.

Notes to Chapters 6–7

37 Presentation by the NVMA to the RCVS Council, 25 May 1939, *Veterinary Record,* 51 (1939), 763–761.
38 *Veterinary Record,* 55 (1943), 398–409.
39 *Veterinary Record,* 56 (1944), 280.
40 'Summary of principal conclusions and recommendations', second report of the Loveday Committee, *Veterinary Record,* 56 (1944), 133.

CHAPTER 7

1 *Veterinary Record,* 54 (1942), 439.
2 *Veterinary Record,* 56 (1944), 134.
3 RAVC, '200 years of history', <http://www.army.mod.uk/ documents/general/RAVC_History.pdf> accessed 30 August 2012.
4 Agriculture Act 1947; J. Martin, *The Development of modern agriculture: British farming since 1931* (Palgrave Macmillan: Basingstoke, 2000).
5 G. Arthur, *Veterinary Record,* 65 (1953), 352.
6 *Veterinary Record,* 57 (1945), 455.
7 Ibid. 561.
8 Ibid. 553.
9 *Veterinary Record,* 58 (1946), 393.
10 Ibid. 546.
11 Ibid.
12 Ibid. 547.
13 *Veterinary Record,* 59 (1947), 291.
14 NVMA comment, *Veterinary Record,* 59 (1947), 457.
15 *Veterinary Record,* 59 (1947), 359.
16 C. C. S. Newton, 'The Sterling Crisis of 1947 and the British Response to the Marshall Plan', *Economic History Review* , 37 (1984), 381–400.
17 *Veterinary Record,* 60 (1948), 381.
18 Ibid. 382.
19 *Veterinary Record,* NS 6 (1926), 523.
20 A. Gardiner, 'Small animal practice in British veterinary medicine, 1920–1952', PhD Thesis (Manchester University, 2010).
21 Ibid.
22 *Veterinary Record,* NS 8 (1933), 149–151.
23 *Veterinary Record,* 49 (1937), 896.
24 Gardiner, 'Small animal practice'.
25 *Veterinary Record Supplement* (20 December 1947), 112.
26 BVA council report, *Veterinary Record,* 60 (1948).
27 *Report of the Committee on Licenses under Section 7 of the Veterinary Surgeons Act 1948* (HMSO: London, 1952).
28 Gardiner, 'Small animal practice'.

Notes to Chapters 7–8

29 *Veterinary Record,* 67 (1955), 706.
30 BVA *Annual Report* 1936.
31 *Veterinary Record,* NS 12 (1932), 1004.
32 *Veterinary Record,* 63 (1951), 756.
33 P. N. Humphreys, *Veterinary Record,* 66 (1954), 554.
34 F. B. Halpin, Ibid. 702.
35 D. J. Skinner, Ibid. 721.
36 Ibid. 702.
37 *Veterinary Record,* 67 (1955), 707.
38 *Veterinary Record,* 60 (1948), 10.
39 Ibid. 307.
40 Ibid. 312.
41 Ibid.
42 Ibid. 376.
43 Ibid. 388.
44 Ibid. 360.
45 Ibid. 311.
46 *Report of the Committee on Veterinary Practice by Unregistered Persons,* Cmd 6611 (HMSO: London, 1945).
47 Hansard report, in *Veterinary Record,* 60 (1948), 28–29.
48 *Veterinary Record,* 60 (1948), 330.
49 Ibid. 352.
50 *Veterinary Record,* 61 (1949), 283.
51 Ibid. 82.
52 *Veterinary Record,* 64 (1952), 496.
53 *Veterinary Record Supplement* (2 April 1955), 7; *Veterinary Record Supplement* (18 June 1955), 83.
54 Veterinary Record, 61 (1949), 233.
55 Ibid. 329.
56 Tributes to H. Steele-Bodger, *Veterinary Record,* 64 (1952), 56.
57 *Veterinary Record,* 78 (1966), 114–116.
58 Ibid. 151.
59 *Veterinary Record,* 79 (1966), 1.
60 *Veterinary Record,* 79 (1966), 888.

CHAPTER 8

1 *Veterinary Record,* 49 (1937), 150–155.
2 *Veterinary Record,* 58 (1946), 590.
3 *Veterinary Record,* 66 (1954), 83.
4 Hansard, HC (series 5) vol. 523, cols 513–38 (12 Feb. 1954).
5 *Veterinary Record,* 66 (1954), 459.
6 *Veterinary Record,* 69 (1957), 640.
7 Ibid. 665.

Notes to Chapters 8–9

8   Ibid. 686.
9   Ibid. 674.
10 Ibid. 695.
11 Ibid. 722.
12 Ibid. 723.
13 *Veterinary Record,* 75 (1963), 872.

CHAPTER 9

1   *Veterinary Record,* 73 (1961), 873–877.
2   *Veterinary Record,* 72 (1960), 815.
3   *Veterinary Record,* 56 (1944), 467.
4   *Report of the Committee of Inquiry into Recruitment for the Veterinary Profession* (Northumberland Committee), Cmnd 2430 (HMSO: London, 1964), 20.
5   *Veterinary Record,* 74 (1962), 436.
6   Ibid. 1173.
7   Ibid.
8   Ibid. 1166.
9   *Veterinary Record,* 75 (1963), 998.
10 Ibid. 479.
11 Ibid. 1308.
12 MAF files, National Archive, quoted by A. Woods in 'Factory farming, the ownership of animal health and the delivery of veterinary preventive medicine in Britain c1945–75' (in press).
13 *Veterinary Record,* 75 (1963), 100.
14 Ibid. 126.
15 Woods, 'Factory farming'.
16 *Veterinary Record,* 84 (1969), 423.
17 Ibid. 317.
18 Woods, 'Factory farming'.
19 BVA *Annual Report* 1974–75, 46.
20 National Archive 287/01, *Report of the working party set up to consider a nationalised veterinary service.* MAF 1963
21 Sir Michael Swann at the BVA congress, 1975 *Veterinary Record,* 97 (1975), 237.
22 *Veterinary Record,* 77 (1965), 180.
23 EB conversations with J. C. MacKellar 1974–1978.
24 Veterinary Defence Society files.
25 *Veterinary Record,* 68 (1956), 613.
26 *Veterinary Record,* 69 (1957), 117.
27 BSAVA *50ᵗʰ Anniversary booklet,* 6.
28 BSAVA 2010 *Report.*
29 *Veterinary Record,* 72 (1960), 721.

Notes to Chapters 9–10

30 *Veterinary Record,* 79 (1966), 471.
31 Report in *Veterinary Times,* April 1976.
32 E.g. BVA News, in *Veterinary Record,* 122 (1989), 531.
33 *Veterinary Record,* 81 (1967), 543.
34 EB conversations with Mary Brancker, various dates.
35 *Veterinary Record,* 103 (1978), 265.
36 *Veterinary Record,* 89 (1971), 118.
37 *Veterinary Record,* 59 (1947), 359.
38 J. Prior's address to BVA council, *Veterinary Record,* 89 (1971), 1.
39 *Veterinary Record,* 93 (1973), 270–271.
40 A. M. Taylor, in an interview with A. Woods 2008.
41 *Veterinary Record,* 93 (1973), 564–566.
42 BVA *Annual Report* 1973–74, 31.
43 *Veterinary Record,* 96 (1975), 570.
44 J. O'Donohue, L. Goulding, G. Allen, 'Consumer price inflation since 1750', *Economic Trends,* 604 (2004), 38–46.
45 *Veterinary Record,* 97 (1975), 265.
46 BVA *Annual Report* 1977–78, 12.
47 M. Nelson, J. Tandy, *The Great Haxby, Veterinary Surgeon Extraordinaire* (BVA Animal Welfare Foundation: London, 2007).
48 BVA evidence to the Duke of Northumberland's committee of enquiry: recruitment to the veterinary profession and the development of postgraduate studies, BVA *Annual Report* 1963, 67.
49 *Report of the Committee of Inquiry into Recruitment for the Veterinary Profession* (Northumberland Committee), Cmnd 2430 (HMSO: London, 1964), 45.
50 *Veterinary Record,* 76 (1964), 1003.
51 *Veterinary Record,* 78 (1966), 591–596.

CHAPTER 10

1 *Veterinary Record,* 97 (1975), 217.
2 *Report of the Committee of Inquiry into the Veterinary Profession* (Swann report), Cmnd 6143 (HMSO: London, 1975).
3 *Veterinary Record,* 97 (1975), 237.
4 N. Snodgrass, address at BVA Congress 1975, *Veterinary Record,* 97 (1975), 283–285.
5 W. I. McIntyre, *Veterinary Record,* 97 (1975), 285.
6 *Veterinary Record,* 97 (1975), 287.
7 Ibid. 289.
8 SPVS evidence to Swann Committee, RCVS Trust archive.
9 Swann report, 12.
10 RCVS *Annual Report* 2010.
11 *Veterinary Record,* 97 (1975), 458.

Notes to Chapters 10–11

12 BVA interim observations on the report of the Committee of Inquiry into the Veterinary Profession, *Veterinary Record,* 98 (1976), 360–369.
13 *Veterinary Record,* 101 (1977), 415.
14 Ibid. 430.
15 BVA *Annual Report* 1978–79, 22.
16 BVA *Annual Report* 1980–81, 44.
17 *Manpower Review of the Veterinary Profession in the UK* (1985) MAFF.
18 *Veterinary Record,* 122 (1988), 4.
19 Adapted from *Veterinary Record,* 122 (1988), 451.
20 *Veterinary Record,* 124 (1989), 73.
21 Ibid. 74.
22 Ibid. 256.
23 Ibid. 381.
24 Ibid. 563.
25 Ibid. 445.
26 Teaching and Higher Education Act 1998.
27 RCVS *Annual Report* 2010

CHAPTER 11

1 A report of the banquet is published in *Veterinary Record,* 110 (1982), 285–289.
2 *Veterinary Record,* 110 (1982), 279–284.
3 Ibid. 519–523.
4 Ibid. 523–525.
5 Ibid. 526–528.
6 Ibid. 255.
7 *Veterinary Record,* 83 (1968), 388.
8 Ibid. 568.
9 EB conversations with BVA members 1973–74.
10 EB conversations with P. B. Turner.
11 Report of an inquiry into the misappropriation of BVA funds, 1984 (Confidential); summarised in BVA *Annual Report* 1983–84, 3.
12 NVMA *Annual Report* 1919–1920.
13 *Veterinary Record,* 116 (1985), 624.
14 Ibid. 471–476.
15 BVA News, in *Veterinary Record,* 123 (1988), 446.
16 *Veterinary Record,* 124 (1989), 541.
17 Ibid. 67.
18 *Veterinary Record,* 139 (1996), 56.
19 *Veterinary Record,* 142 (1998), 416.
20 BVA Executive papers, 1997 annex 14a.
21 *Veterinary Record,* 143 (1998), 63.

Notes to Chapters 11–12

22 *Veterinary Record,* 147 (2000), 90.
23 *Veterinary Record,* 148 (2000), 731.
24 *Veterinary Record,* 149 (2001), 335.
25 *Veterinary Times,* 32 no. 29 (2001).
26 *Off the Record,* October 2002, 2.
27 EB conversations with staff members.
28 J. Baird, BVA chief executive, 1986–2002, in conversation with the author, June 2010.
29 *Veterinary Record,* 151 (2002), 247.
30 Ibid. 275, 336, 364, 396.
31 Ibid. 428.
32 Report, *Veterinary Record,* 151 (2002), 431.
33 *Veterinary Record,* 152 (2003), 5.
34 *Veterinary Times,* 32 no. 30 (2002).
35 N. Paull, interviewed 2011.

CHAPTER 12

1 *Veterinary Record,* 121 (1987), 118.
2 Ibid. 553.
3 *Veterinary Record,* 122 (1988), 118, 144, 167.
4 Ibid. 264.
5 *Veterinary Record,* 146 (2000), 203.
6 Ibid. 295; *Veterinary Record,* 147 (2000), 3–6, 443.
7 Ibid. 4.
8 *Veterinary Record,* 146 (2000), 539.
9 Council report, *Veterinary Record,* 147 (2000), 83.
10 EB interview with David Catlow, 2011.
11 EB interview with David Catlow, 2011.
12 Letter to stakeholders from Director, Veterinary Services, Animal Health, 7 March 2011.
13 RCVS council report, *Veterinary Record,* 142 (1998), 261.
14 *Veterinary Record Supplement* 4 January 1954, 7–9.
15 *Veterinary Record,* 66 (1954), 418.
16 *Veterinary Record Supplement*, 18 September 1954, 106.
17 *Veterinary Record Supplement*, 16 January 1954, 7–9.
18 *Veterinary Record,* 66 (1954), 418.
19 *Veterinary Record,* 67 (1956), 636.
20 *Veterinary Record,* 97 (1975), 486.
21 Ibid. 75.
22 *Veterinary Record,* 98 (1976), 242.
23 *Veterinary Record,* 99 (1976), 39.
24 BVA *Annual Report* 1979–80, 32.
25 Hansard, quoted in *Veterinary Record,* 106 (1980), 111.

Notes to Chapters 12–13

26 BVA *Annual Report* 1979–80, 31.
27 *Veterinary Record,* 112 (1983), 419.
28 *Veterinary Record,* 130 (1992), 214.
29 Ibid. 213.
30 Ibid. 496.
31 *Veterinary Record,* 132 (1993), 420.
32 Address at BVA congress, *Veterinary Record,* 130 (1992), 403.
33 *Veterinary Record,* 133 (1993), 78.
34 Ibid. 77.
35 *Veterinary Record,* 135 (1994), 417.
36 Ibid. 489.
37 Ibid. 559.
38 Hansard, HC (series 5) vol. 292, cols 372–386 (12 March 1997).
39 *Veterinary Record,* 140 (1970), 443.
40 Jill Nute, public health veterinarian, personal communication, 2010.

CHAPTER 13

1   K. Waddington, ' "To stamp out so terrible a malady": Bovine
    tuberculosis and tuberculin testing in Britain, 1890–1939', *Medical
    History,* 48 (2004), 29–48; Peter Atkins, 'The pasteurisation of
    England: the science, culture and health implications of milk
    processing, 1900–1950', in J. Phillips, D. Smith (eds), *Food, science,
    policy and regulation in the 20th century* (Routledge: London, 2000),
    37–51.
2   *Veterinary Record,* 5 (1935), 352.
3   Waddington, 'So terrible a malady'; M. French, J. Phillips, 'Conflicts
    of interest: milk regulation, 1875–1938', in *Cheated not poisoned?
    Food regulation in the United Kingdom, 1875–1938* (Manchester
    University Presss, Manchester, 2000), 158–184; MAFF, *Animal
    Health: A Centenary* (HMSO: London, 1965).
4   *Proceedings* (1924), 17.
5   *Proceedings* (1928), 20.
6   *Proceedings* (1927), 32.
7   P. J. Atkins, 'Lobbying and resistance with regard to policy on bovine
    tuberculosis in Britain 1900–1939: an inside/outside model', in F.
    Condrau, M. Worboys (eds), *Tuberculosis then and now.* (McGill-
    Queen's University Press: Montreal, 2010), 189–212.
8   BVA *Annual Report* 1981–82, 22.
9   *Report by the independent scientific review group on bovine
    tuberculosis in cattle and badgers* (Krebs Report) (MAFF
    publications: London, 1997).
10 *Veterinary Record,* 142 (1998), 257.

Notes to Chapter 13

11 *Badgers and bovine tuberculosis*, reference HC 233, (HMSO: London, 1999).
12 *Veterinary Record*, 143 (1998), 206.
13 Ibid. 28.
14 *Veterinary Record*, 154 (2004), 482.
15 *Veterinary Record*, 156 (2005), 221.
16 Ibid. 293.
17 Ibid. 296.
18 *Veterinary Record*, 157 (2005), 590.
19 *Veterinary Record*, 156 (2005), 556.
20 M. Gilbert and others, *Nature*, 435 (2005), 491–496.
21 *Nature*, 439 (2006), 843–846.
22 <http://archive.defra.gov.uk/foodfarm/farmanimal/diseases/atoz/tb/partnership/documents/prmt_advice201206.pdf> accessed 27 September 2012.
23 *Veterinary Record*, 158 (2006), 418.
24 *Bovine tuberculosis: The scientific evidence: Final report of the independent group on cattle tuberculosis* (HMSO: London, 2007).
25 Wyn Grant, 'Intractable policy failure: the case of TB and badgers', *British Journal of Politics and International Relations*, 11/4 (2009), 557–573.
26 DEFRA figures.
27 Consultation statement, Minister of Agriculture, 10 September 2010.
28 W. A. Watson, 'Epidemiology and control of Aujeszky's disease in Great Britain', *Rev. sci. tech. OIE* 5/2 (1986), 362–378.
29 D. Basinger (former National Pig Advisor, MAFF), 'Politico-Economic aspects of Aujeszky's disease control in Great Britain, 1953–1989', *Pig Veterinary Society Journal*, 24 (1990), 102–120.
30 *Veterinary Record*, 112 (1983), 185.
31 *Veterinary Record*, 112 (1983), 86.
32 R. G. A. Douglas, former president Pig Veterinary Society, personal communication, 2011.
33 *Veterinary Record*, 112 (1983), 236.
34 Ibid. 534.
35 Ibid. 596.
36 Government memorandum of response to the third report from the Agricultural Committee.
37 *Veterinary Record*, 117 (1985), 1.
38 *Veterinary Record*, 120 (1987), 170.
39 *Veterinary Record*, 124 (1989), 384.
40 BVA *Annual Report* 1962, 9.
41 *Veterinary Record*, 74 (1962), 1137.
42 MAFF *Annual Report* 1965.
43 DEFRA statistics.

Notes to Chapters 13–14

44 A. Woods, 'A historical synopsis of farm animal disease and public policy in 20ᵗʰ century Britain', *Philosophical Transactions of the Royal Society: Biological Sciences,* 366 (2011), 1943–1954.

45 *Veterinary Record,* 109 (1981), 393.

46 Report, 'Brucellosis and the veterinary surgeon', *Veterinary Record,* 98 (1976), 253–262.

47 *Veterinary Record,* 112 (1988), 566.

48 Ibid. 497.

49 P. van Zwanenberg, E. Millstone, *BSE: Risk, science and governance* (OUP: Oxford, 2005).

50 *Veterinary Record,* 138 (1996), 381.

51 Ibid. 426.

52 Phillips, J. Bridgeman, M. Ferguson-Smith, *Report of the inquiry into BSE and variant CJD in the United Kingdom* (HMSO: London, 2000).

53 BVA *Annual Report* 1998.

CHAPTER 14

1 T. Corley and A. Godley, 'The Veterinary Medicines Industry in Britain, 1900–2000', *Economic History Review,* 64 (2011), 832–54.

2 R. Bud, *Penicillin: Triumph and tragedy* (OUP: Oxford, 2007).

3 *Report of the Joint Committee on the use of antibiotics in animal husbandry and veterinary medicine 1969* (Swann Report, Cmnd 4910).

4 *Veterinary Record,* 88 (1971), 236.

5 *Veterinary Record,* 99 (1976), 379.

6 Ibid. 377.

7 *Veterinary Record,* 89 (1971), 587.

8 *Veterinary Record,* 101 (1977), 62.

9 Ibid. 349.

10 Ibid. 489.

11 *Veterinary Record,* 101 (1977), 506.

12 *Veterinary Record,* 103 (1978), 121.

13 Ibid. 148.

14 *Veterinary Record,* 110 (1982), 291.

15 Ibid. 310.

16 Ibid. 432.

17 *Veterinary Record,* 112 (1983), 389.

18 *Veterinary Record,* 168 (2011), 60.

19 *Report of the Independent Research Group appointed to review the procedures by which prescription medicines for veterinary use are classified and sold in the UK and the impact current practices may be having on availability and prices* (HMSO: London, 2001).

Notes to Chapter 14

20 Veterinary Medicines Directorate briefing document, quoted in *Veterinary Record,* 146 (2000), 537.
21 Provisional conclusions of the Competition Commission, *Veterinary Record,* 151 (2002), 338.
22 *Veterinary Record,* 152 (2003), 481.
23 Ibid. 484.
24 *Veterinary Record,* 151 (2002), 433.
25 *Veterinary Record,* 156 (2005), 291.
26 Quoted in *Veterinary Record,* 152 (2002), 481.
27 *Veterinary Medicines: A report on the supply within the United Kingdom of Prescription Only Medicines* (HMSO: London, 2003).
28 D. Catlow, interviewed May 2011.
29 A. Woods, 'The history of veterinary ethics in Britain, c1870–2000', in C. Wathes (ed.), *Proceedings of the first international conference on veterinary ethics* (Wiley Blackwell, 2012, in press).
30 A. Gardiner, 'Small animal practice in British veterinary medicine, 1920–1952', PhD Thesis (Manchester University, 2010).
31 EB interview with J. Tandy, 2011.
32 Tandy's concern to improve the technical facilities in practices led him to become an instrumental figure in the foundation of the British Veterinary Hospitals Association in 1972; he was president of the BVA in 1980–81.
33 *Report on the supply of veterinary services in relation to restrictions on advertising,* Monopolies Commission (1976), Cmnd 6572.
34 *Veterinary Record,* 99 (1976), 114.
35 Ibid. 461.
36 Ibid. 445.
37 *Veterinary Record,* 101 (1977), 62.
38 *Veterinary Record,* 115 (1984), 180.
39 *Veterinary Record,* 116 (1985), 16–18.
40 RCVS council meeting report, *Veterinary Record,* 116 (1985), 297.
41 *Veterinary Record,* 116 (1985), 224.
42 Letter to the *Veterinary Record,* 116 (1985), 378.
43 *Veterinary Record,* 116 (1985), 356.
44 Ibid. 677.
45 *Veterinary Record,* 10 (1897), 171.
46 Catriona Blake, *The charge of the parasols: Women's entry to the medical profession* (Women's Press: London, 1990).
47 EB conversations with Mary Brancker, 2000.
48 Maureen Aitken's article, 'Women in the veterinary profession' *Veterinary Record,* 134 (1994), 546–551, gives an account of the situation up to 1994.
49 *Veterinary Record,* NS 14 (1934), 364.
50 Ibid. 61.

Notes to Chapters 14–15

51 *Veterinary Record,* 132 (1993), 521.
52 Obituary, *The Independent,* 7 September 2001.
53 Obituary, *The Times,* 24 July 2010.
54 Obituary, *The Independent,* 4 March 1993.
55 *Veterinary Record,* 67 (1956), 638.
56 Aitken, 'Women in the veterinary profession'.
57 James Herriot, *All creatures great and small* (St Martins Press: New York, 1972).
58 RCVS evidence to Swann Committee, 1973.
59 RCVS *Annual Report* 2010.
60 *Veterinary Record,* 123 (1988), 556.
61 Ibid. 630.
62 *Veterinary Record,* 124 (1989), 314.
63 Maureen Aitken, *Veterinary Record,* 134 (1994), 548.
64 RCVS *Facts* 2010.
65 This study, by Anne Lincoln, seeks to explain feminisation of the veterinary profession – a summary can be found at <https://www.avma.org/News/JAVMANews/Pages/101215l.aspx> accessed 27 September 2012.
66 A. E. Lincoln, 'The shifting supply of men and women to occupations: feminisation in veterinary education', *Social Forces,* 88 (2010), 1969–1998.
67 Interview with R. M. Stevenson, 2010.
68 For accounts of women's experience in the profession see: M. Aitken, *Veterinary Record,* 134 (1994), 346–351; P. Riveson, *JAVMA,* 212 (1998), 182–184; M. Brancker, *In Practice* (September 2002), 474–478; M. Cameron, ibid. (March 2003), 166–167; M. Aitken, ibid. (May 2003), 292–293; J. Nute, ibid. (July/August 2003), 430–432; S. Dyson, ibid. (September 2003), 503–505.
69 J. L. Tomlin and others, 'Influences on the decision to study veterinary medicine: variation with sex and background', *Veterinary Record,* 166 (2010), 747–748.

CHAPTER 15

1 A. Woods, 'Is prevention better than cure?: The rise and fall of veterinary preventive medicine, c1950–80', *Social History of Medicine* (2012 in press).
2 Address to the BVA congress 1983, *Veterinary Record,* 114 (1983), 306.
3 In fact, it would be forced to commit massive funding to the management of BSE (which emerged in 1987) and the worst ever epidemic of foot-and-mouth disease in 2001.
4 DEFRA Agricultural Census.
5 Farm Practices Survey, DEFRA.

Notes to Chapter 15

6 R. Wilson at BVA council, *Veterinary Record,* 147 (2000), 729.
7 EFRACom *Report on Vets and Veterinary Services* (2003) HC 03.
8 <http://archive.defra.gov.uk/foodfarm/farmanimal/diseases/ vetsurveillance/strategy/documents/strategydoc.pdf> accessed 27 September 2012.
9 *Veterinary Record,* 155 (2004), 157.
10 Philip Lowe, *Unlocking potential: A report on veterinary expertise in food animal production* (DEFRA: London, 2009).
11 Nicky Paull, BVA president 2010.
12 RCVS Survey of the profession 2006.
13 'The franchise operation', *Veterinary Record,* 116 (1985), 252–253.
14 S. W. F. Holloway, *Royal Pharmaceutical Society of Great Britain 1841–1991* (Pharmaceutical Press: London, 1991).
15 *RCVS News,* November 1997.
16 *Veterinary Record,* 143 (1998), 291.
17 Address to the BVA congress, *Veterinary Record,* 159 (2006), 578.
18 *Veterinary Record,* 148 (2001), 419.
19 Council reports, *Veterinary Record,* 147 (2000), 90; *Veterinary Record,* 146 (2000), 540.
20 Report, *Veterinary Record,* 146 (2000), 416, 483.
21 Report, *Veterinary Record,* 148 (2001), 4.
22 P. Jinman, past president BVA and RCVS, interview 29 March 2011.

SELECT BIBLIOGRAPHY

Bartrip, P., *Themselves writ large: The British Medical Association 1832–1996* (BMJ Publishers: London, 1996)

Bud, Robert, *Penicillin: Triumph and tragedy* (OUP: Oxford, 2007).

D'Arcy Thompson, Ruth, *The remarkable Gamgees: A story of achievement* (Ramsay Head: Edinburgh, 1974).

Hobday, F., *Fifty years a veterinary surgeon* (Hutchinson: London, 1938).

Holloway, S. W. F., *Royal Pharmaceutical Society of Great Britain, 1841–1991: A political and social history* (Pharmaceutical Press: London, 1991).

Jones, Susan, *Valuing animals: Veterinarians and their patients in modern America* (Johns Hopkins: Baltimore, 2003).

MAFF, *Animal health, a centenary 1865–1965: A century of endeavour to control animal disease* (HMSO: London, 1965).

Martin, John, *The development of modern agriculture: British farming since 1931* (Palgrave Macmillan: Basingstoke, 2000).

Pattison, Iain, *John McFadyean, a great British veterinarian* (J. A. Allen: London, 1981).

Pattison, Iain, *The British veterinary profession 1791–1948* (J. A. Allen: London, 1984).

Phillips, J. Bridgeman, M. Ferguson-Smith, *Report of the inquiry into BSE and variant CJD in the United Kingdom* (HMSO: London, 2000).

Pugh, L., *From farriery to veterinary medicine, 1785–1795* (Heffer: Cambridge, 1962).

Snow, S., *Operations without pain: The practice and science of anaesthesia in Victorian Britain* (Palgrave Macmillan: Basingstoke, 2005).

Waddington, Ivan, *The medical profession in the industrial revolution* (Gill & Macmillan: Dublin, 1984).

Woods, A., *A manufactured plague?: The history of foot and mouth disease in Britain* (Earthscan: London, 2004).

Worboys, Michael, *Spreading germs: Disease theories and medical practice in Britain, 1865–1900* (CUP: Cambridge, 2000).

Zwanenberg, P. van, and Millstone, E., *BSE: Risk, science and governance* (OUP: Oxford, 2005).

APPENDICES

British Veterinary Association (BVA) Presidents

Formerly National Veterinary Association (NVA) and National Veterinary Medical Association (NVMA)

1882	G. Fleming	1910	T. Salusbury Price
1883	Thomas Greaves	1911	W. Woods
1884	Harry Oliver	1912	William Hunting
1885	T. Walley	1913	O. Charnock Bradley
1886	J. Meckinder	1914	O. Charnock Bradley
1887	W.M. Williams	1915	O. Charnock Bradley
1888	W.M. Pritchard	1916	O. Charnock Bradley
1889	T.H. Simcocks	1917	O. Charnock Bradley
1890	J. Wortley Axe	1918	O. Charnock Bradley
1891	J. McCall	1919	O. Charnock Bradley
1892	Edwin Faulkner	1920	O. Charnock Bradley
1893	William Hunting	1921	O. Charnock Bradley
1894	J.M. Parker	1922	H. Sumner
1895	W. Bower	1923	H.J. Dawes
1896	J.F. Simpson	1924	Arthur Gofton
1897	A.W. Mason	1925	J. Basil Buxton
1898	W.H. Boyle	1926	G.H. Wooldridge
1899	Matthew Hedley	1927	J.W. McIntosh
1900	J.R.U. Dewar	1928	O. Charnock Bradley
1901	J. M'Fadyean	1929	G.P. Male
1902	F.W. Garnett	1930	P.J. Simpson
1903	Charles Allen	1931	P.J. Simpson
1904	R.C. Trigger	1932	P.J. Simpson
1905	W.O. Williams	1933	W. Nairn
1906	W. Shipley	1934	J.F. Craig
1907	R. Roberts	1935	J.R. Barker
1908	George Bowman	1936	Robert Simpson
1909	James Macqueen	1937	Donald Campbell

1938	W.J.B. deVine	1975	R.N. Smith
1939	H.W. Steele-Bodger	1976	J. A. Parry
1940	H.W. Steele-Bodger	1977	D.L. Haxby
1941	W.R. Wooldridge	1978	M.J.R. Stockman
1942	W.R. Wooldridge	1979	S.D. Gunn
1943	R.C.G. Hancock	1980	John Tandy
1944	W.M.C. Miller	1981	T.E. Gibson
1945	G.N. Gould	1982	Neal King
1946	W.M. Mitchell	1983	J.L. Crooks
1947	L. Guy Anderson	1984	J.T. Blackburn
1948	R.F. Montgomerie	1985	B. D. Hoskin
1949	J.W. Bruford	1986	B.T. Wells
1950	S.F.J. Hodgman	1987	M.A. Wright
1951	A.J. Wright	1988	Walter Beswick
1952	A.M. Graham	1989	J.S.M. Bower
1953	A. Thomson	1990	D.F. Wishart
1954	A. Robertson	1991	Howard Hellig
1955	E. Wilkinson	1992	F.J.O. Anthony
1956	E.R. Callender	1993	R.C. Young
1957	J. McC. Ingram	1994	C.P. DeVile
1958	H.F. Hebeler	1995	R.M. Stevenson
1959	S.L. Hignett	1996	K.A. Linklater
1960	Sidney Jennings	1997	E.A. Chandler
1961	A.G. Beynon	1998	K.B. Baker
1962	J.B. White	1999	G.R.E. Evans
1963	D.L. Hughes	2000	J.D. Tyson
1964	D.F. Oliver	2001	A. Scott
1965	A. Steele-Bodger	2002	P.C. Jinman
1966	F.V. John	2003	T.C.R. Greet
1967	Mary Brancker	2004	R.M. McCracken
1968	P.D.S. Pugh	2005	Freda M. Scott-Park
1969	J.H. Parsons	2006	D.F. Catlow
1970	P.D.S. Pugh	2007	J.D. Blayney
1971	Nigel Snodgrass	2008	Nicola J. Paull
1972	A.M. Taylor	2009	W.J. Reilly
1973	J.C. Mackellar	2010	P.H. Locke
1974	W.D. Tavernor		

BVA DIVISIONS

TERRITORIAL DIVISIONS

Ayrshire Veterinary Association
Central Veterinary Society
Cornwall Veterinary Association
Cotswold Veterinary Association
Dumfries and Galloway Division
East Midlands Veterinary Association
Eastern Counties Veterinary Society
Sussex Veterinary Society
Hertfordshire and Bedfordshire Veterinary Society
Lakeland Veterinary Association
Lancashire Veterinary Association
Lincolnshire and District Veterinary Association
Mid-West Veterinary Association
North of England Veterinary Association
North of Ireland Veterinary Association
North of Scotland veterinary division
North Wales Division
Royal Counties Veterinary Association
Scottish Metropolitan Division
Shropshire Veterinary Association
South East Midlands Veterinary Association
South Eastern Veterinary Association
Southern Counties Veterinary Society
South Wales Division
Sussex Veterinary Society
Warwickshire Veterinary Association
West of Scotland Division
Western Counties Veterinary Association
Wyvern Veterinary Society
Yorkshire Veterinary Society

SPECIALIST DIVISIONS

Association of Government Veterinarians

Membership is open to all veterinarians permanently in ant part of the UK Civil Service (Formerly Association of State Veterinary Officers).

Association of Veterinarians in Industry

Vets working in commercial appointments, mainly pharmaceutical and allied industries.

Association of Veterinary Students

UK and Dublin students intending to qualify as veterinarians.

Association of Veterinary Teaching and Research Work

Teachers of veterinary science and all engaged in veterinary research.

British Cattle Veterinary Association

Veterinarians involved with cattle interests.

British Equine Veterinary Association

Promotes veterinary and allied sciences relating to the welfare of the horse; a forum for discussion and exchange of ideas.

British Small Animal Veterinary Association

A major association for promotion of all veterinarians concerned with small animals; organises the UK's largest veterinary conference. Registered as a charity.

British Veterinary Hospitals Association

Promotes high standards of patient care through the design, management and equipment of RCVS-approved veterinary hospitals.

British Veterinary Poultry Association

Includes veterinarians in the specialised field of poultry breeding, hatching, welfare and research.

British Veterinary Zoological Society

Covers every aspect of care and welfare of exotic animals, wild animals, zoos, companion avian species.

Fish Veterinary Society

Provides a forum for veterinarians interested in the science and wellbeing of farmed and hobby fish.

Goat Veterinary Society

Promotes interest in and improved knowledge of goats.

Laboratory Animals Veterinary Association

Deals with the veterinary care and all aspects of the welfare of experimental animals.

Pig Veterinary Society

Aims to enhance knowledge and understanding of pig disease and herd health; covers management, husbandry, economics and welfare.

Royal Army Veterinary Corps

Membership is open to serving or retired members of the Royal Army Veterinary Corps who are BVA members.

Sheep Veterinary Society

Aims to promote sheep health and welfare and provide a forum for advice.

Society of Greyhound Veterinarians

Members are concerned with the health and welfare of the racing greyhound.

Society for the Study of Animal Breeding

Seeks to advance knowledge of all aspects of animal breeding and foster discussion on the subject.

Society of Practising Veterinary Surgeons

A major division which provides, advice, information and practical guidance for veterinarians working in general practice.(formerly Society of Veterinary Practitioners).

Veterinary Deer Society

Members are involved with the management and diseases of wild and captive deer.

Veterinary Public Health Association

Concerned with all aspects of the production of food of animal origin and the improvement of animal welfare. Links the BVA and its members with veterinary associations and organisations.

REGIONAL BRANCHES

Scottish Branch

Brings together BVA divisional representatives to assist in obtaining a consensus view on matters affecting in Scotland.

Welsh Branch

Brings together BVA disisional representatives to assist in obtaining a consus view on matters affecting Wales

Appendices

OTHER BVA GROUPS

Overseas Group

A committee which links the BVA and its members with associations, organisations and individuals throughout the developing world. The BVA Overseas Division, now disbanded, represented members in the former Colonial Service.

Young Vets Group

Made up of graduates up to their eighth qualified year; they are entitled to discounts on subscriptions, insurance, CPD benefits and support meetings.

OTHER VETERINARY ASSOCIATIONS

Commonwealth Veterinary Association

Comprised of national veterinary associations of most Commonwealth countries. It aims to improve animal health, welfare and professional standards in the 52 member countries.

Federation of Veterinarians of Europe

Its 36 member countries represent the interests of practitioners, state veterinary officers, hygienists and vets involved in education, research and industry. The FVE monitors and seeks to influence EC legislation as it affects the profession. The BVA, with the RCVS, maintains a delegation to the FVE.

World Veterinary Association

International organisation established in 1863 representing some 100 national veterinary associations. Dedicated to supporting the aims and activities of the organisations it represents.

FINANCIAL STATUS AND MEMBERSHIP

Year	NVA Balance £	NVA Members	RCVS Members
1884	37	221	2,610
1885	72	264	2,707
1886	101	310	2,800
1887	13	303	2,858
1888	411	295	2,928
1889	94	282	2,995
1890	*	274	2,747
1891	219	280	2,747
1892	299	291	2,734
1893	168	302	2,912
1894	144	321	(3,120
1895	157	293	(3,120
1896	196	274	3,179
1897	172	286	3,232
1898	126	274	3,303
1899	*	*	3,363
1900	161	402	3,417
1901	102	417	3,431
1902	172	409	3,382
1903	182	387	3,365
1904	180	364	3,374
1905	391	382	3,411
1906	191	377	3,428
1907	287	373	3,434
1908	174	373	3,382
1909	*	*	3,329
1910	245	365	3,372
1911	see note 38	356	3,423
1912	94	358	3,417
1913	132	362	3,441
1914	11	356	3,408
1915	121	*	3,425
1916	*	*	3,409
1917	*	*	3,401
1918	171	*	3,381
1919	11	376	3,359

Following name change to NVMA and rise in subscription from 10s. 6d. to £2 2s to include the *Veterinary Record*:

Year	NVMA Balance £	NVMA Members	RCVS Members
1920	*	c360	3,346
1921	*	1,205	3,320
1922	365	1,256	3,276
1923	786	1,434	3,277
1924	1,910	1,493	3,364
1925	999	1,518	3,499
1926	2,564	1,532	3,507
1927	5,346	1,590	3,496
1928	5,567	1,614	3,486
1929	6,023	1,622	3,476
1930	6,501	1,631	3,448
1931	6,528	1,622	3,433
1932	6,452	1,663	3,393
1933	6,325	1,662	3,379
1934	6,436	1,647	3,409
1935	6,827	1,707	3,440
1936	7,172	1,799	3,526
1937	7,381	1,878	3,545
1938	7,547	2,050	3,597
1939	7,553	2,122	3,659
1940	7,418	2,180	3,722
1941	7,387	2,239	3,855
1942	8,339	2,360	3,983
1943	10,062	2,540	4,123
1944	10,997	2,620	4,225
1945	11,116	2,810	4,313

Basis of NVA accounting changed in 1911
* data missing
Sources: NVA and NVMA Annual Reports; RCVS Annual Reports and RCVS registers, 'Finances of the Association', *Veterinary Record*, 58 (1945), 523.

INDEX

Agricultural Development and Advisory Service 171–172, 185, 202–203
   and see National Agricultural Advisory Service
Agricultural Research Council 199–200
Alder, Martin 73
Alderman, Henrietta 226
Allcock, James 272, 274
Allen, Charles 35
Almond, N. 30
Alston Edgar, Professor F. W. 18
Anaesthetics 13, 25, 158–159
Anderson, John 153, 215
Anderson, L. Guy 129–130, 135, 140, 144–145
Anderson, Professor Ian 101
Andrews, Dr Anthony H. 221, 264
Animal Diseases Research Association 81, 84, 87
Animal Health Trust 35, 122–123, 175, 181
Annett, Professor H. E. 40
Anthony, Francis 244–245
Armour, Professor Sir James 72
Armstrong, H. E. 16
Army veterinary surgeons 34
   World War I 47–48, 50, 52, 58, 84
   World War II 116, 127
Association of British Abattoir Owners 241
Association of Meat Inspectors 241
Association of Veterinary Practice Managers 309
Association of Veterinary Teachers and Research Workers 205
Aujeszky's disease 257–261
Baird, James H. 219–220, 222, 225, 227
Balerno, Lord 212
Bang, Professor B. 37
Banham, George Amos 6, 7, 9, 12–13, 19–21
Bennett, Professor Richard 304
Bentley, H. M. 293–294
Beswick, Walter 206–208
Beynon, A. G. 262
Biggs, T. 10
Blackburn, Trevor 282–283
Blackmore, D. K. 69
Blackwells 69
Bleby, Professor John 222–223
Bloy, W. H. 31

Index

BMJ Group 73
Board of Agriculture 29–30, 34, 49
Boden, Edward 70, 73
Bombay Veterinary College 7
Borrie, Sir Gordon 283
Bourne, Professor John 251, 253–256
Bovine spongiform encephalopathy 100, 246, 264–268, 309
Bower, William 29
Boyd Orr, John 131
Bradshaw, Ben 301
Brambell committee on intensive livestock husbandry 172–173
Brancker, Mary 97, 119, 180–182, 290
British Cattle Veterinary Association 177, 179, 222, 266, 314
British Equine Veterinary Association 72, 177, 179
British Medical Association 2, 6, 8, 73, 128, 155, 170, 217, 234
British Sheep Veterinary Association 177
British Small Animal Veterinary Association 35, 73, 79, 175–178, 192, 291, 314
British Veterinary Association:
    and anaesthetics 158–159
    and Aujeszky's disease 258–261
    and BSE 264–268
    and foot-and-mouth disease 95–99, 101
    and preventive medicine 119, 163–164, 166–172, 202–203
    and Supplementary Veterinary Register 145–146, 149–151, 153
    and tuberculosis 248–257
    and veterinary education 191–196, 205
    and veterinary nursing 142
    and welfare 173–174
    attitude to advertising 271–5, 279–284
    centenary 211–214
    general secretaries 215–216
    journals 66–73 *and see Veterinary Record*
    Mansfield Street 155–156, 158, 220
    meat hygiene policy 233–247
    presidents 97, 99, 142, 144–146, 152, 158, 164–165, 167–168, 175, 179, 180–187, 189–190, 203, 206, 212, 216, 218, 227–228, 232, 235, 244–245, 253–254, 262, 275, 277, 282, 290–291, 295, 297
    reorganisation 217–227
British Veterinary Nursing Association 73
Brittlebank, Colonel J. W. 59, 217, 249
Brodie, J. S 278
Brown Animal Sanatory Institute 6
Brown, George 148–150
Brown, J. K. 98
Brown, William. R. 61, 65
Bruce, H. R. 2
Brucellosis 119, 186, 229–231, 263–264

Brydon, R. 34
Buckley, J. 219
Bullock, Fred 214
Burroughs Wellcome & Co 84, 95, 118, 176
Buxton, Professor J. Basil 63, 83
BVA Animal Welfare Association 79, 174
Bywater, H. E. 156
Cabot, Daniel 113
Campbell, Donald 108–110, 113
Carter, Henry 98, 281
Catlow, David 223, 232
Cave, Professor T. W. 38
Central Veterinary Medical Society 39
Champion report on licensing of veterinary surgeons 141–142
Chandler, Ted 253
Chapman, M. J. 207
Charnock Bradley, Professor Orlando 38–40, 46–47, 61–62, 81–82
Chipperfield, T. A. R. 146
Chiron award 181
Clark, James 33
Clarke, W. Roger 61
Cox, J. H. 10
Crooks, John 194
Crookshank, E. M. 18
Cust, Aileen 35–36, 285–287
Dale, Sir Henry 128
Dalling, Professor Sir Thomas 84, 117, 119
Dalrymple–Champneys award 181
Dalrymple–Champneys, Sir Weldon 181
Davidson, Viscountess 158–159
Dawes, H. W. 149
De la Warr, Earl 128–129
Deans Rankin, J. 161
DEFRA 101, 233, 247, 256, 277–278, 299–301, 304
Department of the Environment, Food and Rural Affairs *see* DEFRA
DeVile, Paul 221, 245
Devonshire, Duke of 291
Dewar, Professor J. R. U. 30, 33
Dewar, Professor J. W. 23
Dick, William 1
Dickin, Maria 138
Dingle, P. J. 161
Dollar, John A. W. 26, 34
Dollar, T. A. 3, 12, 15, 26, 27
Dorrell, Stephen 265
Dunston, John 31
Eddy, R. G. 201–203, 310

Index

Edwards, A. M. 293
Edwards, J. T. 66
Environmental Health Officers Association 236, 238–241, 244
 and see Institute of Environmental Health Officers
Equine Veterinary Journal 72
Eschericia coli 246
Evans, Eifion 232
Farm Animal Welfare Advisory Committee 174
Farm Livestock Emergency Service 117
Farmers Weekly 106, 111
Faulkner, E. 16, 17, 24
Fenner, Peggy 259, 298
Fenwick Jones, D. 166
Fergusson, Sir Ronald 110
Ferrers, Earl 211, 213
Fitzwygram Prize 6
Fitzwygram, F. W. J. 11
Fleming, George 3–4, 7–8, 14, 16
Fletcher, Alex 282–283
Food Standards Agency 247, 267
Foot-and-mouth disease 74, 90–101, 171, 180, 224
Fowl pest *see* Newcastle disease
Francis, Josephine 70–71
Gamgee, John 11, 14, 15
Gamgee, Joseph 11
Gamgee, Sampson 11
Garnett, F. W. 34, 46, 52
Garnett, Miss M. 91
General Medical Council 3
Gibson, Dr Tom 211–213
Godfrey, Professor Charles 253
Gofton, Arthur 85, 249
Gordon, W. S. 66
Gorman, Professor Neil 226
Gorton, Professor Bernard 82
Gould, George N. 118, 129–133, 146, 165
Gowers, Sir Ernest 94–96
Gowland Hopkins, Sir Frederick 102, 104, 120
Gray, Henry 37, 43, 75–77
Greaves, Thomas 9
Green, Roger 179, 219
Greenough, P. R. 160–161
Greig, J. Russell 87
Griffith, Dr. 42
Grubb, H. R. 69, 71
Gummer, John 242, 265
Gunn, Dixon 190, 217

Hancock, R. G. C. 120–122
Harrison, V. A. 169
Harvey, F. T. 32
Haxby, D. L. (Don) 99; 189–190
Heard, Terry 259
Hebeler, H. F. 150
Hedley, Matthew 32
Hellig, Howard 223, 246
Henderson, Dr Sir William 200
Henderson, G. N. 68; 176
Herriot, James *see* Wight, J. A. (Alf)
Hickman, Colonel John 177
Hicks, R. J. 37
Hignett, P. J. 212
Hignett, Sam 118, 177–178
Hill, Dr Charles 128
Hobday, Professor Sir Frederick 32, 34, 112–113, 287
Hodgman, John 176
Hogg, Douglas 246, 266
Hoskin, Brian 217
Howard, P. J. 143
Hudson, R. A. 118
Hughes, D. L. 66
Hunter, John 11
Hunting, Charles 14, 16
Hunting, William 7, 11, 14–19, 23–26, 32, 34–36, 41–42, 44–45, 61, 157
    death 43, 60
Hurndall, J. Sutcliffe. 12, 19, 21
In Practice 71–72
Institute of Animal Pathology 83
Institute of Environmental Health Officers 243
International Sheep Dog Society 177
James, Professor Philip 267
Jennings, Sidney 164–165
Jinman, Peter 222, 225–277
John McFadyean 81
Johnson, Dr Barry 226
Jones, Bruce V. 176
Jones, David M. 214
Jones, Leonard 88
Jopling, Michael 260
Joshua, Joan 68, 176, 290
Journal of Small Animal Practice 73
Journal of the Association of Veterinary Students 73
Kay, Hugh 169
Kelland, Sir John 109–111
Kennel Club 177

Index

King, James 31
King, Neal 216, 297, 310
Kinghorn, J. F. 146
Knight, Fred 65, 113, 116, 214–215
Krebs, John 251, 255
Krebs report on bovine TB 251
Lambert, J. D 19
Lancaster, D. C. 68
Lane, Dick 214
Livesey, G. H. 38, 42–43, 81
Llewellyn Jones, H. 88
Lloyd, John S. 34, 38
Local veterinary associations 5, 8
Local veterinary inspectors 99, 163, 166, 169, 172, 180, 186, 188, 198, 229–233, 247, 264, 298, 303
Loveday, Dr Thomas 128
Loveday committee on veterinary education 123–125, 128–129, 147, 171, 204, 207
Lowe, Professor Philip 301–303
MacArthur, D. A. 294
McCall, James 10, 23
McCracken, Dr Bob 254
McFadyean, Sir John 6, 22, 24, 29, 30, 34, 36, 48, 59, 139, 249–250
McFarlane, J. 41
MacGillivray, E. A. 18
McIntyre, Professor W. I. 199–200
MacKellar, J. C. 175
McPhail, J. 33
McQueen, Professor J. 27, 29, 39
Malcom, John 21, 22, 27, 60
Male, G. P. 42, 86
Marsh, Sir John 275–276
Martin, E. E. 35
Maxwell, Captain Robert, 69
Meat Hygiene Service 106, 233, 245, 247, 266
Medicines, supply and sale 53, 55–56, 163, 166, 168, 172, 224, 269–278
Meldrum, Keith 229, 243
Mettam, A. E. 35
Middleton Perry, E. 84
Miller, Professor W. C. 117, 129
Ministry of Agriculture and Fisheries 74, 94, 96, 108, 117–118, 123, 133–136, 141, 168
Ministry of Agriculture, Fisheries and Food 98–99, 101, 151, 164–165, 170, 180, 187, 200, 216, 230–232, 240, 243, 261–262
Mitchell, Charles 66–69
Molloy, Lord 208
Monckton, Sir Walter 128

Montgomerie, Dr R. F. 95
Moore, Sir John 84
Moredun Institute 81, 87
Morley, Elliot 277
Morrison, W. S. 106, 108
Napley, Sir David 212
National Agricultural Advisory Service 167, 170–171
National Air Raid Precautions for Animals Committee 116–117
National Canine Defence League 141
National Disease Information Service 300
National Farmers Union 117–119, 128, 130, 164, 169–170
National Institute for Medical Research (Medical Research Council) 93
National Veterinary Association 8–45, 54, 57–59, 154–155, 242
     presidents 7–9, 18, 21, 23–25, 29, 31, 34, 38–39, 41–43, 46–47, 61
National Veterinary Congress 1882 7, 8
National Veterinary Medical Association 59, 60–61, 63–64, 70, 74, 77–89, 104,
     106, 108–109, 112–113, 116–118, 123–125, 128, 130, 132–142, 214, 239
     objects 78
     changes name to British Veterinary Association 142–143
     presidents 61, 65–66, 68, 80, 83, 85–86, 108–110, 113–114, 116, 119–121, 123,
     128–129, 131, 133, 135, 139–140, 143
     general secretaries 214–215
New Veterinary College 13–14, 35, 38
Newcastle disease 261–262
Nicholls, Chrissie 229
Norfolk, Duke of 128
Northumberland committee on recruitment into the veterinary profession
     191, 193–194
Nugent, G. R. H. 159
Olver, Harry 28
Our Dumb Friends League 141
Page, Dr Ewan 209
Paice, Jim 257
Pallin, W. 25
Parker, J. M. 27
Parry, John 189–190, 203
Parsons, John 197
Paull, Nicky 228
Peart, (Lord) T. F. (Fred) 96, 175, 212, 238
Penberthy, John 7, 22, 27
People's Dispensary for Sick Animals 137–141, 150
Pig Disease Eradication Fund 260–261
Porter, Alistair 208, 212
Pringle, Major-General R. 47, 50
Prior, James 185–186
Pritchard, Professor 21
Professional fees 42–43, 54–56, 84

Index

Protection of Animals (Anaesthetics) Act 1954 158–159
Provincial Medical and Surgical Association 2
Pugh, David 183
Pugh, Professor L. P. 183
Queen Elizabeth II 211, 213
Raison, Timothy 211
RCVS News 306
Rees, Howard 258
Reid, John 97, 197
Research in Veterinary Science 68–70, 73
Richardson, John 217
Riddock, J. 33
Riley committee on veterinary education 204–208
Riley, Sir Ralph 209
Rinderpest 1
Ritchie, Sir John 165
Roberts, R. 13
Robertson, Professor Alexander 142, 144, 197
Roy, C. S. 6
Royal College of Veterinary Surgeons:
    aims 77
    and a national veterinary service 168
    and advertising 89, 144, 230, 279–284
    and corporate practice 304, 306
    and sale of medicines 270
    and veterinary nursing 142
    disciplinary committee hearing 162
    Licensed Veterinary Inspectors 233
    premises 154
    presidents 29, 38, 288, 310
    principal 6
    recruitment during World War I 48–50
    register and licensing 1–4; 36, 63; 123–126, 138–139, 142, 145, 147–149, 152, 208, 294, 299
    support for NVA 311
Royal Pharmaceutical Society 271
Royal Society for the Prevention of Cruelty to Animals 10, 137–139, 141, 150
Royal Veterinary College 1, 7, 13, 17, 34, 39, 83
Runciman, J. G. 7
Salaries 42, 47–48, 86–87, 130–134, 136, 199–200
Sampson, S. 58
Sanatorium 138
Scott, Andrew 225, 275, 278
Scott, T. G. & Son 71
Scott-Park, Dr Freda 291
Scudamore, Jim 232
Share-Jones, Professor J. 51–52

Shepherd, E. K. 292
Shepherd, Gillian 244
Sheridan, John 305–306, 308
Shillito, Charles 216–217
Sibley, Dick 222
Silkin, John 190, 203, 239
Simcocks, T. H. 19, 21
Simon, J. R. 2
Simpson, P. J. 139, 143
Simpson, Professor J. F. 29, 30
Simpson, Robert 123; 155
Singleton, W. Brian 175, 197
Slocock, Sidney 38
Smith, Lt. Gen. Frederick 18, 41
Snodgrass, Nigel 197–198, 214, 217, 283
Soames, Christopher 165
Society of Practising Veterinary Surgeons 79, 88, 105, 144, 150, 201, 205
Society of Veterinary Practitioners *see* Society of Practising Veterinary
    Surgeons
Society of Women Veterinary Surgeons 290, 294
Soul, Peter 246
Soulsby, Lord (Lawson) 307
Soutar, Dr H. S. 128
SPVS Bulletin 73
Stableforth, A. W. 66
Stamp, Lord 158–159
State Veterinary Service 99, 100, 102–103, 106–110, 163, 185–188, 231, 259, 263,
    312
Steel, J. H. 7
Steele-Bodger, Alasdair 151–152, 272, 275
Steele-Bodger, Harry W. 104–105, 114–119, 155, 290
    death 150–151
Stevens, A. J. 200–201
Stevenson, R. M (Bob) 265–266, 295
Stockman, Sir Stewart 36–37, 38, 46, 48, 81, 90–93
Stodart, Lord 204, 208–209
Storie-Pugh, Dr Peter 183–185, 215
Straiton, E. C. (Eddie) 160–162
Strang, Dr Gavin 196, 246
Sumner, H. 40
Supplementary Veterinary Register 145–146, 149–151, 153
Swann, Sir Michael 171–172, 196–199, 203–204
Swann committee on antibiotics in agriculture 269–271
Swann committee on veterinary profession and education 171–172, 196–200,
    204, 209
Swine fever 29, 30, 35
Swinnerton-Dyer, Sir Peter 209–210

Index

Tail docking 10
Tandy, John 213, 219, 274, 279–280
Taylor, Angus 185–187
Taylor, H. 40
Tennant, Major 29
Thompson, Des 266
Thompson, Donald 261
Thomson, A. 235
Thornton, H. 234
Torney, Tom 259
Townson, H. W. 86
Townson, R. F. 146
Tuberculosis 10, 22, 27, 30–32, 38, 42, 89, 102, 165, 248–257
Turner, Pat B. 69, 215–216
Turner, Trevor 214
Uvarov, Olga 125, 288–289
Vaccination 18, 26, 53, 176, 263
Vandepeer, Sir Donald 109–110, 132, 135–136
Veterinarian 14, 19
Veterinary Defence Society 175
Veterinary education 16–17, 35–37, 40–41, 76, 101, 122–125, 193–194, 204–210
Veterinary Formulary 73
Veterinary Investigation Service 88
Veterinary Journal 14, 16, 19
Veterinary Nursing Journal 73
Veterinary Practitioners League *see* Society of Practising Veterinary
    Surgeons 88
Veterinary Record: 22, 25, 32, 76, 80, 82, 91, 107, 109–110, 112–114, 128, 152,
    156, 178–179, 196, 224, 229, 244, 254, 261, 271, 277, 284
    acquisition by NVMA 58–64
    advertising 130, 132, 134, 157, 273, 280, 312
    correspondence 19, 41, 57, 99, 145–146, 160–161, 175, 225, 256, 285, 292–
    294
    cost 189
    cover 28, 45, 70, 157
    editors 7, 11, 14–19, 23–26, 32, 34–36, 41–45, 60–61, 65–70, 73, 157, 229
    launch 14–16, 26
    moves to BMA House 73, 158
    NVA annual meeting 36
    on salaries 133–134
    World War I 52–53, 56–58
Veterinary Surgeons Act 1881 2–4, 130, 138
Veterinary Surgeons Act 1948 141, 145–150, 313
Veterinary Surgeons Act 1966 151–153
Vogel, Colin 214
Walker, Peter 239–240
Wallace Hoare, E. 25

Walsby, J. B. 189
Walster, Chris 308
Ware, Stephen 221
Wells, Bernard 282
Whalley, Professor W. 10, 13–14
White, J. B. 167–168
Whitelaw, Sir William 211
Wight, J. A. (Alf) 162, 194, 292
Wilkins, J. H. 68
Wilkinson, Edward 160, 235
Willey, Fred 159
Williams, Beatrice 292–293
Williams, Derek 71
Williams, John 246
Williams, Tom 131–132, 135–136, 147, 149
Williams, W. O. 13, 21, 23, 31, 35–36
Wilson, Peter 54
Winstanley, Lord 212
Women vets 1, 35, 97, 145, 161–162, 180–181, 194, 201, 285–296, 314
Wood, Peter 69, 71
Woodrow, C. E. 176
Woods, William 41
Wooldridge, Dr W. R. (Reg) 35, 66, 117, 119–122, 125–126, 165, 234
Wooldridge, G. H. 83
Wooldridge, G. W. 35, 38, 58
World War I 47–58, 248, 311
World War II 116–120, 122–128, 181, 183, 312
Wortley Axe, Professor J. 22, 35
You and Your Vet 284
Young, R. C. 227
Zuckerman, Lord 250
Zuckerman report on bovine TB 250

Lightning Source UK Ltd.
Milton Keynes UK
UKOW041809020613

211632UK00002B/20/P